T0321375

Dynamical Biostatistical Models

Chapman & Hall/CRC Biostatistics Series

Published Titles

Published Titles

Bayesian Modeling in Bioinformatics
Dipak K. Dey, Samiran Ghosh,
and Bani K. Mallick

**Benefit-Risk Assessment in
Pharmaceutical Research and
Development**
Andreas Sashegyi, James Felli,
and Rebecca Noel

**Biosimilars: Design and Analysis of
Follow-on Biologics**
Shein-Chung Chow

Biostatistics: A Computing Approach
Stewart J. Anderson

**Causal Analysis in Biomedicine and
Epidemiology: Based on Minimal
Sufficient Causation**
Mikel Aickin

**Clinical and Statistical
Considerations in Personalized
Medicine**
Claudio Carini, Sandeep Menon,
and Mark Chang

Clinical Trial Data Analysis using R
Ding-Geng (Din) Chen and
Karl E. Peace

Clinical Trial Methodology
Karl E. Peace and
Ding-Geng (Din) Chen

**Computational Methods in
Biomedical Research**
Ravindra Khattree and
Dayanand N. Naik

Computational Pharmacokinetics
Anders Källén

**Confidence Intervals for Proportions
and Related Measures of Effect Size**
Robert G. Newcombe

**Controversial Statistical Issues in
Clinical Trials**
Shein-Chung Chow

**Data Analysis with Competing Risks
and Intermediate States**
Ronald B. Geskus

**Data and Safety Monitoring
Committees in Clinical Trials**
Jay Herson

**Design and Analysis of Animal
Studies in Pharmaceutical
Development**
Shein-Chung Chow and
Jen-pei Liu

**Design and Analysis of Bioavailability
and Bioequivalence Studies,
Third Edition**
Shein-Chung Chow and
Jen-pei Liu

**Design and Analysis of Bridging
Studies**
Jen-pei Liu, Shein-Chung Chow,
and Chin-Fu Hsiao

**Design and Analysis of Clinical Trials
for Predictive Medicine**
Shigeyuki Matsui, Marc Buyse,
and Richard Simon

**Design and Analysis of Clinical Trials
with Time-to-Event Endpoints**
Karl E. Peace

**Design and Analysis of Non-Inferiority
Trials**
Mark D. Rothmann, Brian L. Wiens,
and Ivan S. F. Chan

**Difference Equations with Public
Health Applications**
Lemuel A. Moyé and
Asha Seth Kapadia

**DNA Methylation Microarrays:
Experimental Design and
Statistical Analysis**
Sun-Chong Wang and
Arturas Petronis

Published Titles

DNA Microarrays and Related Genomics Techniques: Design, Analysis, and Interpretation of Experiments
David B. Allison, Grier P. Page,
T. Mark Beasley, and Jode W. Edwards

Dose Finding by the Continual Reassessment Method
Ying Kuen Cheung

Dynamical Biostatistical Models
Daniel Commenges and
Hélène Jacqmin-Gadda

Elementary Bayesian Biostatistics
Lemuel A. Moyé

Empirical Likelihood Method in Survival Analysis
Mai Zhou

Exposure–Response Modeling: Methods and Practical Implementation
Jixian Wang

Frailty Models in Survival Analysis
Andreas Wienke

Generalized Linear Models: A Bayesian Perspective
Dipak K. Dey, Sujit K. Ghosh,
and Bani K. Mallick

Handbook of Regression and Modeling: Applications for the Clinical and Pharmaceutical Industries
Daryl S. Paulson

Inference Principles for Biostatisticians
Ian C. Marschner

Interval-Censored Time-to-Event Data: Methods and Applications
Ding-Geng (Din) Chen, Jianguo Sun,
and Karl E. Peace

Introductory Adaptive Trial Designs: A Practical Guide with R
Mark Chang

Joint Models for Longitudinal and Time-to-Event Data: With Applications in R
Dimitris Rizopoulos

Measures of Interobserver Agreement and Reliability, Second Edition
Mohamed M. Shoukri

Medical Biostatistics, Third Edition
A. Indrayan

Meta-Analysis in Medicine and Health Policy
Dalene Stangl and
Donald A. Berry

Mixed Effects Models for the Population Approach: Models, Tasks, Methods and Tools
Marc Lavielle

Modeling to Inform Infectious Disease Control
Niels G. Becker

Modern Adaptive Randomized Clinical Trials: Statistical and Practical Aspects
Oleksandr Sverdlov

Monte Carlo Simulation for the Pharmaceutical Industry: Concepts, Algorithms, and Case Studies
Mark Chang

Multiple Testing Problems in Pharmaceutical Statistics
Alex Dmitrienko, Ajit C. Tamhane,
and Frank Bretz

Noninferiority Testing in Clinical Trials: Issues and Challenges
Tie-Hua Ng

Published Titles

Optimal Design for Nonlinear Response Models
Valerii V. Fedorov and Sergei L. Leonov

Patient-Reported Outcomes: Measurement, Implementation and Interpretation
Joseph C. Cappelleri, Kelly H. Zou, Andrew G. Bushmakin,
Jose Ma. J. Alvir, Demissie Alemayehu, and Tara Symonds

Quantitative Evaluation of Safety in Drug Development: Design, Analysis and Reporting
Qi Jiang and H. Amy Xia

Randomized Clinical Trials of Nonpharmacological Treatments
Isabelle Boutron, Philippe Ravaud, and David Moher

Randomized Phase II Cancer Clinical Trials
Sin-Ho Jung

Sample Size Calculations for Clustered and Longitudinal Outcomes in Clinical Research
Chul Ahn, Moonseong Heo, and Song Zhang

Sample Size Calculations in Clinical Research, Second Edition
Shein-Chung Chow, Jun Shao, and Hansheng Wang

Statistical Analysis of Human Growth and Development
Yin Bun Cheung

Statistical Design and Analysis of Clinical Trials: Principles and Methods
Weichung Joe Shih and Joseph Aisner

Statistical Design and Analysis of Stability Studies
Shein-Chung Chow

Statistical Evaluation of Diagnostic Performance: Topics in ROC Analysis
Kelly H. Zou, Aiyi Liu, Andriy Bandos, Lucila Ohno-Machado, and Howard Rockette

Statistical Methods for Clinical Trials
Mark X. Norleans

Statistical Methods for Drug Safety
Robert D. Gibbons and Anup K. Amatya

Statistical Methods for Immunogenicity Assessment
Harry Yang, Jianchun Zhang, Binbing Yu, and Wei Zhao

Statistical Methods in Drug Combination Studies
Wei Zhao and Harry Yang

Statistics in Drug Research: Methodologies and Recent Developments
Shein-Chung Chow and Jun Shao

Statistics in the Pharmaceutical Industry, Third Edition
Ralph Buncher and Jia-Yeong Tsay

Survival Analysis in Medicine and Genetics
Jialiang Li and Shuangge Ma

Theory of Drug Development
Eric B. Holmgren

Translational Medicine: Strategies and Statistical Methods
Dennis Cosmatos and Shein-Chung Chow

Chapman & Hall/CRC Biostatistics Series

Dynamical Biostatistical Models

Daniel Commenges

University of Bordeaux, France

Hélène Jacqmin-Gadda

University of Bordeaux, France

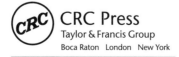

CRC Press
Taylor & Francis Group
Boca Raton   London   New York

CRC Press is an imprint of the
Taylor & Francis Group, an **informa** business

A CHAPMAN & HALL BOOK

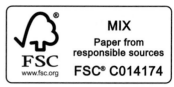

CRC Press
Taylor & Francis Group
6000 Broken Sound Parkway NW, Suite 300
Boca Raton, FL 33487-2742

International Standard Book Number-13: 978-1-4987-2967-3 (Hardback)

Visit the Taylor & Francis Web site at
http://www.taylorandfrancis.com

and the CRC Press Web site at
http://www.crcpress.com

Contents

Preface

In the continuous development of statistics, models for the analysis of longitudinal data took a particularly important place, especially in biostatistics. The Biostatistics team of Bordeaux within the Public Health Institute (ISPED) and successive INSERM units (currently Research Center of Epidemiology and Biostatistics) contributed to this development in terms of research and teaching. This book aims at describing the methods available to date with a pedagogical concern and dissemination among applied statisticians. We hope it will be a tool for teaching biostatistics at the master's degree level, a reference for PhD students in biostatistics or epidemiology, and will also be useful to statisticians engaged in data analysis of time-dependent data. This book is not an encyclopedia covering any topic in statistics or even in biostatistics, an ambition that could not be achieved. With the exception of a chapter summarizing the main results of statistical inference, the book focuses on models for longitudinal data at large, that is to say, repeated measures of quantitative or qualitative variables and events history (including survival and multistate models), and a chapter about the dynamic approach to causal inference.

The work is accompanied by the development of a set of software that will allow applying most of the advanced methods such as multistate models and joint models. Most of the methods may be applied using the SAS or R software.

One feature of this book is that it is a collective work, the fruit of research and teaching experience of a team whose members have worked together for years. With this shared experience of the eight authors, the book is homogeneous both in general vision and in notations.

Acknowledgments

We gratefully acknowledge the researchers who provided the data sets used in this book to illustrate the different methods described: Prof. J.F. Dartigues and Dr. P. Barberger-Gateau (University of Bordeaux) for Paquid cohort; Prof. H. Sandler (CEDARS-Sinai Medical Center, Los Angeles), Dr. D. Hamstra (University of Michigan, Ann Arbor), and Prof. J. Taylor (University of Michigan, Ann Arbor) for the cohort of patients treated for prostate cancer at the University of Michigan; Dr. A. Hernandez and the clinical documentation department of the Bellvitge Hospital for the cohort of patients with colorectal cancer at Barcelona University Hospital (Spain); Prof. G. Chêne and Dr. C. Fagard (Unit of clinical trials, Bordeaux), Prof. J.M. Molina (Saint-Louis Hospital, Paris), Prof. F. Raffi (Nantes University Hospital), and Prof. C. Leport (Bichat Hospital, Paris) as well as National Research Agency for AIDS (ANRS) for ALBI clinical trial and APROCO cohort. We also thank K. Leffondré for stimulating discussions, and L. Ferrer and A. Rouanet for their suggestions during the reading of the manuscript.

Daniel Commenges and Hélène Jacqmin-Gadda
Bordeaux

List of Figures

List of Tables

Co-authors

Alioum Ahmadou
Inserm, Biostatistics Team
Bordeaux University, ISPED
France

Pierre Joly
Inserm, Biostatistics Team
Bordeaux University, ISPED
France

Benoit Liquet
Inserm, Biostatistics Team
Bordeaux University, ISPED
France

Cécile Proust-Lima
Inserm, Biostatistics Team
Bordeaux University, ISPED
France

Virginie Rondeau
Inserm, Biostatistics Team
Bordeaux University, ISPED
France

Rodolphe Thiébaut
Inserm, Biostatistics Team
Bordeaux University, ISPED
France

Notations

General

By convention, a vector is a column vector.

n is the size of a sample, that is the number of subjects, except for grouped or longitudinal data where N is the number of subjects and n_i the number of measures by group or subject.

$Y, X, Z, \ldots$: random variables with values in $\mathbb{R}$ or $\mathbb{R}^p$.

$\beta^\top$: β transposed

Symbols for vectors or matrices are not in bold character: context allows distinguishing them from scalar quantities.

$y, x, z, \ldots$: real values that random variables can take, or generic values.

a, b, c, u, v, w: random effects.

c: latent classes.

$f_Y^\theta(y)$: probability density function of the random variable Y in y; in a model it is indexed by a parameter θ. We will use $f^\theta(y)$ or $f(y)$ for short, but not $f(Y)$, which is the density taken in Y, that is the likelihood for observation Y.

$f_{Y|X}^\theta(y|x)$: conditional density.

$F_Y(y)$: cumulative distribution function (or $F(y)$ if not ambiguous).

$\Lambda(t)$: 1) compensator for counting processes; 2) latent process.

$\mathcal{N}(\mu, \sigma^2)$: Gaussian distribution with expectation μ and variance σ^2.

$\mathcal{N}(\mu, B)$: Gaussian distribution with expectation μ and variance matrix B.

χ_q^2: Chi-square distribution with q degrees of freedom.

$I_{\{Y=X\}}$: indicator function: $I_{\{Y=X\}} = 1$ if $Y = X$ and 0 otherwise.

Regression models

Y: variable to be explained; X, Z explanatory variables.

$\theta, \beta, \gamma, \ldots$ and other small Greek letters: parameters (scalars or vectors); θ means in general the vector of all the parameters.

$X_i^\top \beta$ or $\beta^\top X_i$: linear predictor for i; sometimes expressed with Z_i in place of X_i.

$\mathcal{L}(\theta)$: likelihood.

$L(\theta)$: log-likelihood.

log: natural logarithm.

$\hat{\theta}$: estimator of θ. The true value is denoted by θ^* or to simplify notation by θ.

$\mathrm{var}(\hat{\theta})$: variance-covariance matrix (short: variance matrix) of $\hat{\theta}$.

Survival and multistate models

T: time of occurrence of the event of interest.

C: right-censoring time.

$\tilde{T} = \min(T, C)$: follow-up time.

$\delta = I_{\{T \leq C\}}$: Indicator of uncensored observation of the event.

$S(t) = 1 - F(t)$: survival function.

$\alpha(t)$: hazard function.

$A(t)$: cumulative risk function.

$\alpha_{ij}(t)$: transition intensity from state i to state j.

1

Introduction

1.1 General presentation of the book

We could sketch a brief history of biostatistical modeling as follows. Analysis of variance dominated until about 1970; it essentially allows analyzing the influence of qualitative factors on quantitative observations. In the seventies, several major developments occurred: the development of regression models for binary data and survival data (Cox, 1972), unification of regression models within generalized linear models (Nelder and Wedderburn, 1972) and unification of linear models with random effects (Harville, 1977). In the eighties we saw the development of nonlinear mixed-effect models and the application of linear and non-linear models to longitudinal data. A deeper understanding of survival data was also developed and this topic was rigorously studied using the theory of counting processes; the first realistic applications of multistate models in epidemiology appeared. The application of the theory of counting processes to survival models was initiated by Aalen (1978); Andersen et al. (1993) present a remarkably complete account of the theory and its applications. In the mid-nineties, the theory of linear and non-linear mixed-effect models and that of survival data as well were matured. In each of the two domains, multivariate models were proposed, to model the evolution of several repeated quantitative variables or risk of occurrence of several events. The first joint models for simultaneous analysis of repeated quantitative data and events were developed in the late nineties; thus, the two major pathways of model development joined. In the beginning of the 21st century, theory and applications of these models have continued to develop, with particular attention to more complex patterns of incomplete observations such as left-censoring, interval-censoring and cases of informative censoring.

This book presents the main statistical models for the analysis of longitudinal data in general. This term *longitudinal data* actually covers two types of data: firstly, repeated measurements of quantitative or qualitative variables often called "longitudinal data" (in a strict sense), and secondly the time of occurrence of events which are usually censored (called "survival data"). A common feature of these data is that their collection requires longitudinal monitoring; similarly, modeling requires taking into account the time factor (hence the term dynamic models). Typically, these data are collected in cohort studies. For example, in the Paquid cohort study on cognitive aging (Dartigues et al., 1992), cognitive abilities of the subjects were measured at each visit using psychometric tests, and the age of occurrence of events such as dementia, Alzheimer's disease or death was also recorded. In the field of human immunodeficiency virus (HIV), monitoring infected patient in observational studies and in clinical trials provides repeated measurements of biological markers such as the concentration of CD4 + T cells (CD4 counts) or viral load; it also allows recording the occurrence of various clinical events (opportunistic diseases, death . . .).

The book describes advanced regression models which include the time dimension, such as mixed-effect models, survival models, multistate models, and joint models for repeated measures and time-to-event (the reader is assumed to be familiar with standard regression models, such as linear or logistic regression models). It also explores the possibility of unifying these models through a stochastic process point of view. Beyond inference techniques, what should come in the first place is the issue of interpretation of the results. Data are collected, and models are used for analysis, to answer questions of interest (mainly epidemiological questions in this book). The query is often about causal relations. This is the main reason in fact why dynamical models are interesting. Not all dynamical models can be interpreted as causal but integrating time in the models is a first step towards this aim.

The two main inferential approaches are the frequentist and the Bayesian approaches. In this book, only the frequentist approach will be developed, although Bayesian inference is also possible. A recent account of the Bayesian methods is given by Lesaffre and Lawson (2012). For parametric models, the frequentist approach most often relies on the maximum likelihood approach. For nonparametric or semi-parametric models, the likelihood and some of its variants such as partial likelihood and penalized likelihood (which has a link with the Bayesian approach) will also be described.

The theoretical and numerical aspects of frequentist inference for these models are developed. The practical aspects are not neglected since the modeling strategy is discussed as well as methods for testing the assumptions and assessing the fit of the data. Each method is illustrated with applications to real data, emphasizing the task of interpreting the results; essential elements for implementing the methods in the SAS and/or R softwares are given in the Appendix.

1.2   Organization of the book

The first chapter is the introduction, the last two sections of which present the notation and three examples of datasets which will be analyzed by different methods. The core of the book is divided into two parts: Part I includes Chapters 2-4 which present the conventional methods for analysis of longitudinal and survival data, and can be skipped by readers already familiar with these methods. Part II includes Chapters 5-8 which present more advanced dynamic models that may be considered as extensions of these conventional methods. They have been more recently developed and are still active areas of research. Part II also includes Chapter 9 which explores the causality issue from a dynamic point of view.

Chapter 2 summarizes the main methods of inference (estimation, and model selection) used in other chapters. Chapter 3 presents the conventional methods of analysis of survival data: estimation of the survival function, proportional hazards model and accelerated failure time model; it also gives elements of the theory of counting processes which allows describing the additive model and briefly present the degradation models. Chapter 4 discusses the main models for longitudinal data, that is mainly mixed-effect models (linear, generalized linear, nonlinear models), but also the marginal models and the Generalized Estimating Equation approach. The problem of incomplete data in longitudinal studies is then discussed. Chapter 5 describes extensions of mixed models to treat curvilinear data (including measures with floor and ceiling effect), multivariate longitudinal data and heterogeneous longitudinal data using latent class mixed models. Chapter 6 discusses more advanced topics in survival analysis, such as relative survival, competing risks, frailty models and cure models. Chapters 7 and 8 tackle more complex models: Chapter 7 introduces multistate models and Chapter 8 describes joint models for longitudinal data and time-to-event. Chapter 9 presents a dynamical approach to causality: it includes a theoretical presentation of influences between stochastic processes and developments in both conventional epidemiological multistate or joint models and mechanistic models based on differential equations. The most theoretical developments in this chapter (Sections 9.2 and 9.3) may be skipped by readers mainly interested by applications and practical aspects of causality. Finally, the Appendix shows the R and SAS codes that were used to treat the book examples. Several R packages have been developed specifically for the proposed methods in this book; their detailed manuals are deposited on the CRAN.

1.3 Notation

Random variables and observable processes are noted by Roman capitals alphabet. When studying the theoretical properties of statistics, *observations* are considered as random elements. These random elements take particular values (outputs) when we have *data*. Random effects are denoted by lower-case letters of the Roman alphabet. Lower-case letters are used to represent generic (or dummy) variables, such as the argument of a density or an integration variable. Sample sizes are denoted by n or N. Model parameters are denoted by Greek letters. A list of the main notation is given at the beginning of the book.

1.4   Presentation of examples

Three main examples are used throughout the book; they are taken from studies of brain aging, HIV infection and cancer. Each of these studies can address several epidemiological questions and raises several methodological issues.

1.4.1   Dementia: the PAQUID study

The main objective of Paquid is the study of cognitive aging, dementia and frailty in the elderly (Dartigues et al., 1992). It is based on a cohort of 3,777 subjects aged 65 and over living at home in Dordogne and Gironde (two departments of southwest France) at the date of entry into the cohort which started in 1988-1989. Subjects were visited by a psychologist in their homes at baseline and every two or three years for 20 years (1, 3, 5, 8, 10, 13, 15, 17 and 20 years after baseline); they completed a questionnaire on socio-demographic characteristics, lifestyle, personal and family medical history, health events since the last visit and also completed a battery of cognitive tests, scales of dependence and of depressive symptomatology. Following each interview, participants who met the DSM-III-R criteria of dementia or had lost at least 3 points to a global cognitive test (Mini Mental State Examination) received a visit from a neurologist to make a diagnosis of dementia and Alzheimer's disease. Information on the death or admission to an institution were also collected. Data analysis of Paquid raises many methodological issues addressed in this book.

Repeated measures of cognitive tests allow describing cognitive decline with age using methods of analysis of longitudinal data that take into account the within-subject correlation (Chapters 4 and 5). As in most cohorts, particularly those involving the elderly, follow-up is often incomplete. Some participants refuse to answer certain questions, refuse visits, decide to leave the study or die. Analytical methods must be used to treat these types of incomplete data, avoiding selection bias that might be associated with the observation process (see Section 4.5 and Chapter 8). Furthermore, cognition is measured by a battery of psychometric tests; the score at these tests are highly correlated and present different measurement characteristics (including floor and ceiling effects, unequal sensitivity to change over the entire observable range of cognitive ability, etc.). The linear Gaussian model is rarely appropriate in this situation, and extensions have been proposed to address these measurement characteristics (Section 5.1). To avoid describing brain aging using a single arbitrarily chosen cognitive test, models for multivariate longitudinal data (Section 5.2) can be used. Finally, since the elderly population is very heterogeneous, the latent class models are useful for estimating the different profiles of cognitive aging (Section 5.3).

One of the main objectives of Paquid is the identification of risk factors of onset of dementia or Alzheimer's disease, requiring methods of analysis of survival data (Chapters 3, 6 and 7). A thorough analysis of the event histories collected in the Paquid study raises several difficulties. On one hand, since age is the main risk factor for dementia, it is often preferable to use age as the baseline time in the analyses, rather than the duration of follow-up in the study. The subjects are included in the analysis only if they were non-demented at entry into the study: this produces left-truncated observations (see Section 3.3.2). On the other hand, the age of onset of dementia is censored by interval since the diagnosis can be made only at visiting times (every two or three years), and it is not possible to identify *a posteriori* the date of onset of the disease. Finally, the analysis of the risk of dementia should take into account the competing risk of death (see Section 6.2 and Chapter 7). More generally, various events are collected in Paquid: dementia, death, admission to an institution, dependence, etc. The analysis of hazards of transitions between these states can be done with multistate models (Chapter 7). Multistate models allow studying the natural history and risk factors of normal and pathological aging. In all these analyses, the choice of the baseline time is an important issue: age, duration of follow-up, time since an exposure measurement, time since the entry into a state.

Dementia is defined as a decline in memory and at least one other cognitive function with an impact on the activities of daily living. The risk of dementia is strongly correlated to changes in cognitive test scores. To describe the natural history of dementia or provide tools for early diagnosis, it is necessary to jointly model the risk of dementia and cognitive decline using joint models that combine a mixed model for longitudinal data and a survival model. This is developed in Chapter 8.

1.4.2 AIDS: the ALBI trial

The ALBI ANRS 070 trial is a randomized clinical trial comparing three strategies for antiretroviral therapy based on dual therapy with inhibitors of reverse transcriptase (Molina et al., 1999). At baseline, patients infected with HIV started either a treatment combining zidovudine (AZT) and lamivudine (3TC), or a treatment combining stavudine (d4T) and didanosine (ddI). After 12 weeks of treatment, a group of patients that began with ddI + d4T changed to AZT + 3TC. A total of 151 patients were enrolled in the trial: 51 in the AZT + 3TC group, 51 patients in the ddI + d4T group, and 49 patients in the alternating combinations. Patients were followed during six months. The assessment of the response to the antiretroviral treatments was carried out by measuring the number of CD4+ T-cells (target cells of the virus and the major players in the immune response) and plasma HIV viral load. These measurements were carried out every month. The measurement of plasma viral load has a detection limit. Above the detection limit, viral load can be accurately quantified. Below the detection limit, it is known that the viral load is below the threshold, but we cannot have a precise quantification. Statistically, this produces left-censored measures.

The initial analysis of the trial found a superiority of ddI + d4T combination with a decrease in plasma viral load and CD4 growth more pronounced at 6 months compared to the other two groups. These findings do not use all the repeated observations of viral load and CD4 counts. Yet the analysis of all these data allows us to compare the dynamic of markers between treatment groups, explaining the final outcome at 6 months. We present in this book an analysis of the longitudinal data using a standard linear mixed model (Chapter 4) and a mechanistic model (Chapter 9).

1.4.3 Colorectal cancer

In Chapter 6 we will illustrate advanced survival analyses using cancer data. The data come from a prospective cohort of patients diagnosed with colorectal cancer and treated at the University Hospital of Hospitalet in Barcelona, Spain (González et al., 2005). The patients were diagnosed with colorectal cancer between January 1996 and December 1998 and were actively followed up until 2002. Interest lies particularly in the duration between readmissions. The sample contains a total of 861 readmission events for 403 patients included in the analyses. Several readmissions may occur for the same patient, which warrants the use of survival models with random effects (or frailty models) (Section 6.3.3). Individual characteristics are the stage of the tumor measured by the DUKES score, comorbidity measured by the Charlson score, gender and chemotherapy. Information on the patient's death was collected, which also allows us to illustrate the use of multivariate survival models with recurrent events and death (Section 6.4.1). The whole data file is available in the R package `Frailtypack`.

Part I

Classical Biostatistical Models

2

Inference

2.1 Generalities on inference: the concept of model

In this chapter we recall the main results for the maximum likelihood approach which is the main inference approach used in this book. We also recall the main model choice criteria, and also effective algorithms for maximizing the likelihood.

The central issue in statistics is that we have observations from some probability law which is unknown. Inference is the art of saying something about this unknown probability law. Consider the problem where we observe Y; let f_Y^* be the unknown true density of Y. A *model* is a family of distributions, generally characterized by a family of densities $\{f_Y^\theta\}$, $\theta \in \Theta$. The family of densities is indexed by a parameter θ which takes its values in a set Θ. A model is parametric if Θ is included in $\mathbb{R}^p$ for some p. The model is well specified if $f_Y^* \in \{f_Y^\theta\}$: that is to say if there exists $\theta^* \in \Theta$ such that $f_Y^* = f_Y^{\theta^*}$ (θ^* is the true parameter value). In many statistical texts, the distinction is not clear between the true value θ^* and other possible values of θ which indexes the distributions in the model. For simplifying the notation, one often says that one wishes to estimate θ in the model $\{f_Y^\theta\}$, $\theta \in \Theta$, when one should say that one wishes to estimate θ^*.

If f^* does not belong to $\{f_Y^\theta\}$, then the model is misspecified.

2.2 Likelihood and applications

2.2.1 The likelihood

The likelihood is a fundamental tool for statistical inference. The method of maximum likelihood is very useful not only for constructing estimators of the parameters of statistical models that have good asymptotic properties (lack of bias and efficiency), but also to build tests on these parameters in many situations. In other words, when the number of observations n is sufficiently large, the estimators and tests derived from the likelihood are the best.

Definition 1 (Likelihood) *Let* $Y = (Y_1, \ldots, Y_n)$ *be random variables and* *denote the joint density f_Y^θ depending on a parameter vector $\theta = (\theta_1, \ldots, \theta_p)$ belonging to a parameter space Θ. The likelihood is defined by :*

$$\mathcal{L}(\theta; Y) = f_Y^\theta(Y).$$

Here, $f_Y^\theta(\cdot)$ generally is the joint probability density function (p.d.f.), which is a probability only for discrete variables. Note the distinction between the p.d.f. $f_Y^\theta(\cdot)$ and the likelihood $f_Y^\theta(Y)$ which is the p.d.f. of Y taken in Y (or more precisely *composed* with the random variable Y); in applications, Y will be replaced by its observed value. The idea behind the likelihood is that we observe $Y = (Y_1, \ldots, Y_n)$ and the value of θ^* is unknown. It is therefore natural to consider the possible values of this function for different values of θ and for observation Y.

When $Y_i, i = 1, \ldots, n$ are independent, we have $f_Y^\theta(Y) = \prod_{i=1}^n f_{Y_i}^\theta(Y_i)$. The likelihood is then written as the product of likelihoods for each observation:

$$\mathcal{L}(\theta; Y) = \prod_{i=1}^n f_{Y_i}^\theta(Y_i).$$

Definition 2 (Maximum Likelihood Estimator) *The maximum likelihood estimator (MLE) $\hat{\theta} = T(Y)$ of the parameter θ is the value of θ that maximizes the likelihood $\mathcal{L}(\theta; Y)$:*

$$\sup_{\theta \in \Theta} \mathcal{L}(\theta; Y) = \mathcal{L}(\hat{\theta}; Y).$$

Conceptually, it is necessary to distinguish the *estimator* $\hat{\theta} = T(Y)$, which is a random variable, and its realization $\hat{\theta} = T(y)$ the estimate, even if we use the same notation $\hat{\theta}$ for both quantities.

In general, it is easier to maximize the natural logarithm of the likelihood $L(\theta; Y) = \log \mathcal{L}(\theta; Y)$, called the "log-likelihood" that has the same maximum as the likelihood; log will denote the natural logarithm. Under the assumption of independence of Y_i, the log-likelihood is the sum of the individual log-likelihoods:

$$L(\theta; Y) = \log \mathcal{L}(\theta; Y) = \sum_{i=1}^n \log f_{Y_i}^\theta(Y_i) = \sum_{i=1}^n L_i(\theta; Y_i).$$

We assume that $L(\theta; Y)$ is differentiable at θ. The vector (or function) score $U(\theta)$ is the first derivative of the log-likelihood with respect to the parameter vector $\theta = (\theta_1, \ldots, \theta_p)^\top$.

$$U(\theta) = U(\theta; Y) = \begin{pmatrix} \frac{\partial L(\theta; Y)}{\partial \theta_1} \\ \vdots \\ \frac{\partial L(\theta; Y)}{\partial \theta_p} \end{pmatrix}.$$

For independent observations, we have: $U(\theta; Y) = \sum_{i=1}^{n} U_i(\theta; Y_i)$, where $U_i(\theta; Y_i) = \frac{\partial L(\theta; Y_i)}{\partial \theta}$ is the individual score. Since the MLE maximizes $L(\theta; Y)$, the derivative of $L(\theta; Y)$ must be null in $\hat{\theta}$. The MLE must satisfy the score equation:

$$U(\theta; Y) = 0.$$

In regular cases, there is one and only one solution to this equation, which thus defines the MLE $\hat{\theta}$, so we have $U(\hat{\theta}; Y) = 0$. Solving the score equation is a way to find the MLE, as shown in Example 1. Example 2 shows a case where the score is not defined for any value of θ and where the MLE cannot be found by solving the score equation.

Example 1 *Consider the observations $Y_i, i = 1, \ldots, n$, i.i.d. from $\mathcal{N}(\mu, \sigma^2)$. Let $\theta = (\theta_1, \theta_2)^\top = (\mu, \sigma^2)^\top$. The likelihood is:*

$$\mathcal{L}(\theta; Y) = \mathcal{L}(\mu, \sigma^2; Y) = \prod_{i=1}^{n} \frac{1}{\sqrt{2\pi\sigma^2}} \exp\left(-\frac{(Y_i - \mu)^2}{2\sigma^2}\right),$$

and the log-likelihood is given by:

$$L(\theta; Y) = L(\mu, \sigma^2; Y) = -\frac{n}{2}\log(2\pi\sigma^2) - \frac{\sum_{i=1}^{n}(Y_i - \mu)^2}{2\sigma^2}.$$

To determine the MLE of μ and σ^2, one must compute the derivatives of $L(\mu, \sigma^2; Y)$ with respect to these parameters:

$$\frac{\partial L(\mu, \sigma^2; Y)}{\partial \mu} = \frac{\sum_{i=1}^{n}(Y_i - \mu)}{\sigma^2}$$

and

$$\frac{\partial L(\mu, \sigma^2; Y)}{\partial(\sigma^2)} = -\frac{n}{2\sigma^2} + \frac{\sum_{i=1}^{n}(Y_i - \mu)^2}{2\sigma^4}$$

Solving these score equations:

$$\frac{\partial L(\hat{\mu}, \hat{\sigma}^2; Y)}{\partial \mu} = \frac{\sum_{i=1}^{n}(Y_i - \hat{\mu})}{\hat{\sigma}^2} = 0$$

$$\frac{\partial L(\hat{\mu}, \hat{\sigma}^2; Y)}{\partial(\sigma^2)} = -\frac{n}{2\hat{\sigma}^2} + \frac{\sum_{i=1}^{n}(Y_i - \hat{\mu})^2}{2\hat{\sigma}^4} = 0$$

allows obtaining the MLE

$$\hat{\mu} = \bar{Y} = \frac{\sum_{i=1}^{n} Y_i}{n}$$

and

$$\hat{\sigma}^2 = \frac{\sum_{i=1}^{n}(Y_i - \bar{Y})^2}{n}.$$

Example 2 *Suppose that observations $Y_1, \ldots, Y_n$ are i.i.d. and have a uniform distribution on interval $[0, \theta]$, for $\theta > 0$. The likelihood writes:*

$$\mathcal{L}(\theta) = \mathcal{L}(\theta; Y) = \prod_{i=1}^{n} \frac{1}{\theta} I_{\{0 \le Y_i \le \theta\}} = \theta^{-n} I_{\{0 \le Y_1, \ldots, Y_n \le \theta\}} = \theta^{-n} I_{\{\theta \ge \max(Y_1, \ldots, Y_n)\}}.$$

We have that $\mathcal{L}(\theta) = 0$ for $\theta < \max(Y_1, \ldots, Y_n)$ and $\mathcal{L}(\theta)$ is a decreasing positive function of θ for $\theta \ge \max(Y_1, \ldots, Y_n)$. It is clear that $\mathcal{L}(\theta)$ is not continuous, hence not differentiable in θ: we cannot use the score equation to find the MLE. On the other hand, we have that $\mathcal{L}(\theta) = 0$ for $\theta < \max(Y_1, \ldots, Y_n)$ and is equal to θ^{-n} (a decreasing function) for $\theta \ge \max(Y_1, \ldots, Y_n)$; hence the MLE of θ is:

$$\hat{\theta} = \max(Y_1, \ldots, Y_n).$$

Invariance property of MLE

One of the very nice properties of MLE is the *invariance* under reparameterization. This property can be stated as follows: if $\hat{\theta}$ is the MLE of θ and g a bijective function, then $g(\hat{\theta})$ is the MLE of $g(\theta)$.

To illustrate this property, consider variables $Y_i, i = 1, \ldots, n$, i.i.d. according to an exponential distribution with parameter $\lambda > 0$; the density function of Y_i is:

$$f(y; \lambda) = \begin{cases} \lambda e^{-\lambda y}, & y \ge 0 \\ 0, & y < 0 \end{cases}$$

and $E(Y_i) = \mu = \frac{1}{\lambda}$. The log-likelihood is defined by $L(\lambda; Y) = n \ln \lambda - \lambda \left(\sum_{i=1}^{n} Y_i \right)$, and we deduce the MLE $\hat{\lambda} = \frac{n}{\sum_{i=1}^{n} Y_i}$. The invariance property implies that the MLE of $\mu = g(\lambda) = \frac{1}{\lambda}$ is equal to $\hat{\mu} = \frac{1}{\hat{\lambda}} = \frac{\sum_{i=1}^{n} Y_i}{n}$.

Similarly in Example 1, knowing the MLE of the variance σ^2, one can deduce by the invariance property, the MLE of the standard deviation $\sigma = g(\sigma^2) = \sqrt{\sigma^2}$:

$$\hat{\sigma} = \sqrt{\frac{\sum_{i=1}^{n} (Y_i - \bar{Y})^2}{n}}.$$

2.2.2   Asymptotic properties of the MLE

Maximum likelihood estimators have very interesting statistical properties, especially in terms of bias, convergence and asymptotic distribution. The likelihood theory also allows constructing tests that have asymptotically all the good properties (in terms of respect of Type I error and power). In practice, these estimators and these tests have good properties for large enough n. Although the likelihood theory can also be used for misspecified models, for the sake of simplicity we assume in this section that the model is well specified.

The first property is that of the consistency of MLE, that is the MLE tends to the true value of the parameter when n increases, assuming that the number of parameters remains fixed. The essential condition is that the maximum on θ of $E_*[\log f_Y^\theta(Y)]$ be *well separated*, see Van der Vaart (2000); here E_* denotes the expectation under the true distribution. This condition is satisfied in the classical models that are discussed in this book. Intuitively a model is well separated if one cannot find values of θ that are not in the vicinity of the maximum and give values $E_*[\log f_Y^\theta(Y)]$ arbitrarily close to the maximum.

Theorem 1 (Consistency of MLE) *If the maximum on θ of $E_*[\log f_Y^\theta(Y)]$ is well separated, the MLE $\hat\theta = \hat\theta(Y_1, \ldots, Y_n)$ of parameter θ is consistent, that is, it tends in probability towards the true value of θ as n tends to infinity.*

Asymptotic normality of the MLE can be obtained under conventional regularity conditions on the function $\log f_Y^\theta(y)$ (Van der Vaart, 2000): (i) it is three times continuously differentiable; (ii) it is integrable on the parameter space Θ, an open set of $\mathbb{R}^p$ as well as its first, second and third derivatives; (iii) the support of the log-likelihood function does not depend on θ; (iv) there exists a neighborhood of the true value of θ in which the third derivative of the log-likelihood is uniformly bounded. Before giving the theorem, we define the Fisher information matrix.

Definition 3 (Fisher information matrix) *Fisher information matrix $I(\theta)$ is the negative of the expectation of the second derivative of the log-likelihood with respect to θ.*

$$I(\theta) = -E_\theta\left(\frac{\partial^2 L(\theta; Y)}{\partial\theta\partial\theta^\top}\right).$$

We note also:

$$H(\theta) = -\frac{\partial^2 L(\theta; Y)}{\partial\theta\partial\theta^\top}$$

We have $I(\theta) = E_\theta[H(\theta)]$. $H(\theta)$ is called *observed Fisher information matrix*.

The variance of the score is equal to $E_\theta[\frac{\partial L(\theta)}{\partial\theta}\frac{\partial L(\theta)}{\partial\theta}^\top] = E_\theta[H(\theta)] = I(\theta)$. One can also define the information matrix as being the variance of the score. The equality between the two quantities holds only if the model is well specified.

Example 3 *Consider again Example 1. Recall that the log-likelihood is:*

$$L(\mu, \sigma^2; Y) = -\frac{n}{2}\log(2\pi\sigma^2) - \frac{\sum_{i=1}^n (Y_i - \mu)^2}{2\sigma^2}$$

The score vector is:

$$U(\mu, \sigma^2; Y) = (U_\mu, U_{\sigma^2})^\top$$

with

$$U_\mu = \frac{\partial L(\mu, \sigma^2; Y)}{\partial \mu} = \frac{\sum_{i=1}^n (Y_i - \mu)}{\sigma^2}$$

and

$$U_{\sigma^2} = \frac{\partial L(\mu, \sigma^2; Y)}{\partial (\sigma^2)} = -\frac{n}{2\sigma^2} + \frac{\sum_{i=1}^n (Y_i - \mu)^2}{2\sigma^4}$$

The second derivative of the log-likelihood is:

$$\frac{\partial^2 L(\mu, \sigma^2; Y)}{\partial \mu \partial \mu} = -\frac{n}{\sigma^2}$$

$$\frac{\partial^2 L(\mu, \sigma^2; Y)}{\partial \mu \partial (\sigma^2)} = -\frac{\sum_{i=1}^n (Y_i - \mu)}{\sigma^4}$$

$$\frac{\partial^2 L(\mu, \sigma^2; Y)}{\partial (\sigma^2) \partial (\sigma^2)} = \frac{n}{2\sigma^4} - \frac{\sum_{i=1}^n (Y_i - \mu)^2}{\sigma^6}$$

Given that $\mathrm{E}(Y_i - \mu) = 0$ *and that* $\mathrm{E}(Y_i - \mu)^2 = \sigma^2$, *it follows that:*

$$
\begin{aligned}
I(\mu, \sigma^2) &= -\mathrm{E} \begin{pmatrix} \frac{\partial^2 L(\mu, \sigma^2; Y)}{\partial \mu \partial \mu} & \frac{\partial^2 L(\mu, \sigma^2; Y)}{\partial \mu \partial (\sigma^2)} \\ \frac{\partial^2 L(\mu, \sigma^2; Y)}{\partial \mu \partial (\sigma^2)} & \frac{\partial^2 L(\mu, \sigma^2; Y)}{\partial (\sigma^2) \partial (\sigma^2)} \end{pmatrix} \\
&= -\mathrm{E} \begin{pmatrix} -\frac{n}{\sigma^2} & -\frac{\sum_{i=1}^n (Y_i - \mu)}{\sigma^4} \\ -\frac{\sum_{i=1}^n (Y_i - \mu)}{\sigma^4} & \frac{n}{2\sigma^4} - \frac{\sum_{i=1}^n (Y_i - \mu)^2}{\sigma^6} \end{pmatrix} = \begin{pmatrix} \frac{n}{\sigma^2} & 0 \\ 0 & \frac{n}{2\sigma^4} \end{pmatrix}.
\end{aligned}
$$

It can be verified that the variance of the score is $I(\mu, \sigma^2)$. *The score for* μ *is* $\frac{\sum_{i=1}^n (Y_i - \mu)}{\sigma^2}$. *It is easy to see that the variance of* U_μ *(which is the first term of the diagonal of* I*) is* n/σ^2. *Then we can verify that the covariance (off-diagonal terms) is zero. In fact, this covariance is* $\mathrm{E}(U_\mu U_{\sigma^2})$ *and is a sum of terms of the form* $\mathrm{E}(Y_i - \mu)(Y_j - \mu)$ *and* $\mathrm{E}(Y_i - \mu)^3$ *which are all zero (for independence of* Y_i *and symmetry of the normal density). Calculating the variance of* U_{σ^2} *involves the moment of order 4 of the normal law and one can verify the equality* $\mathrm{var}(U_{\sigma^2}) = n/2\sigma^4$.

To properly define the relevant asymptotic distribution of $\hat{\theta}$ let us define the *individual information matrix* $I_i(\theta) = -\mathrm{E}_\theta \left(\frac{\partial^2 L_i(\theta; Y)}{\partial \theta \partial \theta^\top} \right)$, where L_i is the individual log-likelihood. In the i.i.d. case, the matrices $I_i(\theta)$ are the same for all i and one can write for example: $I_i(\theta) = I_1(\theta)$ for all i. We then have $I(\theta) = \sum_{i=1}^n I_i(\theta) = nI_1(\theta)$.

Theorem 2 (Asymptotic normality of MLE) *Under standard conditions of regularity and when the size n of the sample tends to infinity, we have the convergence in distribution:*

$$\sqrt{n}(\hat{\theta} - \theta) \xrightarrow{d} \mathcal{N}(0, I_1^{-1}(\theta))$$

Interpretation: The distribution of the maximum likelihood estimator $\hat{\theta} = \hat{\theta}(Y_1, \ldots, Y_n)$ converges to a normal distribution with expectation equal to the true value of θ and variance the inverse of the Fisher information matrix evaluated at θ.

$$\hat{\theta} \xrightarrow{d} \mathcal{N}(\theta, I^{-1}(\theta)).$$

Remark: The theorem states the convergence in a rigorous way. In the statement of a convergence, the limit does not depend on n. Therefore the interpretation of the asymptotic distribution of $\hat{\theta}$ itself is considered rather as an approximation. To compute this approximation when θ is unknown, one can replace θ by $\hat{\theta}$ in the above expression; the information matrix itself involves an expectation which is often difficult to compute. So, most often the information matrix is replaced by the *observed* information matrix H. Thus, the distribution of $\hat{\theta}$ is most often approximated by $\mathcal{N}(\hat{\theta}, H^{-1}(\hat{\theta}))$.

So asymptotically, the MLE $\hat{\theta}$ has all the right properties. Its expectation is equal to the true value of θ, the variance $I^{-1}(\theta)$ reaches the Cramer-Rao bound: no unbiased estimator has a smaller variance than $I^{-1}(\theta)$. So the MLE is asymptotically unbiased and *efficient*. Moreover, its distribution is normal.

Example 4 *Take again example 3. The inverse of the individual Fisher information matrix is equal to:*

$$I_i^{-1}(\mu, \sigma^2) = \begin{pmatrix} \sigma^2 & 0 \\ 0 & 2\sigma^4 \end{pmatrix}.$$

Indeed, $I(\mu, \sigma^2)$ being a diagonal matrix, its inverse is a diagonal matrix obtained by taking the inverse of the diagonal elements.

The asymptotic normality of $\hat{\theta} = (\hat{\mu}, \hat{\sigma}^2)^{\top}$ can be written:

$$\sqrt{n} \begin{pmatrix} \hat{\mu} - \mu \\ \hat{\sigma}^2 - \sigma^2 \end{pmatrix} \xrightarrow{d} \mathcal{N}\left(\begin{pmatrix} 0 \\ 0 \end{pmatrix}, \begin{pmatrix} \sigma^2 & 0 \\ 0 & 2\sigma^4 \end{pmatrix} \right)$$

One retrieves thus well-known results:

- $E(\hat{\mu}) = \mu$ *and* $\mathrm{var}(\hat{\mu}) = \frac{\sigma^2}{n}$: $\hat{\mu}$ *is an unbiased estimator of μ and $\mathrm{var}(\hat{\mu})$ tends to 0 when n tends to infinity.*

- $E(\hat{\sigma}^2) = \frac{n-1}{n}\sigma^2$ *and* $\mathrm{var}(\hat{\sigma}^2) = \frac{2\sigma^4}{n}$: *when n tends to infinity, $\hat{\sigma}^2$ tends to σ^2 (asymptotically unbiased) and $\mathrm{var}(\hat{\sigma}^2)$ tends to 0.*

- *For n large enough, the law of $\hat{\mu}$ is approximately $\mathcal{N}(\mu, \frac{\sigma^2}{n})$. One can use this property for constructing a hypothesis test for μ when the size n is large enough.*

Another convergence result which has a more theoretical than practical importance, concerns the asymptotic distribution of the score.

Theorem 3 (Asymptotic normality of the score) *Under standard conditions of regularity and when the size n of the sample tends to infinity, the distribution of score $U(\theta)$ evaluated at the true value of θ tends to a normal distribution with zero expectation and variance equal to the Fisher information matrix.*

$$n^{-1/2}U(\theta) \xrightarrow{d} \mathcal{N}(0, I_1(\theta))$$

As before we can interpret this result by saying that the asymptotic distribution of the score is normal with zero mean and variance equal to the Fisher information matrix $I(\theta)$.

Example 5 *Let $Y_1, \ldots, Y_n$ i.i.d. variables with a Poisson distribution of parameter $\lambda > 0$, with $\lambda = \mathrm{E}(Y_i) = \mathrm{var}(Y_i)$. The log-likelihood is:*

$$L(\lambda) = \log(\lambda)\left(\sum_{i=1}^{n} Y_i\right) - n\lambda - \sum_{i=1}^{n} \log(Y_i!).$$

The score is:

$$U(\lambda) = \frac{\partial L(\lambda)}{\partial \lambda} = \frac{\sum_{i=1}^{n} Y_i}{\lambda} - n.$$

The Fisher information matrix is:

$$I(\lambda) = -\mathrm{E}_\lambda\left(\frac{\partial^2 L(\lambda)}{\partial \lambda^2}\right) = -\mathrm{E}_\lambda\left(-\frac{\sum_{i=1}^{n} Y_i}{\lambda^2}\right) = \frac{n}{\lambda}.$$

We deduce that $\hat{\lambda} = \frac{\sum_{i=1}^{n} Y_i}{n}$ and $\mathrm{var}(\hat{\lambda}) = I^{-1}(\lambda) = \frac{\lambda}{n}$. Moreover for n large enough, the distribution of $\hat{\lambda}$ is approximately $\mathcal{N}(\lambda, \frac{\lambda}{n})$.
Moreover, one can verify that $\mathrm{E}(U) = 0$ and that $\mathrm{var}(U) = \mathrm{E}(U^2) = I = \frac{n}{\lambda}$.

Estimation of the asymptotic variance of $\hat{\theta}$ The asymptotic variance of $\hat{\theta}$ is equal to $I^{-1}(\theta)$. Calculating $I^{-1}(\theta)$ however is not immediate, on the one hand because the calculation of an expectation is not always obvious, and secondly because the true value θ is not known. We can estimate the variance of $\hat{\theta}$ by $\widehat{\mathrm{var}}(\hat{\theta}) = I^{-1}(\hat{\theta})$. In practice, when the estimate of θ is obtained by a numerical algorithm, the estimator of the variance of $\hat{\theta}$ is approached by the observed information matrix evaluated at $\hat{\theta}$, $H(\hat{\theta})$.

Asymptotic normality of the MLE $\hat{\theta}$ implies that every component $j = 1, \ldots, p$, $\hat{\theta}_j$, approximately follows a normal distribution $\mathcal{N}(\theta_j, \widehat{\mathrm{var}}(\hat{\theta}_j))$ when n is sufficiently large. This allows constructing a $100(1-\alpha)\%$ confidence interval for θ_j :

$$\left[\hat{\theta}_j \pm |z_{\alpha/2}| \sqrt{\widehat{\text{var}}(\hat{\theta}_j)} \right]$$

where $z_{\alpha/2}$ is the value such that $\text{P} \left[Z < z_{\alpha/2} \right] = \alpha/2$, with $Z \sim \mathcal{N}(0,1)$.

2.2.3 Asymptotic tests

The asymptotic results also allow constructing tests. Three asymptotic tests are commonly used: Wald test, score test and likelihood ratio test.

The Wald test is most often used to test the hypothesis that a single parameter is equal to a particular value θ_j^0 (often zero). The Wald test statistic is $\frac{\hat{\theta}_j - \theta_j^0}{\sqrt{\widehat{\text{var}}(\hat{\theta}_j)}}$ and this has asymptotically a standard normal distribution under the null hypothesis. Wald test can be extended to test a vector of parameters although is rarely used so.

More generally, consider the problem of testing $\boldsymbol{\theta}_2 = \boldsymbol{\theta}_2^0$, where $\boldsymbol{\theta}_2$ is a sub-vector of θ. The p-vector of parameters can be decomposed as: $\theta = (\boldsymbol{\theta}_1, \boldsymbol{\theta}_2)^{\top}$ with $\boldsymbol{\theta}_1 = (\theta_1, \ldots, \theta_{p-k})$ and $\boldsymbol{\theta}_2 = (\theta_{p-k+1}, \ldots, \theta_p)$ with dimension $(p-k)$ and k, respectively. The score and the information matrix and its inverse can be partitioned as:

$$U(\theta) = (\boldsymbol{U}_1(\theta), \boldsymbol{U}_2(\theta))^{\top},$$

where $\boldsymbol{U}_1(\theta) = \frac{\partial L(\theta)}{\partial \boldsymbol{\theta}_1}$ and $\boldsymbol{U}_2(\theta) = \frac{\partial L(\theta)}{\partial \boldsymbol{\theta}_2}$;

$$I(\theta) = \left(\begin{array}{cc} I_{11}(\theta) & I_{12}(\theta) \\ I_{21}(\theta) & I_{22}(\theta) \end{array} \right);$$

$$I^{-1}(\theta) = \left(\begin{array}{cc} V_{11}(\theta) & V_{12}(\theta) \\ V_{21}(\theta) & V_{22}(\theta) \end{array} \right) = V.$$

The complete model has p parameters $\theta = (\theta_1, \ldots, \theta_p)^{\top}$; the restricted model has $(p-k)$ parameters $\boldsymbol{\theta}_1 = (\theta_1, \ldots, \theta_{p-k})^{\top}$, the other k parameters are fixed under the null hypothesis. We note $(\hat{\boldsymbol{\theta}}_1, \hat{\boldsymbol{\theta}}_2) = (\hat{\theta}_1, \ldots, \hat{\theta}_{p-k}, \hat{\theta}_{p-k+1}, \ldots, \hat{\theta}_p)$ the MLE in the complete model and $(\tilde{\boldsymbol{\theta}}_1, \boldsymbol{\theta}_2^0) = (\tilde{\theta}_1, \ldots, \tilde{\theta}_{p-k}, \theta_{p-k+1}^0, \ldots, \theta_p^0)$ the MLE in the restricted model.

The Wald test relies on the fact that the asymptotic variance of the marginal distribution of $\hat{\boldsymbol{\theta}}_2$ is V_{22}. By conventional results of matrix calculus we have $V_{22} = [I_{22} - I_{21}I_{11}^{-1}I_{12}]^{-1}$. As for the score test, taking I_{22} as the asymptotic variance leads to a conservative test; we have to take account of the conditioning on $\boldsymbol{U}_1(\hat{\boldsymbol{\theta}}_1, \boldsymbol{\theta}_2^0) = 0$; we must use the corrected formula $V_{22}^{-1} = I_{22} - I_{21}I_{11}^{-1}I_{12}$ (see Cox and Hinkley, 1979, Section 9.3).

The three test statistics are:

- **Wald test**:

$$X_W = (\hat{\boldsymbol{\theta}}_2 - \boldsymbol{\theta}_2^0)^{\top} [V_{22}(\hat{\boldsymbol{\theta}}_1, \hat{\boldsymbol{\theta}}_2)]^{-1} (\hat{\boldsymbol{\theta}}_2 - \boldsymbol{\theta}_2^0)$$

- **Score test:**

$$X_S = U_2(\tilde{\boldsymbol{\theta}}_1, \boldsymbol{\theta}_2^0)^\top [V_{22}(\tilde{\boldsymbol{\theta}}_1, \boldsymbol{\theta}_2^0)] U_2(\tilde{\boldsymbol{\theta}}_1, \boldsymbol{\theta}_2^0)$$

- **Likelihood ratio test:**

$$X_L = -2[L(\tilde{\boldsymbol{\theta}}_1, \boldsymbol{\theta}_2^0) - L(\hat{\boldsymbol{\theta}}_1, \hat{\boldsymbol{\theta}}_2)]$$

The three test statistics have asymptotically a χ_k^2 distribution under the null hypothesis. The Wald test requires only fitting the complete model; the likelihood ratio test requires fitting both restricted and complete models; the score test requires fitting only the restricted model.

The three tests are asymptotically equivalent. In practice they may give slightly different results, but a large discrepancy may indicate numerical problems (due to an inaccurate computation of the log-likelihood and its derivatives). These tests are described in more details for instance in Kalbfleisch and Prentice (2002).

2.3 Other types of likelihoods and estimation methods

The method of maximum likelihood is the main route for frequentist parametric or non-parametric inference. However, there are other types of likelihoods and other estimation methods that can be interesting, especially to eliminate or reduce the impact of nuisance parameters. Nuisance parameters are parameters that appear in the model but which are not the parameters of interest. It is outside the field of this book to detail all these methods but we define them here quickly and some of them are used in specific contexts in the book.

2.3.1 Other types of likelihood

The likelihood that we talked about in the previous section is the complete likelihood. A non-exhaustive list of other types of likelihood is as follows.

- Conditional likelihood: if there is the factorization $f_{Y,X}^{\theta,\gamma} = f_{Y|X}^{\theta} f_X^{\gamma}$, where θ is the parameter of interest and γ a nuisance parameter, we can use the conditional likelihood $f_{Y|X}^{\theta}(Y|X)$. An interesting example has been given by Kalbfleisch (1978) who showed that permutation tests are obtained as score tests from a likelihood conditional on the order statistics.

- Marginal likelihood: in other cases, it is the marginal density of Y which depends only on the parameter of interest θ. One can then use the marginal likelihood $f_Y^{\theta}(Y)$; in this approach we pretend not having observed X. An interesting application has been given by Kalbfleisch (1978) who showed that rank tests can be obtained as score test from a likelihood marginal with respect to the order statistics; that is, we pretend not having observed the exact values of the variables but only their rank.

- Partial likelihood: it may happen that the likelihood can be factored in a way that can be exploited to eliminate nuisance parameters. A function that is the product of some of these factors, usually those that do not depend on some nuisance parameters, is called "partial likelihood"; the best known partial likelihood has been proposed by Cox for the proportional hazard model (see Section 3.5.2).

- Restricted likelihood: this likelihood is used in linear mixed-effect models because it allows correcting the bias of the estimators of variances. It is a likelihood of a transformed vector which does not depend on the explanatory variables, and as such it is a kind of marginal likelihood; it will be presented in Section 4.1.3.2.

- Profile likelihood: for each value of θ one can define the MLE of γ, $\hat{\gamma}(\theta)$. Replacing in the likelihood γ by $\hat{\gamma}(\theta)$, one obtains a function depending only on θ, called "profile likelihood."

- Penalized likelihood: one can add a penalty to the log-likelihood. The penalized likelihood is used in particular for obtaining smooth non-parametric estimators of hazard functions or transition intensities. Here, non-smooth trajectories have a larger penalty than smooth ones.

- Pseudo-likelihood: in some cases of complex dependence of observations (spatial analysis for example), the likelihood may be very difficult to compute: the idea is to keep only terms that express simple conditional densities; in some cases the estimators based on the maximization of such a pseudo-likelihood have good properties.

2.3.2 Other methods of inference

2.3.2.1 Other estimation methods

There are systematic methods to build estimators that are not based on the likelihood. A non-exhaustive list is as follows.

- Method of moments: to estimate the parameters of a distribution, the method of moments is to find the parameter value that gives the same first moments (expectation and variance if there are two parameters) as the empirical distribution. However, this method does not guarantee the asymptotic efficiency and is not general.

- Method of least squares: the least squares estimator minimizes $\sum_{i=1}^{n}\{Y_i - E_\theta(Y_i)\}^2$; this method only allows estimating the parameters that model the expectation of observed variables; it is not general.

- Estimating equations: an estimating equation has the form $\sum_{i=1}^{n} \psi_\theta(Y_i) = 0$ where ψ_θ is a known function. The estimator that solves this equation can be convergent if $E\{\psi_\theta(Y_i)\} = 0$. The estimators proposed for the survival models in the formalism of the counting processes come from an extension of this approach.

- Generalized Estimating Equations (GEE): estimating equations were generalized to the case where observations are not independent.

- M-estimators: an M-estimator is defined as maximizing a function of the form: $\sum_{i=1}^{n} \phi_\theta(Y_i)$ where ϕ_θ is a known function. The theory is quite general and includes maximum likelihood estimators and least squares estimators as particular cases. There is also a strong link with the estimating equations because if ϕ_θ is differentiable at θ, the M-estimators satisfy an estimating equation.

- Pseudo-values: this approach proposed by Andersen and Perme (2010) allows making simple regression analyses in complex cases with incomplete data; an example of application is given in Section 7.9.2.

2.3.2.2   Methods for variance estimation and tests

There are methods which are not directly estimation methods but can be used to correct bias or estimate variances, or to construct robust tests. The main methods are the following.

- Resampling methods: these include the *bootstrap* (Efron and Tibshirani, 1994), as well as permutation (Good, 2000) and randomization tests (Edgington, 1995).

- Delta method: assume that $\hat{\theta}$ is a consistent estimator of θ (which may be a vector) with variance Σ. Consider the case where we wish to estimate $g(\theta)$, where $g(\cdot)$ is a once-differentiable function. We can estimate it by $g(\hat{\theta})$ and approximate its variance by $\frac{\partial g(\theta)}{\partial \theta}^\top \Sigma \frac{\partial g(\theta)}{\partial \theta}$; see DasGupta (2008), Section 3.4 for a rigorous development. In the Poisson example, an estimator of λ is $\hat{\lambda} = \frac{\sum_{i=1}^{n} Y_i}{n}$ and $\text{var}(\hat{\lambda}) = I^{-1}(\lambda) = \frac{\lambda}{n}$. We can estimate $1/\lambda$ by $1/\hat{\lambda}$ and since $\frac{\partial g(\lambda)}{\partial \lambda} = -1/\lambda^2$, we can estimate the variance by $\frac{1}{n\hat{\lambda}^3}$.

- Simulation from the distribution of estimators: if we want to compute the variance of $g(\hat{\theta})$ it may be very difficult to use the delta method in complex cases: it is then possible to compute it by simulation, generating a large number of realizations from the distribution of $\hat{\theta}$ and computing the empirical variance of this sample. This method has been used by Aalen et al. (1997); see also Mandel (2013).

2.4   Model choice

For prediction or decision, we will have worse results when using $f_Y^{\hat{\theta}}$ rather than the true distribution f_Y^*. The *risk* incurred will be large if $f_Y^{\hat{\theta}}$ is far from f_Y^*. For a well-specified model, $f_Y^{\hat{\theta}}$ can depart from f_Y^* because of the statistical variability of the estimator $\hat{\theta}$; this is the statistical risk. For a misspecified model, there exists in general a value θ_0 of the parameter such that $f_Y^{\theta_0}$ has the minimum risk in the model. This minimum risk can be called the *misspecification risk*. When one uses $f_Y^{\hat{\theta}}$, the total risk is the sum of the statistical risk and the misspecification risk. There are different ways of defining the risk. One can use distances between distributions. The most commonly used risk however is the Kullback-Leibler divergence. The Kullback-Leibler divergence between f_Y^{θ} and f_Y^* is: $\mathrm{KL}(f_Y^{\theta}; f_Y^*) = \int \log\{\frac{f_Y^*(y)}{f_Y^{\theta}(y)}\} f_Y^*(y)\, dy$. This concept comes from information theory, and can be used to justify inference based on likelihood.

2.4.1   Akaike criterion: AIC

In the case where $\hat{\theta}$ is the MLE in a parametric model ($\theta \in \mathbb{R}^p$), Akaike (1973) proposed the AIC criterion (An Information Criterion, or Akaike Information Criterion) which estimates Kullback-Leibler risk, up to additive and multiplicative constants (that do not depend on the model):

$$\mathrm{AIC} = -2L(\hat{\theta}) + 2p. \tag{2.1}$$

In a modeling work, it is common (and useful) to try several models which are thus in competition. One will prefer the model with the smallest risk, and in practice with the smallest AIC. These models can be misspecified, they can be nested or not. A model $\mathcal{M}_1$ is nested in $\mathcal{M}_2$ if $\mathcal{M}_1 \subset \mathcal{M}_2$ (all the distributions of $\mathcal{M}_1$ are in $\mathcal{M}_2$). If $\mathcal{M}_1$ is indexed by the parameter $\theta^1 \in \mathbb{R}^p$, it is common that the model $\mathcal{M}_2$ is indexed by $\theta^2 = (\theta^1, \theta_{p+1})$, that is $\mathcal{M}_2$ has one more parameter than $\mathcal{M}_1$. It is easy to see that the maximum log-likelihood for $\mathcal{M}_2$ is always larger than that of $\mathcal{M}_1$. If however the difference is small, the AIC for $\mathcal{M}_2$ may be larger because of the penalty $2(p+1)$, rather than $2p$. For nested models, a likelihood ratio test can be done for testing the hypothesis that the true distribution is in the smallest model. The philosophy of model choice is however different from that of tests (test results are often interpreted in an explanatory way, while model choice is more oriented toward prediction). Akaike criterion can be used if the models are not nested. Commenges et al. (2008) have shown that a normalized difference of Akaike criteria, D, estimates a difference of Kullback-Leibler risks. Moreover the asymptotic distribution of D can also be estimated.

Other criteria have been proposed. The most serious competitor of Akaike criterion is the Bayesian Information Criterion (BIC) proposed by Schwarz

(1978):

$$\text{BIC} = -2L(\hat{\theta}) + \log(n)p, \tag{2.2}$$

which differs from AIC by the penalty term $\log(n)$ (where log is the natural logarithm), leading in general to larger penalization for additional parameters than AIC. Although the construction of the BIC uses a Bayesian argument, BIC is essentially used in a frequentist framework.

2.4.2 Cross-validation

If $\hat{\theta}$ is not the MLE, one can no longer use AIC. Cross-validation is more general and can be applied when $\hat{\theta}$ is not the MLE, and also when the assessment risk is not the Kullback-Leibler risk. The idea leading to cross-validation is natural. The first step comes from the idea of external cross-validation. It consists in estimating the parameter using a training sub-sample and in assessing its performances using another sub-sample, called "validation sample." The easiest way to do it is to split the original sample in two sub-samples; however, both sub-samples are smaller than the original sample, which is detrimental to both training and validation. The idea of cross-validation is to remove a small part of the original sample for constituting a validation sample, to repeat this operation and to compute the mean of the different criteria. For instance, one can split the sample into five parts, each of the five sub-samples being used successively as a validation sample. This would be called a "five-fold cross-validation." More generally we can use a v-fold cross-validation. It is better to take v large, and the extreme case is $v = n$, that is the validation sample is reduced to one observation, but the criterion is the mean of the n values obtained. This is the "leave-one-out cross-validation."

Up to an additive constant which is the entropy of f_Y^*, the Kullback-Leibler risk is equal to $\mathrm{E}_* \{ -\log f_Y^{\hat{\theta}}(Y) \}$. The "Leave-one-out" cross-validation for estimating this risk is:

$$\text{CV}(\hat{\theta}) = -n^{-1} \sum_{i=1}^{n} \log f_Y^{\hat{\theta}_{-i}}(Y_i),$$

where $\hat{\theta}_{-i}$ is the MLE on the sample $\bar{\mathcal{O}}_{n|i}$, that is the original sample from which observation i has been removed. This criterion has good properties for estimating $\mathrm{E}_* \{ -\log f_Y^{\hat{\theta}}(Y) \}$ and it is asymptotically equivalent to AIC in the parametric case.

The drawback of cross-validation is that it is necessary to perform the analysis several times, v times for a v-fold cross-validation. When $v = n$ and when the likelihood is numerically difficult, the computation time can be excessive. This is why approximation formulas have been proposed. AIC can itself be considered as an approximation. Other formulas have been proposed, in particular for selection estimators based on penalized likelihood: the general information criterion (GIC) (Konishi and Kitagawa, 1996; Commenges et al., 2007). A universal approximated cross-validation formula for regular risk functions has been proposed by Commenges et al. (2015).

2.5 Optimization algorithms

2.5.1 Generalities

Optimization algorithms play an important role in statistical inference, and especially for inference based on the maximum likelihood. They can also be used in Bayesian inference when we want to calculate the estimator of the "maximum a *posteriori*." The optimization algorithms are used in many other areas, but we focus on the problem of maximum likelihood, and we further assume that θ takes values in $\mathbb{R}^p$ and $L(\theta)$ is a continuous function that is twice differentiable in θ. In simple cases, mainly in Gaussian linear models, one can compute the maximum likelihood estimators analytically. In most non-linear models, there is no analytical solution and one uses iterative algorithms. As is conventional in optimization theory, we present the problem as a minimization problem and we are working on minus the log-likelihood. Therefore, we have to find the value $\hat{\theta}$ that minimizes $-L(\theta)$. Iterative algorithms start with an (initial) value $\theta^{(0)}$ of the parameter, and most algorithms are "descending": given a value of $\theta^{(k)}$ in iteration k, they find a value of $\theta^{(k+1)}$ such that $-L(\theta^{(k+1)}) < -L(\theta^{(k)})$. If $-L$ has a minimum bound, descent algorithms converge. Under some additional conditions, $L(\theta^{(k)})$ converges to $L(\hat{\theta})$ and $\theta^{(k)}$ converges $\hat{\theta}$. In practice, we must stop after a finite number of iterations. So we need a stopping criterion.

Some difficulties may arise:

- Existence of several minima. This can happen but it is rare for the log-likelihood. It can be shown that under certain conditions in the i.i.d. case at least, the probability that there is only one minimum tends to 1 when n tends to infinity. An empirical way to verify if the algorithm did not converge to a local minimum is to start the algorithm from different initial values.

- Significant numerical errors in the computation of $L(\theta)$. If the likelihood is complex, including in particular the numerical computation of integrals, numerical errors accumulate, especially in the calculation of the derivatives. If this is combined with an almost flat parametric surface, it becomes difficult to find a good descent direction. The algorithm may fail, or not be able to give a sufficiently accurate value of $\hat{\theta}$. Studying the accuracy of the computation can again be done by starting from several different initial values.

- Lack of a good stopping criterion. It is very important to have a good stopping criterion. The risk is to stop the algorithm before convergence. Here again, experiments with different initial values is a way of knowing if the algorithm has converged with sufficient accuracy. Two conventional stopping criteria are the difference of log-likelihood values or the norm of the difference of $\theta^{(k)}$ between two iterations. A better test is based on the norm of the gradient in the metric of the Hessian (see Section 2.5.2).

There are many algorithms. We focus on the most effective and the most widely used in statistics. We will not speak of the simplex algorithm of Nelder and Mead (1965) which has the advantage of not using the derivatives of the function, but which is not the most efficient.

2.5.2   Newton-Raphson and Newton-like algorithms

2.5.2.1   Newton-Raphson

The most efficient algorithms use the derivatives of the function to be minimized. The simplest is the gradient (or steepest descent) algorithm which proceeds by searching the smallest value in the direction of the gradient: $-\frac{\partial L(\theta)}{\partial \theta} = -U(\theta)$. For this research it is necessary to have an optimization algorithm in one dimension (line-search). However, a much more effective algorithm is the Newton-Raphson algorithm, which uses in addition the second derivative of the function to minimize (the Hessian), $-\frac{\partial^2 L(\theta)}{\partial \theta^2} = H(\theta)$. The displacement is:

$$\theta^{(k+1)} = \theta^{(k)} + H^{-1}(\theta^{(k)})U(\theta^{(k)}). \tag{2.3}$$

This formula is derived from a quadratic approximation of the surface to minimize.

One difficulty with this method is the need to calculate the first and second derivatives. It is often difficult to calculate them analytically, but there are simple and efficient algorithms to compute them numerically. An advantage of this approach in statistical inference is that it provides a direct estimate of the variance of the maximum likelihood estimators $\hat{\theta}$. Indeed, if the model is well specified, the asymptotic variance of $\hat{\theta}$ is $I(\theta^*)^{-1}$, where $I(\theta^*) = \mathrm{E}_*[H(\theta^*)]$ is the Fisher information matrix (θ^*: true value of the parameter); $H(\hat{\theta})$ is an estimator of $I(\theta^*)$.

Another advantage is the existence of a good stopping criterion. Indeed an extremum is characterized by $U(\hat{\theta}) = 0$. So, a good convergence test must be based on an estimate of the slope at the current point, that is to say on a norm of $U(\theta^{(k)})$. The good metric for this norm is specified by H, because we can show that $U(\theta)H^{-1}(\theta)U(\theta)$ has invariance properties. Moreover, if we divide this expression by p, it can be interpreted as an approximation of the numerical error report on the statistical error, or also as a relative distance to the minimum (rdm) (Commenges et al., 2006):

$$\mathrm{rdm}(\theta^{(k)}) = p^{-1}U(\theta^{(k)})^\top H^{-1}(\theta^{(k)})U(\theta^{(k)}).$$

This criterion retains the same interpretation for different problems (e.g., change of units). We certainly hope that the numerical error is less than the statistical error and thus the stopping criterion will be rdm $< c$ where c must be less than 1. The smaller rdm, the better the convergence. In practice, $c = 10^{-1}$ ensures a reasonably good convergence.

However, the Newton-Raphson algorithm may be unstable. If the quadratic approximation is not good, formula (2.3) may give a bad result. Stability can be increased while maintaining the same direction of movement, but by searching for the optimal distance in that direction. However, even with this change, if the initial value is far from the maximum, one can be in a non-convex region in which the Hessian is non-invertible, making it impossible to apply formula (2.3). There are more robust versions.

2.5.2.2 Marquardt algorithm

One calls algorithms "Newton-like" when the displacement is:

$$\theta^{(k+1)} = \theta^{(k)} + \omega_k G^{-1}(\theta^{(k)}) U(\theta^{(k)}). \tag{2.4}$$

The Gradient and Newton-Raphson algorithms are particular cases obtained respectively by setting $G = I_d$, where I_d is the identity matrix, and $G = H$. The first choice is not very efficient and the second may fail if H is not positive-definite. The optimal ω_k is found by line-search.

Marquardt algorithm (Marquardt, 1963) uses a matrix G obtained by adding to H a definite positive matrix. The simplest form is: $G(\theta^{(k)}) = H(\theta^{(k)}) + \lambda_k I_d$ and λ_k is updated in order that $G(\theta^{(k)})$ be positive-definite; if H is positive-definite around the maximum, λ_k is smaller and smaller and G is almost equal to H near the maximum. This algorithm has a much more stable behavior than the Newton-Raphson algorithm in complex problems.

2.5.2.3 BHHH and BFGS algorithms

Berndt, Hall, and Hall (1974) have proposed $G(\theta^{(k)}) = \sum_{i=1}^{n} U_i(\theta^{(k)}) U_i^{\top}(\theta^{(k)})$, defining an algorithm known as BHHH, the initials of the four authors of this paper. This is a general minimization algorithm, but in statistics it can be justified by the relationship between the matrix G so defined and the Hessian. On the one hand, for the least squares estimators, the Hessian takes precisely this form. On the other hand, $I(\theta^*) = \mathrm{E}_*[H(\theta^*)] = \mathrm{E}_*[U(\theta^*)(U(\theta^*))^{\top}]$. Thus, if $\theta^{(k)}$ is close to θ^*, we have $G(\theta^{(k)}) \approx H(\theta^{(k)})$. The BHHH algorithm therefore uses a matrix G which is always positive-definite and, at least near the maximum, is close to H, and therefore produces an effective direction. An additional advantage is that it only requires the calculation of the first derivatives, a significant time savings compared to the calculation of H.

On the other hand, far from the maximum, $G(\theta^{(k)})$ may be different from $H(\theta^{(k)})$, because $U(\theta^{(k)}) \neq 0$. A version (called Robust Variance Scoring or RVS) which aims at improving this algorithm was proposed by Commenges et al. (2006). It uses:

$$G(\theta^{(k)}) = \sum_{i=1}^{n} U_i(\theta^{(k)})U_i^{\top}(\theta^{(k)}) - \eta_k n^{-1} U(\theta^{(k)})U^{\top}(\theta^{(k)}).$$

Another type of algorithm is the quasi-Newton family whose principle is to approximate H by incremental update using the difference of gradients $U(\theta^{(k+1)}) - U(\theta^{(k)})$ between two successive iterations. The most famous (and most effective) algorithm is the BFGS (Broyden-Fletcher-Goldfarb-Shanno) algorithm (Fletcher, 2013). It is available in the R package `Optimix`.

2.5.3 EM algorithm

As we have seen, the numerical computation of the likelihood can be complicated: the main complication is the need to calculate numerical integrals used to calculate expectations. The presence of expectations in the likelihood often comes from incomplete (that is, missing or censored) observations. The most common case of incomplete observations is the case of censored observations. Right-censoring in general does not lead to major complications in the calculation, but this is not true for the left-censoring and interval-censoring. In the case of random effects models, we can also consider that we have incomplete observations. This case is different from the case of censoring because, by definition, the random effects are never observed. However, in formal terms these two cases are similar and in both cases we can use the EM algorithm which consists of two steps: "E" for "expectation" and "M" for "maximization." This algorithm proposed by Dempster et al. (1977), uses the fact that the likelihood for complete data is often simple to calculate. As the observations are in fact incomplete, they must be completed in a stage where the log-likelihood is replaced by its expectation given the observations and the current value of the parameters; this is step "E". This expectation is maximized in the "M" step. E and M steps are iterated until convergence.

Let $Y = (Y_1, \ldots, Y_n)$ an i.i.d. observed sample. The complete data are: $X = (X_1, \ldots, X_n)$, where $X_i = (Y_i, Z_i)$. Interesting cases for the EM algorithm are those where the likelihood of the complete data is simpler than that for the observed data. If $X = (Y, Z)$ was observed, $L(\theta; X) = f_{Y,Z}^{\theta}(Y, Z)$ would be easy to compute, hence to maximize. The observed likelihood is $\mathcal{L}(\theta; Y) = f_Y^{\theta}(Y)$ where $f_Y^{\theta}(Y) = \int f_{Y,Z}^{\theta}(y, z) \; dz$, thus involving an integral, or a sum in the discrete case. In the EM algorithm we replace $\mathcal{L}(\theta; X)$ which cannot be easily computed, by its expectation conditional on the observations, and computed at the current value of the parameter $\theta^{(k)}$. This is the "E" step:

$$Q(\theta|\theta^{(k)}) = E_{\theta}\{\mathcal{L}(\theta; X)|Y\}.$$

In the "M" step, this expression is maximized on θ, leading to the new parameter value $\theta^{(k+1)}$:

$$\theta^{(k+1)} = \mathrm{argmax}_\theta Q(\theta|\theta^{(k)}).$$

Steps "E" and "M" are iterated until convergence. Louis' formula (Louis, 1982) allows computing the Hessian of the log-likelihood at convergence.

Properties:

- the likelihoood increases at each iteration (this is a descent algorithm)

- $\theta^{(k)}$ converges to a local maximum of $L(\theta; Y)$

- if the maximum is unique, $\theta^{(k)}$ converges to the MLE, $\hat{\theta}$.

There are a number of variants of the EM algorithm. These variants have been introduced because the EM algorithm is often slow. In a generalized EM, the maximization step is replaced by a faster choice $\theta^{(k+1)}$ such that $Q(\theta^{(k+1)}|\theta^{(k)}) > Q(\theta^{(k)}|\theta^{(k)})$. The "E" step often raises difficulties because computation of expectations often implies to compute numerical integrals. It has been proposed to achieve this step by simulation, leading to the stochastic EM (SEM) algorithms. It was also proposed to use a stochastic approximation algorithm (Robbins and Monro, 1951) to accelerate both steps leading to the Stochastic approximation EM (SAEM) (Kuhn and Lavielle, 2004).

Advantages and drawbacks: The main advantage is that the steps of maximization of expectation are often simplified compared to the direct computation. The disadvantages are: slowness of the algorithm (in its original formulation); unreliable stopping criterion, because it is based solely on the norm of $\theta^{(k+1)} - \theta^{(k)}$ and computation of the Hessian (needed for estimators of the variances) by another method (Louis' formula).

Example 6 (Mixture of distributions) *The model is:*

$$f_Y^\theta(y) = \sum_{m=1}^M \pi_m f_Y^{\gamma_m}(y),$$

with $\sum_{m=1}^M \pi_m = 1$. For example, $f_Y^{\gamma_m}(y)$ is the probability density of the normal law $\mathcal{N}(\mu_m, \sigma_m^2)$. The log-likelihood of the sample Y is: $L(\theta; Y) = \sum_{i=1}^n \log\{\sum_{m=1}^M \pi_m f_Y^{\gamma_m}(Y_i)\}$, which can be considered as "difficult" to maximize by a Newton-type algorithm. The computation of first and second derivatives of the log-likelihood needed in a Newton algorithm may appear laborious (in fact this difficulty is often exaggerated because these derivatives can be computed numerically).

The EM algorithm can be applied by considering that the complete data include the class, Z_i, whose distribution is $f_{Z_i}(m) = P(Z_i = m) = \pi_m$. If one observes $Z_i = m$, the likelihood is $\pi_m f^{\gamma_m}(Y_i)$, where f^{γ_m} is interpreted as the conditional density of Y given $Z = m$. The complete likelihood is thus:

$$\mathcal{L}(\theta; X) = \Pi_{i=1}^n \Pi_{m=1}^M \{\pi_m f^{\gamma_m}(Y_i)\}^{c_{im}},$$

with $c_{im} = 1_{\{Z_i = m\}}$ and the log-likelihood:

$$L(\theta; X) = \sum_{i=1}^{n} \sum_{m=1}^{M} c_{im} \{\log \pi_m + \log f^{\gamma_m}(Y_i)\}.$$

The "E" step yields:

$$Q(\theta|\theta^{(k)}) = E_\theta\{L(\theta; X)|Y\} = \sum_{i=1}^{n} \sum_{m=1}^{M} E_\theta^k(c_{im})\{\log \pi_m + \log f^{\gamma_m}(Y_i)\},$$

and one finds, using Bayes Theorem, $\pi_{i,m}^{(k)} = E_\theta^{(k)}(c_{im}) = \dfrac{\pi_m^{(k)} f_X^{\gamma_m^{(k)}}}{\sum_{l=1}^{M} \pi_l^{(k)} f_X^{\gamma_l^{(k)}}}$. *The*

"M" step maximizes $Q(\theta|\theta^{(k)})$. The condition $\frac{\partial Q(\theta|\theta^{(k)})}{\partial \pi_l}$ allows obtaining after

some algebra: $\pi_l^{(k+1)} = \dfrac{\sum_{i=1}^{n} \pi_{li}^{(k)}}{n}$. *It still remains to maximize over γ_m.*

3

Survival analysis

3.1 Introduction

Survival analysis is the study of a time from a given origin to the occurrence of a particular event for one or several groups of individuals. Historically, the event was death but this was extended to other types of events. The event of interest can be death from a specified cause, or the appearance of a disease, or the disappearance of symptoms.

Survival analysis is used in the context of longitudinal studies such as cohorts or clinical trials. A main issue is the difficulty to completely observe all the times of events. For example, when the studied event is death, time of occurrence of the event is not observed for the subjects still alive at the end of the study. This type of incomplete observation is called "right-censoring."

The random variable studied is the time of occurrence of the event of interest and is called "survival time". This time is in fact a duration, that is the time elapsed from a given origin to the occurrence of the event.

The choice of the origin (time 0) depends on the event of interest. In some cases the choice is obvious, in other cases several possibilities exist. The event defining the time-origin can be the birth of the subject if we study the age at which the event of interest occurs, the beginning of an exposure, a surgical operation, the beginning of a treatment, the entrance in the study. The time-origin can thus vary from one subject to another in terms of calendar time. The interpretation of the results and the results themselves can be different according to the choice of the origin.

In survival analysis, it is common to estimate the probability to be still "alive" at any time. This probability is the survival function. A well-known non-parametric estimator of the survival function is the Kaplan-Meier estimator presented in Section 3.4. We can compare the survival functions of several groups of subjects by the log-rank test.

These topics will be developed after Section 3.2.2 dedicated to definitions and Section 3.3 introducing the incomplete data which are one of the characteristics of the survival data.

Regression models can be used to analyze the effect of explanatory variables on the survival. A logistic regression model can be used to study the association between the explanatory variables and the probability of occurrence of the event. In this case, the binary variable is "to have or not undergone the event before a given time t_e ". This simple approach however induces a loss of information because only a dichotomous version of the exact times of occurrence of the event is used. Moreover, it cannot be used in the presence of censored observations (see Section 3.3). For survival analysis, the most popular regression model is the Cox model, presented in Section 3.5.

3.2 Event, origin and functions of interest

3.2.1 Choice of the event of interest

A precise definition of the event of interest is necessary. If we study the mortality, the definition is generally clear. On the other hand, if we study the appearance of a disease we must specify the diagnostic criteria; also we may distinguish between the beginning of the disease and its diagnosis. If the time elapsed between the two events is short, it can be suited to choose as date of event, the date of diagnosis. If this time can be long, it may be necessary to take it into account in analyses. Furthermore it is common that the event is in fact a composite event, as for example "relapse or death," and in this case the time of event is the time corresponding to the occurrence of the first event in the chronological order.

3.2.2 Choice of the time-origin

There are basically three types of choices of time-origin (or time-scale). When we choose as origin the birth of the subject, the survival time is the age of the subject. This choice is adapted as soon as we study an event for which we know *a priori* that the hazard strongly depends on age; this is the case for the appearance of the first tooth, or the occurrence of a chronic disease, or death.

The second choice of time-scale corresponds to an origin appropriate to the subject, other than birth; for example, if one studies the duration of remission of leukemic patients after bone-marrow transplant, the event which defines the origin is obviously bone-marrow transplant. Other examples of events defining time-origin are infection by a virus, start of a treatment, start of an exposure, entry into an institution. The entry in the study is relevant as time-origin only if it corresponds to a particular event for the subjects.

The third type of time-scale is defined by a time-origin which is a common calendar date for all the subjects such as a natural disaster, a war, the implementation of new practices or a new law, etc.

3.2.3   Functions in survival analysis

The survival time is a positive random variable that we denote T. We assume here that T is a continuous variable taking any value on $\mathbb{R}^+$; in some applications it may be more adapted to consider that T is a discrete variable. The distribution of T may be characterized by several functions defined on $\mathbb{R}^+$.

- The probability density function $f(t)$:

$$f(t) = \lim_{\Delta t \to 0^+} \frac{\mathrm{P}(t \leq T < t + \Delta t)}{\Delta t}.$$

  We suppose here that this limit exists for every t.

- The cumulative distribution function $F(t)$:

$$\begin{aligned} F(t) &= \int_0^t f(u)du \\ &= \mathrm{P}(T \leq t). \end{aligned}$$

  $F(t)$ is the probability of occurrence of the event before or at t.

- The survival function $S(t)$ is the probability to be still "alive" in t:

$$\begin{aligned} S(t) &= \mathrm{P}(T > t) \\ &= 1 - F(t). \end{aligned}$$

  The survival function is a non-increasing function and we have $S(0) = 1$ and $\lim_{t \to +\infty} S(t) = 0$.

- The hazard function $\alpha(t)$:

$$\begin{aligned} \alpha(t) &= \lim_{\Delta t \to 0^+} \frac{\mathrm{P}(t \leq T < t + \Delta t \mid T \geq t)}{\Delta t} \\ &= \frac{f(t)}{S(t)}. \end{aligned}$$

  $\alpha(t)\Delta t$ is the probability that the event occurs between t and $t + \Delta t$ conditionally on not having occurred before t.

- The cumulative hazard function $A(t)$:

$$A(t) = \int_0^t \alpha(u)du.$$

  We have $\alpha(t) = -\mathrm{d}\log S(t)/\mathrm{d}t$, that is $S(t) = e^{-A(t)}$.

3.3   Observation patterns: censoring and truncation

Event history analysis is characterized by the presence of incomplete observations. Many sampling patterns and observation patterns lead to truncation and censoring.

3.3.1   Censoring

Censoring is a common feature in survival analysis. The most common and the best known is right-censoring. On the contrary, left-censoring is rarely encountered. Interval-censoring is often neglected for simplicity although it often occurs in epidemiological studies.

3.3.1.1   Right-censoring

In survival analysis, all individuals under study may not have undergone the event at the end of the observation period. This kind of incomplete observation is known as "right-censoring." In this case, the survival time is not observed: it is only known that it is greater than a certain time C, called the "censoring variable."

Right-censoring can occur for two different reasons: the event has not occurred at the end of the study, or the subject left the study before the occurrence of the event (subject lost to follow-up). In this last case we must assume *independent censoring* to perform simple inference, as will be shown in Section 3.3.4. Dependent censoring arises for instance if subjects are removed from the study before occurrence of the event because they are in poor health, so that the fact that subjects are censored gives an information on their risk of death. Assuming independent censoring in this case would lead to underestimation of the hazard.

With right-censoring the observations are $(\tilde{T}, \delta)$ where

$$\tilde{T} = \min(T, C),$$

where T is the true survival time and C the time of right-censoring, and δ is an indicator variable

$$\delta = \left\{ \begin{array}{ll} 0 & \text{if } T > C, \\ 1 & \text{otherwise.} \end{array} \right.$$

3.3.1.2   Left- and interval-censoring

A survival time is left-censored when the event has already occurred before we begin to observe the subject. We know only that his survival time T is lower than a certain observed time C. This is a less common case than right-censoring in the literature. Indeed, the criteria of inclusion of most studies exclude subjects who have already undergone the event at the time of inclusion.

A survival time is interval-censored if it is known only to lie in an interval instead of being observed exactly. Interval-censored data occur commonly in cohort studies that entail periodic visits. There is a sequence of N visit-times: $V = (V_0, V_1, \ldots, V_N)$ with $V_0 = 0$, $V_j \leq V_{j+1}$ and $V_{N+1} = +\infty$. The sequence defines a partition of $\mathbb{R}^+$:

$$\bigcup_{j=0}^{N} A_j = \mathbb{R}^+$$

with $A_j = [V_j, V_{j+1}[$. At each visit-time V_j, it is assessed whether the event already occurred or not; thus it is only known that the survival time lies in some interval A_j. An extreme special case of interval-censored data is current status data. In this situation, each subject is observed only once. At that observation time, either the event has already occurred and it is a left-censored observation, or the event has not already occurred and it is a right-censored observation.

As for right-censoring, the issue of independent censoring arises if the V_j's are random variables. A sufficient condition for independent censoring is that the V_j's and T are independent.

3.3.2 Truncation

Truncation corresponds to sampling from a conditional distribution. In survival analysis, it arises when a subject can belong to a sample only if his survival time lies in a given interval. When the event occurred outside this interval the subject cannot be included in the sample. If the left boundary of the interval is not zero, the data are said to be left-truncated; if the right boundary of the interval is not infinite, the data are said to be right-truncated.

There is left-truncation if T is observable only if $T > T_0$, with T_0 independent of T. In some studies, all subjects may not have been observed from the same time-origin. In this case, individuals are observed conditionally on not having undergone the event by the time the follow-up begins. For example, when we study the age of subjects at the occurrence of the event, it is common that the subjects are not followed-up since their birth; there is left-truncation if subjects who experienced the event before the beginning of the follow-up are excluded. This feature distinguishes truncation from censoring. With censoring there is incomplete information about survival times. With truncation, subjects of the study are sampled from a conditional sub-sample, or in other words subjects are selected in a way that depends on the outcome of interest. Data coming from registers provide examples of data which can be both left- and right-truncated.

3.3.3 Risk set

The concept of risk set is important in survival analysis. The risk set at time t is the set of subjects who are at risk to undergo the event at time t, that is the set of subjects "alive" (who have not yet undergone the event) and uncensored just before time t.

With left-truncated data, the risk set at time t is the set of subjects alive and uncensored just before time t and with entry time before time t. We speak here of delayed entry because the subjects are included in the risk set only after their entry time (time of left-truncation).

3.3.4 The likelihood for censored and truncated data

The likelihood was presented in Chapter 2. Censoring and truncation must be taken into account in writing the likelihood.

3.3.4.1 Censoring

If the right-censoring variables are not random, the likelihood, for n subjects with right-censored data, can be written:

$$\mathcal{L} \quad = \quad \prod_{i=1}^{n} f(\tilde{T}_i)^{\delta_i} S(\tilde{T}_i)^{(1-\delta_i)}. \tag{3.1}$$

We can also write:

$$\mathcal{L} \quad = \quad \prod_{i=1}^{n} \alpha(\tilde{T}_i)^{\delta_i} S(\tilde{T}_i), \tag{3.2}$$

with $(\tilde{T}_i, \delta_i), i.i.d., \quad i = 1, \ldots, n$ as defined in Section 3.3.1.1.

If the right-censoring variables are random variables, the likelihood depends on the C_i distribution. If C_i and T_i are independent the likelihood is:

$$\mathcal{L} = \prod_{i=1}^{n} \alpha(\tilde{T}_i)^{\delta_i} S(\tilde{T}_i) \prod_{i=1}^{n} \alpha_C(\tilde{T}_i)^{1-\delta_i} S_C(\tilde{T}_i),$$

where α_C and S_C are the functions of C_i. For inference on T_i we can use the likelihood (3.2) as the censored part provides no information on the distribution of T. In this case the censoring mechanism is said to be independent or sometimes non-informative. Andersen et al. (1993) generalize this concept. They distinguish between the concepts of independent and non-informative censoring, the latter requiring that the model for the censoring variables does not include the same parameters as for the time of interest. This is most often the case, so this distinction is not used so much.

In this chapter we will assume that censoring and truncation are non-informative.

For interval-censored data, the contribution to the likelihood of a subject i for whom the event occurred between T_{1i} and T_{2i} is:

$$\mathcal{L}_i \quad = \quad S(T_{1i}) - S(T_{2i}). \tag{3.3}$$

3.3.4.2 Truncation

Truncation can be taken into account by using a conditional likelihood. In the case of left-truncation, the likelihood of the survival observation given that $\tilde{T}_i$ is greater than T_{0i} is obtained by dividing the likelihood that we would write for the non-truncated case by the probability of not having experienced the event before T_{0i}. Thus, for a right-censored observation $(\tilde{T}_i, \delta_i)$ truncated at T_{0i}, the contribution to the likelihood of a subject i is:

$$\mathcal{L} = \frac{\alpha(\tilde{T}_i)^{\delta_i} S(\tilde{T}_i)}{S(T_{0i})}. \tag{3.4}$$

Right-truncation can be treated the same way. Identifiability problems occur in non-parametric approaches if the risk set is empty for some times; for instance, if all subjects are left-truncated at a given time t_0, the risk sets are empty for $t < t_0$.

3.4 Estimation of the survival function

To estimate the survival function we can use non-parametric or parametric approaches. In this section we begin with the non-parametric Kaplan-Meier estimator; the related non-parametric Nelson-Aalen estimator of the cumulative hazard is presented in Section 3.7.4. Then we turn to parametric and penalized likelihood approaches.

3.4.1 The Kaplan-Meier estimator

The Kaplan-Meier estimator (Kaplan and Meier, 1958), also called product-limit estimator, is the non-parametric maximum likelihood estimator of the survival function $S(\cdot)$. Consider n i.i.d. right-censored observations $(\tilde{T}_i, \delta_i), i = 1, \ldots, n$. Let $t_{(1)} < t_{(2)} < \ldots < t_{(k)}$ the ordered observed times of events; we can define for each time $t_{(j)}, j = 1, \ldots, k$: d_j the number of events and n_j the size of the risk set. The Kaplan-Meier estimator takes the form:

$$\hat{S}(t) = \prod_{j:t_{(j)} \leq t} \frac{n_j - d_j}{n_j}$$

$$= \prod_{j:t_{(j)} \leq t} \left(1 - \frac{d_j}{n_j}\right).$$

By definition $\hat{S}(0) = 1$. The function $\hat{S}(t)$ is a non-increasing step-function, constant between two consecutive times of event, continuous to the right with a jump at every time of event. It is not defined beyond the last time of observation if it corresponds to a right-censored time. $t \in [0, t_{(k)}[$. The asymptotic properties of $\hat{S}(t)$ can be rigorously studied with counting process methods. Andersen et al. (1993) prove its consistency and asymptotic normality which allow approximating its distribution.

Property 1 *For large n, the distribution of $\hat{S}(t)$ can be approximated by $\mathcal{N}\left(S(t), \hat{\sigma}_t^2\right)$ where $\hat{\sigma}_t^2$ is the variance of $\hat{S}(t)$ estimated by Greenwood's formula:*

$$\hat{\sigma}_t^2 = [\hat{S}(t)]^2 \sum_{j:t_{(j)} \leq t} \frac{d_j}{n_j(n_j - d_j)}.$$

The Kaplan-Meier estimator is easily generalized to left-truncated data. In this case the delayed entry must be taken into account in the calculation of the size of the risk sets. It cannot however be used with interval-censored data. The non-parametric maximum likelihood estimator was extended by Peto (1973) and Turnbull (1976) to more general schemes of censoring and truncation.

We may wish to compare the survival functions of two groups (denoted 1 and 2) at a given time t, i.e., test the following null hypothesis: $H_0 : S_1(t) = S_2(t)$. Under H_0, the statistic

$$\frac{(\hat{S}_1(t) - \hat{S}_2(t))^2}{\hat{\sigma}_1^2 + \hat{\sigma}_2^2}$$

has asymptotically a χ^2 distribution with 1 degree of freedom. This does not test the overall equality of survival distributions in the two groups. This more interesting null hypothesis is $H_0 : S_1(t) = S_2(t) \; \forall t$. For testing this hypothesis, we can use the log-rank test; see Kalbfleisch and Prentice (2002) for details. The log-rank test assumes that the times of event are fixed and compares the number of events in each group to the number of expected events calculated under H_0. It is most powerful if the alternative is a proportional hazards model (see Section 3.5). If the two survival functions intersect during the study period, the power of the log-rank test may be very low. It is therefore important to observe the graph of survival functions prior to making the test. The log-rank test is easily generalized to compare $g > 2$ groups. In the latter case, the statistic has asymptotically a χ^2 distribution with $g - 1$ degrees of freedom. To take into account the effect of another covariate that can affect the test result, it is possible to use a stratified log-rank test, also called "adjusted log-rank." However, when we wish to consider more than one covariate, a regression model (see Section 3.5) may be preferable.

3.4.2 Parametric estimators

In the parametric approach it is assumed that the distribution of survival times belongs to a family of distributions, the parameters of which can be estimated by maximizing the likelihood (see Chapter 2). The most common distributions used in survival analysis are the exponential, Weibull and Gamma distributions.

3.4.2.1 The exponential model

The exponential distribution, which depends on a single parameter (γ) strictly positive, assumes that the hazard function is constant over time: $\alpha(t, \gamma) = \gamma$.

Its density function is:
$$f(t, \gamma) = \gamma e^{-\gamma t}.$$

Its cumulative distribution function is:
$$F(t, \gamma) = 1 - e^{-\gamma t}.$$

If the assumption of a constant hazard function is too strong, it is better to use a piecewise exponential distribution, that is a function with constant hazard on time intervals. This generalization of the exponential model is analogous to the "person-years" method which is used to estimate incidence in epidemiology.

3.4.2.2 The Weibull model

The Weibull distribution depends on two positive parameters γ and ρ. The probability density and cumulative distribution functions of the Weibull distribution are:
$$f(t, \gamma, \rho) = \rho \gamma^\rho t^{\rho-1} e^{-(\gamma t)^\rho},$$
$$F(t, \gamma, \rho) = 1 - e^{-(\gamma t)^\rho}.$$

The hazard function is:
$$\alpha(t, \gamma, \rho) = \rho \gamma^\rho t^{\rho-1}.$$

This is a flexible model that has an increasing hazard function if $\rho > 1$, a constant hazard function (exponential model) if $\rho = 1$ and a decreasing hazard function if $0 < \rho < 1$.

3.4.2.3 The Gamma model

The Gamma distribution depends on two positive parameters $(\beta$ and $\xi)$. This is another generalization of the exponential distribution obtained with $\xi = 1$. The density is:
$$f(t, \beta, \xi) = \frac{\beta^\xi t^{\xi-1} e^{-\beta t}}{\Gamma(\xi)},$$

with

$$\Gamma(\xi) = \int_0^\infty s^{\xi-1}e^{-s}ds.$$

Its cumulative distribution function is:

$$F(t,\beta,\xi) \quad = \quad \frac{1}{\Gamma(\xi)}\int_0^{\beta t} s^{\xi-1}e^{-s}ds.$$

3.4.3   Penalized likelihood approach

The non-parametric Kaplan-Meier estimator is a consistent estimator of the survival function. Since this estimator is a step function, it does not allow to directly obtain a smooth estimator of the hazard function. It puts probability masses at the observed times of events; for such a distribution, the cumulative hazard is also a step function (which corresponds to the Nelson-Aalen estimator presented in Section 3.7.4); thus the corresponding hazard function is null everywhere except at times of events. In many situations, hazard functions are expected to be smooth, that is not only continuous but also presenting a very small number of maxima. So the hazard function corresponding to the non-parametric estimators is not consistent in general for the true hazard function. Smoothing methods, such as kernel methods (see Ramlau-Hansen, 1983), can be applied to non-parametric estimators in order to obtain smooth estimators of the hazard function. Kernel methods have the advantage of simplicity but have two drawbacks: the estimator is obtained in two stages and there are edge effects.

The penalized likelihood approach directly provides a smooth estimator of the hazard function without making parametric assumptions. The idea was proposed for density estimation in survival model especially by O'Sullivan (1988). A way of expressing the *a priori* knowledge on smoothness of the hazard function is to penalize the likelihood by a term which takes large value for rough functions. For example, the penalty term may be the square norm of the second derivative of the hazard function ($\int_0^{+\infty} \alpha''^2(u)du$). This implies that $\alpha(\cdot)$ is continuous, twice differentiable and that its second derivative is square integrable. The penalized log-likelihood is thus defined as:

$$pl(\alpha) \quad = \quad L(\alpha) - \kappa \int_0^{+\infty} \alpha''^2(u)du, \qquad (3.5)$$

where L is the full log-likelihood and κ the positive smoothing parameter which controls the trade-off between the fit of the data and the smoothness of the function. Maximization of (3.5) defines the maximum penalized likelihood estimator $\hat{\alpha}(t)$. This estimator cannot be calculated explicitly. However, it can be approximated using splines. The approximation $\tilde{\alpha}(t)$ of $\hat{\alpha}(t)$ can be calculated by a linear combination of cubic M-splines. Cubic M-splines, a variant of B-splines, are piecewise polynomial functions which are combined linearly to approximate a function on an interval. The estimator is approximated by

$$\tilde{\alpha}(t) = \hat{\theta}^{\top} M(t),$$

where $M(t) = (M_1(t), \ldots, M_m(t))^{\top}$ is the vector of values, in t, of m spline functions and θ is the vector of spline coefficients. The vector of spline coefficients $\hat{\theta}$, for fixed κ, is obtained by maximizing $pl(\alpha)$. The number m of spline functions has not a crucial importance in the penalized likelihood approach if m is large enough, because the degree of smoothness is determined by κ (this contrasts with a non-penalized approach where this is the number of splines which determines the degree of smoothness). In theory, the larger m the better the approximation. In practice, however, the number of spline functions must not be too large to avoid numerical problem. One solution is to start with a reasonable number (for example 5 or 7) and add more until the approximated estimator $\tilde{\alpha}(t)$ does not vary. O'Sullivan proposed an approximate cross-validation score to choose the smoothing parameter κ.

An approximate estimator of the survival function is:

$$\tilde{S}(t) = \exp(-\int_0^t \tilde{\alpha}(u)du).$$

A Bayesian technique for generating confidence bands for $\tilde{\alpha}(t)$ was proposed by Wahba (1983). Up to a constant, the penalized log-likelihood pl is a posterior log-likelihood for θ and the penalty term is the prior log-likelihood. Asymptotically, the posterior law is Gaussian, which justifies the estimation of the variance of $\hat{\theta}$ by the Hessian of the penalized log-likelihood:

$$\text{var}(\hat{\theta}) = -\hat{H}^{-1},$$

where H is the Hessian of the penalized log-likelihood. A 95% pointwise confidence bands for $\tilde{\alpha}(t)$ is :

$$\tilde{\alpha}(t) \pm 1,96\tilde{\sigma}_t,$$

where the approximated standard error in t is:

$$\tilde{\sigma}_t = \sqrt{M^{\top}(t)\left[-\hat{H}\right]^{-1} M(t)}.$$

However, this estimator does not take into account the variability due to the choice of the smoothing parameter.

The penalized likelihood approach can be seen as an intermediate approach between the non-parametric approach and the parametric approach. Indeed, on one hand, no parametric assumption is made and, on the other hand, spline functions are used, just as parametric functions. This approach can deal easily, like parametric approaches, with interval-censored data. The only assumption is the smoothness of the hazard function. Choosing the smoothing parameter κ is the difficult part of the method and can be done by approximate cross-validation. The asymptotic properties are difficult to study.

3.5   The proportional hazards model

In this section, the proportional hazards regression model is presented. The Cox model is a semi-parametric approach; parametric models will be presented in Section 3.5.9.

3.5.1   The proportional hazards model

The Cox regression model (Cox, 1972) is perhaps the most widely used regression model in medical research. The idea of the Cox model is to focus on the effect of explanatory variables on the hazard function. The relationship between the hazard function associated to the occurrence of an event and the vector of p explanatory variables $Z = (Z_1, Z_2, \ldots, Z_p)^\top$ is as follows:

$$\alpha(t; Z, \beta) = \alpha_0(t) r(\beta, Z),$$

where $\beta = (\beta_1, \ldots, \beta_p)^\top$ is the vector of regression parameters and $\alpha_0(t)$ is the baseline hazard function. The exponential form $r(\beta, Z) = \exp(\beta_1 Z_1 + \ldots + \beta_p Z_p)$ has become standard. It is an easy way to get a positive risk function without constraint on the coefficients β. The model is then:

$$\alpha(t; Z, \beta) = \alpha_0(t) \exp(\beta^\top Z),$$

where $\alpha_0(t)$ is the hazard function for an individual with all explanatory variables Z_j $(j = 1, \ldots, p)$ at zero (if it makes sense). The model assumes the hazard ratio between subjects i and j (with vectors of explanatory variables Z_i and Z_j) to be constant over time:

$$\begin{aligned}
\frac{\alpha_i(t; Z_i, \beta)}{\alpha_j(t; Z_j, \beta)} &= \frac{\alpha_0(t) \exp(\beta^\top Z_i)}{\alpha_0(t) \exp(\beta^\top Z_j)} \\
&= \frac{\exp(\beta^\top Z_i)}{\exp(\beta^\top Z_j)}.
\end{aligned}$$

It is an assumption which must be checked, as discussed in Section 3.5.8.

3.5.2   The partial likelihood

Cox (1975) proposed to estimate the vector β by maximizing a partial likelihood. This partial likelihood does not depend on $\alpha_0(t)$ which allows estimating β without making any assumption on $\alpha_0(t)$. The Cox model is therefore a semi-parametric proportional hazards model since it includes a vector of parameter β (the parametric part) and a non-parametric part $\alpha_0(t)$.

Partial likelihood is obtained by factorizing the likelihood and by removing the part which involves $\alpha_0(t)$. The remaining part is similar (but not exactly equal) to a conditional probability. Indeed, with $t_{(1)} < t_{(2)} < \ldots < t_{(k)}$ the ordered observed times of events and with $(1), \ldots, (k)$ the indices of the subjects experiencing the events at these times. Using the proportional hazards model assumption, the conditional probability that the subject (i) undergoes the event at $t_{(i)}$, knowing he is at risk at $t_{(i)}$, and assuming there is only one event at that time, is equals to:

$$
\begin{aligned}
p_i &= \frac{\alpha_0(t_{(i)}) \exp(\beta^\top Z_{(i)})}{\sum_{l:\tilde{T}_l \geq t_{(i)}} \alpha_0(t_{(i)}) \exp(\beta^\top Z_l)} \\
&= \frac{\exp(\beta^\top Z_{(i)})}{\sum_{l:\tilde{T}_l \geq t_{(i)}} \exp(\beta^\top Z_l)}.
\end{aligned}
$$

This quantity does not depend on the baseline hazard function $\alpha_0(t)$ which is considered here as a nuisance parameter. The partial likelihood is then obtained as the product of the conditional probabilities calculated at each event time:

$$
\mathcal{L}(\beta, Z) = \prod_{i=1}^{k} p_i = \prod_{i=1}^{k} \frac{\exp(\beta^\top Z_{(i)})}{\sum_{l:\tilde{T}_l \geq t_{(i)}} \exp(\beta^\top Z_l)}. \tag{3.6}
$$

With left-truncated data, entry time must be taken into account in the risk set. Subject l can belong to risk set at time $t_{(i)}$ only if $t_{(i)} \geq T_{0l}$ (in the same way as for Kaplan-Meier estimator).

Partial likelihood (3.6) is valid only when there is only one event at each time (no tie). Several approximations of the partial likelihood have been proposed when there are ties (see Therneau and Grambsch, 2000). Most packages use the Breslow approximation:

$$
\tilde{\mathcal{L}}(\beta, Z) = \prod_{i=1}^{k} \frac{\exp(\beta^\top s_i)}{\left[\sum_{l:\tilde{T}_l \geq t_{(i)}} \exp(\beta^\top Z_l) \right]^{m_i}},
$$

where m_i is the number of subjects having undergone the event at time t_i and s_i is the sum of the vector of explanatory variables for these subjects. All the proposed corrections give good results when the number of ties is not too high. Otherwise, methods suitable for the analysis of grouped data, such as Poisson regression is more appropriate.

The estimators of the regression parameters are defined as values that maximize the partial likelihood. They are obtained by iterative methods such as those presented in Chapter 2. Partial likelihood is not equal to the usual full likelihood but it was established that it has essentially the same properties (Efron, 1977; Andersen and Gill, 1982); the estimators of the maximum partial likelihood are consistent and asymptotically normal.

Property 2 *When $n \to +\infty$:*

i) $\hat{\beta} \xrightarrow{P} \beta$

ii) $\hat{\beta}$ *approximately follows a Gaussian distribution* $\mathcal{N}\left(\beta, \mathcal{I}^{-1}\right)$ *where* $\mathcal{I}^{-1}$ *is the inverse of the Fisher information matrix based on the partial likelihood.*

These properties are used to calculate confidence intervals and build test as described in Chapter 2. The three classical tests, Wald, likelihood ratio and score, can be used.

3.5.3   Parameters interpretation

The Cox model assesses how the baseline hazard is modified by exposure to a particular factor but it does not give an estimator of the hazard function, since this function is considered as a nuisance parameter. An estimator of the hazard function, the Breslow estimator, is presented in Section 3.7.4.

Here $\exp(\beta)$ is the hazard ratio for an increase of 1 unit of the covariate. There is an analogy between the hazard ratio (HR) (the ratio of hazard functions) in the Cox model and the odds ratio (OR) in the logistic model, but the hazard ratio must be understood in terms of instantaneous risk. Indeed, by definition, all subjects will undergo the event if the follow-up time is long enough. If a group is more at risk than another, that is, the hazard ratio is significantly higher than 1, then in this group the survival time will be generally shorter than in the other group.

More specifically, if the covariate is dichotomous $\exp(\beta)$ is the hazard ratio of a subject with $Z = 1$ (exposed) compared to a subject with $Z = 0$ (unexposed). This hazard ratio is assumed to be constant in time. This is a very strong assumption. Several methods for checking this proportional hazards assumption will be discussed in Section 3.5.8. In a model with p explanatory variables $\mathrm{HR}_k = \exp(\beta_k)$ is the hazard ratio associated with the variable Z_k adjusted on all other explanatory variables.

If the covariate Z is a continuous variable, $\exp(\beta)$ is the hazard ratio for a subject where $Z = z + 1$ compared to a subject for who $Z = z$. The hazard ratio depends on the units chosen to measure Z. For a continuous explanatory variable, the log-linearity assumption implies that the hazard ratio is constant for a one-unit increase regardless of the value of the explanatory variable. For example, if we consider age as a continuous covariate, the model will assume the same hazard ratio for an increase of 1 year for age 30 or age 70 years. The log-linearity assumption has also to be checked.

3.5.4   Confidence interval and tests

Since the regression parameter estimators are asymptotically distributed according to a Gaussian distribution, it is easy to calculate asymptotic confidence intervals and to use Wald tests.

The 95% confidence interval of the regression parameter β_k is: $[\hat{\beta}_k \pm 1.96 \times \hat{\sigma}_k]$, where $\hat{\beta}_k$ is the estimator of the parameter β_k and $\hat{\sigma}_k$ is the standard deviation of $\hat{\beta}_k$. In general, it is more interesting to provide the confidence interval of the hazard ratio. Since the hazard ratio is $\exp(\beta)$, its 95% confidence interval can be calculated by:

$$[e^{\hat{\beta}_k - 1.96 \times \hat{\sigma}_k}; e^{\hat{\beta}_k + 1.96 \times \hat{\sigma}_k}].$$

In the Cox model, several tests are available to test the hypothesis "H_0 : $\beta_k = 0$". In general, Wald tests and likelihood ratio tests are used. These tests are detailed in Chapter 2. When the sample is large enough, these two tests are equivalent. They are used to test parameters individually or in groups and compare two nested models.

3.5.5 Example: survival after entry in institution

The subjects are from the Paquid cohort that was presented in Chapter 1. The sample includes 481 subjects who entered an institution for the elderly (nursing homes) during the follow-up of the cohort and continued to be followed after their entry in institution. The event of interest is death and the visit at 15 years of follow-up in the cohort was chosen as the end of the study. We aim at estimating the global survival of subjects from their entry in institution and the association of age, gender and educational level with the death risk.

The mean age of entry in institution is 85.3 years old (minimum 69.8 years old and maximum 102.8 years old). There are 356 women and 125 men. Regarding educational level, 208 subjects had no education or had not validated the primary level, 246 had a validated primary level, and finally 27 had a validated long secondary or higher level. During follow-up, 412 patients died (69 were right-censored, that is still alive at the 15-year follow-up visit). During the follow-up, 298 women and 114 men died.

We estimated a Cox model with the time since the entry in institution as time-scale and 3 explanatory variables: age (continuous variable), educational level (using two dummy variables taking the lowest level of education as the reference class) and sex (coded: 1 for men; 2 for women). The estimators of the hazard ratios, 95% confidence intervals, and p-values of the tests are given in Table 3.1.

TABLE 3.1
Survival analysis using a Cox model of 481 subjects in institution (Paquid study): estimated hazard ratio ($\widehat{HR}$), 95% confidence interval (CI) and p-values.

Variables	$\widehat{HR}$	CI 95%	p-value
Age	1.05	[1.03 ; 1.07]	< 0.0001
Educational level			0.12
level 2	0.83	[0.68 ; 1.01]	
level 3	0.75	[0.47 ; 1.18]	
Sex	0.54	[0.43 ; 0.67]	< 0.0001

Age was significantly associated with the risk of death ($p < 0.0001$) adjusted on the level of education and sex, with a hazard ratio equal to 1.05 per year of age ($\widehat{HR} = 1.05$). For a difference of 5 years the hazard ratio was $\exp(\hat{\beta} \times 5) = \widehat{HR}^5 = 1.27$. The model includes two dummy variables for the educational level. According to confidence intervals, neither parameters (β_2 and β_3) was significantly different from 0. To test globally the factor education, it is necessary to test the null hypothesis "$H_0 : \beta_2 = \beta_3 = 0$" with a Wald test or a likelihood ratio test:

- The Wald test statistic X_W^2 is equal to 4.20. Under H_0, X_W^2 has approximately a χ^2 distribution with 2 degrees of freedom. The p-value is 0.12. So, there is no significant association between the level of education and the risk of death.

- The likelihood ratio test compares the above model and a model without the two dummies variables for education. Under H_0, the test statistic has approximately a χ^2 distribution with 2 degrees of fredom. The values of -2 × log-likelihood are respectively equal to 4298.87 and 4303.06 and the test statistic is therefore 4.19 (p-value= 0.12), very close to the Wald statistic.

Finally, the estimated hazard ratio of women compared to men is 0.54 with a confidence interval $[0.43; 0.67]$. Adjusted for age and level of education, women are less likely to die than men at any time since entry in institution.

3.5.6   The stratified Cox model

To relax the proportional hazards assumption for a categorical covariate, the Cox model may be stratified on the value of the covariate. The stratified Cox model permits different baseline hazard functions in each strata but assumes proportional hazards for the other explanatory variables within each stratum. For a subject i from the stratum k, the hazard function is:

$$\alpha_{0k}(t) \exp(\beta^\top Z_i).$$

The baseline hazard function $\alpha_{0k}(t)$ is common to all subjects of the stratum k. The partial likelihood of the sample is the product of partial likelihoods of each stratum. Stratification allows adjusting on the strata, but it does not provide an estimate of the effect of the variable that defines the strata. With the basic stratified model, the regression parameters are assumed to be the same for each stratum but interactions between covariates and strata may be included for relaxing this assumption.

3.5.7   Time-dependent explanatory variables

Another generalization of the Cox model is to consider time-dependent covariates. Indeed, in some situations, it is interesting to take into account information that will be collected during the follow-up, such as repeated measures of the level of pollution. The proportional hazard model is then written:

$$\alpha(t; Z(t), \beta) = \alpha_0(t) \exp(\beta^\top Z(t)).$$

Note that it is not the "effect" of the variable that varies but the variable itself; extensions of the Cox model to varying coefficient $\beta(t)$ also exist but are more difficult to handle. The partial likelihood properties remain valid for the model with time-dependent covariates. The computation of the partial likelihood, however, requires knowing the value of covariates for all subjects at risk for each event time. This can be a problem for some covariates whose values are only known at some measurement times which may not coincide with event times in the sample. In this case, assumptions (or models) are required to impute values at the times of events. A more sophisticated approach is to use joint models (see Chapter 8).

We must distinguish exogenous (or external) variables and endogenous (or internal) variables. An exogenous variable is a variable whose value is not affected by the occurrence of the event, such as air pollution or outside temperature. Biological markers of disease progression are endogenous variables. Their values are associated with a change in risk of occurrence of the event. For example, for an HIV patient it can be the number of CD4 or the viral load. Endogenous variables raise the problem of causal interpretation discussed in Chapter 9.

3.5.7.1 Endogenous time-dependent explanatory variables and causality

In a clinical trial with primary focus on the effect of a treatment on an event of interest (disease, death, recovery ...), which is fixed at the beginning of the study, biomarkers may change in response to treatment and may mediate the effect of treatment on the event of interest. Accordingly, adjusting on biological markers can mask the effect of treatment. For example, a treatment has an effect on viral load and CD4 count which is the most important factor in the risk of AIDS. In this case, adjusting on CD4 count may severely bias the global effect of treatment on the risk of AIDS. In clinical trial, these markers can be considered as proxies and, in this case, it is of interest to estimate the effect of the treatment on the markers themselves. An interesting case is that of a change of treatment. Treatment is in principle an exogenous variable, but treatment changes often depend on patient health. If the factor that affects treatment is not included in the model, the estimated effect cannot be interpreted causally. For example, if the event of interest is AIDS, antiretroviral treatment can be included as an explanatory variable. In an observational study, it is conceivable that the treatment is most often given to patients who have a low number of CD4. If the model is not adjusted on CD4, one can find that the treatment is deleterious, because treatment is given to the patients most at risk of developing AIDS. This is an indication bias. If this variable is included in the model, the above-mentioned problem of disappearance of the effect of the treatment due to mediation arises. This issue is detailed in Section 9.6.

3.5.8 Model checking: proportional hazards assumption

As explained earlier, the proportional hazards assumption means that the ratio of hazard functions for two fixed different values of the covariates is independent of time.

What is the problem when the proportional hazards assumption is not true? To make it simple, we will assume a binary covariate. The hazard ratio may change over time in a quantitative or qualitative manner. One group is more at risk than another but the hazard ratio is either increasing or decreasing over time. Indeed, it often happens that hazard ratios decrease with time; this can be partly explained by the presence of frailties (see Aalen et al., 2008, Chapter 6). If a group is always more at risk than the other (a situation we call "quantitative change"), there is not a major problem of interpretation and the power of the test of the null hypothesis (no difference between the groups) will not be much affected. The only concern is that the estimate will give an "average" hazard ratio over the period, while the relationship is a bit more complex.

A more problematic situation is when there is a qualitative change of the hazard ratio over time, that is when the hazard ratio crosses the value 1. Then the group with the highest hazard at the beginning of the period has the lowest hazard after a certain time. In this case, not only the effect of the covariate is not properly taken into account, but also we may conclude, incorrectly, that there is no effect of the covariate on the event. Note, however, that the crossing of hazard functions does not imply the crossing of survival functions.

The next sections describe some methods for evaluating the proportional hazards assumption.

3.5.8.1 Graphical check

A simple form of graphical check in the case of the comparison of two groups is to estimate the survival function with a non-parametric estimator for each of the two groups. We can draw the $\ln[-\ln(\hat{S}(t))]$ curves in each group on the same chart (see an example with Figure 3.1) and check that the curves have an approximately constant gap which should be equal to $\hat{\beta}$. A review of graphical methods for checking the proportional hazard assumption can be found in Hess (1995). When using a parametric model, a kernel smoothing or a penalized likelihood approach, it is possible to directly estimate the hazard functions. We can then draw them or their logarithm to visually check the proportional hazard assumption.

The major shortcomings of graphical methods are the subjectivity and the fact that it is difficult to take into account other covariates simultaneously. The advantage are the simplicity of use and availability in software. Furthermore, they allow visualizing the evolution of hazard ratios.

3.5.8.2 Residuals

Several types of residuals have been proposed in survival analysis and many articles and books (Therneau and Grambsch, 2000; Andersen and Keiding, 2006; Klein and Moeschberger, 2003; Hosmer Jr et al., 2011) discuss the use of residuals. In this paragraph we briefly introduce Cox-Snell residuals, martingale residuals and Schoenfeld residuals.

Cox-Snell residuals are used to verify the overall fit of the model (Kalbfleisch and Prentice, 2002). The residual for subject i, is the cumulative hazard estimated at time $\tilde{T}_i$:

$$\hat{A}_i(\tilde{T}_i) = \exp(Z_i^\top \hat{\beta})\hat{A}_0(\tilde{T}_i),$$

where $\hat{A}_0$ is the Breslow estimator of the baseline cumulative hazard described in Section 3.7. If the model is well specified, $(\hat{A}_i(\tilde{T}_i), \delta_i), i = 1, \ldots, n$ behaves like a censored sample from an exponential variable with parameter 1. Indeed $A(T)$ follows an exponential distribution with parameter 1 since its survival function is equal to $\exp(-y)$. The Nelson-Aalen estimator (see Section 3.7.4) of the cumulative hazard function of the Cox-Snell residuals can be compared graphically to the cumulative hazard function of an exponential distribution with parameter 1, which is a straight line passing through 0 and with slope 1. This graphical method, although available in softwares, should be used with caution (Klein and Moeschberger, 2003). Indeed, it only gives a check of the overall adequacy. It is often better to check the proportional hazards assumption variable by variable.

The martingale residuals come from the counting process theory briefly introduced in Section 3.7.3. A test using martingale residuals was developed by Lin et al. (1993) to globally check the proportional hazards assumption. Martingale residuals are also useful for testing the functional form of the effect of a covariate and thus the log-linearity; a test is available with SAS (Allison, 2012). Martingale residuals are defined by:

$$\hat{M}_i = \delta_i - \hat{A}_i(\tilde{T}_i).$$

This denomination comes from the fact that $\hat{M}_i$ is the value of the martingale in the Doob-Meyer decomposition of the counting process N_i (see Section 3.7), taken in $\tilde{T}_i$. The classical property of residuals $\sum_{i=1}^n \hat{M}_i = 0$ holds and the $\hat{M}_i$ are asymptotically independent. It is better to use a smoothing method to interpret a graph of residuals, because there are usually big differences between the values for the censored observations (always negative) and the uncensored ones (often positive).

The Schoenfeld residuals (Schoenfeld, 1982) are defined for the subjects who underwent the event by:

$$Z_i - E_1(\hat{\beta}, T_i),$$

where

$$E_1(\hat{\beta}, T_i) = \sum_{l=1}^{n} p_l(\hat{\beta}, T_i) Z_l$$

is a weighted mean of covariate values of all subjects at risk at time T_i. The weights are

$$p_l(\hat{\beta}, T_i) = \frac{Y_l(T_i) \exp(Z_l^\top \hat{\beta})}{\sum_{j:\tilde{T}_j \geq T_i} \exp(Z_j^\top \hat{\beta})},$$

where $Y_l(t)$ is the "at risk" indicator for subject l which takes the value 1 if the subject is at risk at t, and 0 otherwise. This equation defines a vector of residuals for all covariates. There should not be any correlation between time and residuals. We can check the proportional hazards assumption by visual inspection (Allison, 2012). R software provides a test; with SAS, correlation between time and residuals should be tested. The Schoenfeld residuals also give an indication of the influence of a subject on the estimate of β.

3.5.8.3   Test for interaction between time and the covariate

In order to test the proportional hazards assumption for a covariate, a practical solution is to introduce in the model an interaction between a function of time and the covariate. This method is simple to implement and allows adjusting on other covariates. The idea is then to test the interaction parameter. Many functions of time can be used (Gill and Schumacher, 1987) including the following two examples.

We may add an interaction between time and the covariate in the model, by adding the time-dependent variable $(t \times Z_k)$. We need two cefficients for the effect of Z_k, β_{k1} for the simple effect and β_{k2} for the interaction variable. In this example, the hazard ratio for a deviation of one unit of the covariate Z_k is equal to $\exp[\beta_{k1} + \beta_{k2}t]$. The hazard ratio varies exponentially with time. If we take an interaction with the logarithm of the time, the hazard ratio varies linearly with time. A test of the hypothesis "$H_0 : \beta_{k2} = 0$" is a test of proportional hazards for Z_k.

Another possibility is to assume that the hazard ratio is constant by pieces. This is possible by putting an interaction with a step function of time.

An advantage of this approach is that it also provides a solution to the non-proportionality. We can build non-proportional hazards models simply by adding interactions with a function of time.

Remark: The various tests are for the same null hypothesis (proportional hazards). The tests are powerful if the departure from H_0 is close to the assumed parametric form for the alternative hypothesis (piece-wise constant, linear or exponential hazard ratio). Similarly, graphical methods and residuals-based tests are more or less sensitive to various types of deviation from the proportional hazard hypothesis. It is therefore not surprising that they do not always lead to consistent results. In practice, it is not possible to use all methods but in case of divergent conclusion, it must be considered that the hypothesis is not verified.

3.5.8.4 Solutions

If the proportional hazards assumption does not hold for a covariate, there are several options. The choice depends on whether this covariate is the factor of interest or an adjustment covariate. If this covariate is not the factor of interest, a solution is to stratify the model on this covariate. If it is the factor of interest, stratification is not a good choice because it makes inference difficult. One possibility is to introduce an interaction between time and the covariate, as seen above. In this case, several hazard ratios for different time-periods must be presented in the communication of the results for this covariate. It is also possible to use a model which does not need the proportional hazards assumption, such as the accelerated failure time model (see Section 3.6) and the additive hazards model. The interpretation of the regression parameters are different: rather than a log-hazard ratio, the parameters represent a factor of acceleration of time in accelerated failure time models and an excess of hazard in the additive hazards models. The models which allow time-varying coefficients are more flexible. This is the case of Aalen additive hazards model, and there are also versions of the proportional hazard models with time-varying coefficients.

3.5.8.5 Example

In the example of survival after entry in institution with the delay since the entry into institution (delay) as time-scale, the proportional hazards assumption is checked for age, educational level and gender. Several tests were performed for illustration in this example. As stated previously, it is not advisable to do as many tests in a real study, mainly because this would raise an issue of multiplicity of tests.

   With Schoenfeld residuals, a correlation between a function of time and the residual has been used. With the delay, there is a problem for adequacy with age (p-value = 0.003). With the logarithm of the delay there is a problem also with gender (p-value = 0.004). With interaction between time and covariates, we have similar results: for $\exp(\beta_1 \times Z + \beta_2 \times \text{delay} \times Z)$, we reject the proportionality assumption only for age (p-value = 0.0002), whereas with an interaction with the logarithm of the delay there is also a problem with gender (p-value= 0.005).

   By plotting $\ln[-\ln(\hat{S}(t))]$ for women and men (Figure 3.1) it appears that the difference between men and women tends to decrease over time. For computing a change of the hazard ratio over time, an interaction with the logarithm of the delay was used (therefore a hazard ratio equals to $\exp(\beta_1 \times \text{sex} + \beta_2 \times \ln(\text{delay}) \times \text{sex})$). For a delay of 2 years the esti-

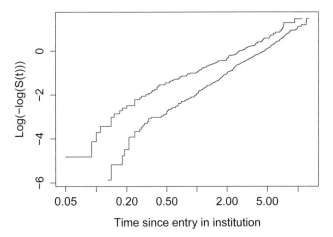

FIGURE 3.1
Functions $\ln[-\ln(\hat{S}(t))]$ to check proportional hazards assumption for gender. Sample of 481 subjects in nursing homes (Paquid study).

mated hazard ratio for women compared to men is equal to 0.57 ([0.46; 0.72]) and for a delay of 6 years 0.81 ([0.56; 1.17]). Regarding age, whatever the method there is a problem of proportionality. For a hazard ratio equal to $\exp(\beta_1 \times \text{age} + \beta_2 \times \text{delay} \times \text{age})$, for a delay of 2 years the estimated hazard ratio for age is equal to 1.04 ([1.02; 1.06]) and 1.10 ([1.07; 1.14]) for a delay of 6 years.

3.5.9 Parametric and penalized likelihood approaches

The semi-parametric Cox model, which has been presented in Section 3.5.2 is the model of choice for estimating the effect of covariates from right-censored and possibly left-truncated data. This model is not always the most suitable, especially when times of events are interval-censored or when an estimate of the baseline hazard function $\alpha_0(t)$ is desired. In these cases, a parametric estimator can be used as those presented in Section 3.4.2 for the hazard function. If one does not wish to make strong assumptions about the shape of the hazard function, it is preferable to resort to the penalized likelihood seen in Section 3.4.3. In both cases, the hazard function and the regression parameters are estimated simultaneously by maximizing the likelihood. To check the proportional hazards assumption, the simplest way is to graphically represent the estimates of hazard functions for different groups defined by the values of the covariates. For a parametric approach, the assumption of a particular distribution needs to be tested too. To overcome this problem, some authors have proposed very general parametric functions (Gallant and Nychka, 1987;

Kooperberg and Clarkson, 1997) but they are currently not easily available in software.

3.6 Accelerated failure time model

The accelerated failure time model is mainly used in reliability, for machine components for example (by the way, the term "failure" comes from reliability theory). In this case we want to study the longevity of components in normal use without spending too much time in the experiments. Therefore these components are exposed to a stress in order to reduce their lifetime. The idea is that under stress conditions, the aging of the component is faster. Assume that the stress is represented by the explanatory variable Z_1, with $Z_1 = 1$ coding for a stress condition, $Z_1 = 0$ otherwise. The model postulates that survival under stress in t is the same as survival in normal condition at te^{β_1}. The survival function can thus be written: $S(t; Z_1, \beta_1) = S_0(te^{\beta_1 Z_1})$. The model can be generalized to take into account a vector Z of discrete or quantitative variables. The expression of the accelerated survival model is:

$$S(t; Z, \beta) = S_0(te^{\beta^\top Z}).$$

It follows (by differentitation and application of relations between survival, density and hazard function) that the hazard is:

$$\alpha(t; Z, \beta) = \exp(\beta^\top Z)\alpha_0(te^{\beta^\top Z}).$$

The class of accelerated failure time models is an alternative to the proportional hazards models. Both classes have an intersection that is the Weibull model: a Weibull proportional hazards model is also a Weibull accelerated failure time model. This is also true of the exponential model (constant hazard) since it is included in the Weibull model. There is no other model that has both properties.

Parametric assumptions for α_0 are often made in the accelerated failure time model. For example, one can choose the hazard function of a Weibull or Gamma distribution. The inference can then be done by maximum likelihood. If one does not make a parametric assumption on α_0, then this is a semi-parametric model, comparable to the Cox model. For this class of models, however, there is no equivalent of the Cox partial likelihood that easily eliminates the nuisance parameter α_0. The inference is more complex both theoretically and numerically (see Kalbfleisch and Prentice, 2002, Chapter 7).

We can also define these models by linear regression of the variable of interest, which may seem very natural. Since the variable T is positive, it is natural to model $Y = \log T$ by a linear regression:

$$Y = \beta^\top Z + \varepsilon,$$

where ε is a zero mean variable; such a model is called *log-linear*. If we assume that ε is normally distributed, we get a log-normal accelerated failure time model that is different from the log-normal proportional hazards model. We obtain the accelerated failure-time (and proportional hazard) Weibull model by assuming that ε is equal to σW, where W has the *extreme value* distribution, with density $f_W(w) = \exp(w - e^w)$. There are simple relationships between the parameters of the log-linear model and those of the proportional hazards model (Kalbfleisch and Prentice, 2002). If we do not make assumptions about the distribution of ε, we find the semi-parametric accelerated failure time model.

3.7   Counting processes approach

The modern approach to event history models uses counting processes theory (Andersen et al., 1993). It allows treating rigorously the increase of information with time. A summary of this approach is given in this section.

We first give a very "heuristic" description of concepts of stochastic processes, filtration, martingale and Doob-Meyer decomposition. For a more thorough description of basic concepts and discrete-time stochastic processes (see Williams, 1991). A process is a set of random variables indexed by t: $N = (N(t), t \geq 0)$; here we assume that time is continuous, which is most often the case in survival analysis.

3.7.1   Counting processes

A univariate counting process N is a non-decreasing process such as $N(0) = 0$; the trajectories are step functions making jumps of magnitude 1. $N(t)$ counts the number of events of interest that occurred before t. The simplest counting process is one for which the event of interest is the death of an individual. The process takes zero up to T, the time when the individual dies, and takes the value of 1 after.

3.7.2   Filtration

A very important concept is that of filtration. To define it, we must first define the concept of sigma-algebra (or sigma-field) generated by a random variable. An algebra is essentially a set of events which is stable by union and intersection; a sigma-algebra is stable for an infinite number of unions (see Williams, 1991, for precise definition). The sigma-algebra generated by a random variable X is the sigma-algebra generated by events $X \in B$ where B is a Borel set of $\mathbb{R}$. If for fixed t, we consider the random variable $N(t)$ where N is a counting process, $N(t)$ is a binary variable. In this case, the sigma-algebra generated by $N(t)$ has four elements: $(\{N(t) = 0\}, \{N(t) = 1\}, \Omega, \emptyset)$, where Ω is the whole space (which can be written $\{N(t) = 0\} \cup \{N(t) = 1\}$) and $\emptyset$ is the empty set. One can consider the sigma-algebra generated by a set of variables, for example:

$$\mathcal{F}_t = \sigma(N(u), 0 \le u \le t).$$

"Observing" a sigma-algebra comes down to knowing which events are realized. For example, if we observe $\mathcal{F}_t$, we know if the event of interest (death of the individual for instance) occurred before t looking whether the event $N(t) = 1$ is true (or has occurred). In this case, the sigma-algebra also contains information on the exact time of death T. On the contrary, if $N(t) = 0$ we only know that $T > t$. A variable X is *measurable* for a sigma-algebra $\mathcal{F}_t$, if the sigma-algebra it generates is included in $\mathcal{F}_t$: $\sigma(X) \subset \mathcal{F}_t$. This is interpreted by saying that if one observes $\mathcal{F}_t$, X is observed. For example, the variable $N(u)$ is measurable for $\mathcal{F}_t$ if $u \le t$ and it is not if $u > t$.

$\mathcal{F}_t$ represents the information on N until t ; since it is clear that information increases with t we can write $\mathcal{F}_s \subset \mathcal{F}_t$ if $s < t$ (all events of $\mathcal{F}_s$ belong to $\mathcal{F}_t$). A filtration is an increasing family of sigma-algebras. The family $\{\mathcal{F}_t : t \ge 0\}$ we have just described is a filtration: the filtration *generated* by the process N.

3.7.3 Martingales and Doob-Meyer decomposition

Then we can define for a given probability law and a given filtration, the concepts of predictable process and martingale. A process C is predictable, if for all t, the variable $C(t)$ is *measurable* for $\mathcal{F}_{t-}$; that is to say, we know the value of $C(t)$ just before t. A martingale is a process $M(t)$ such that $M(0) = 0$ and such that:

$$\mathrm{E}[M(t) \mid \mathcal{F}_s] = M(s), \quad s < t.$$

Here we use the general definition of the conditional expectation for allowing conditioning on a sigma-algebra. If Y and X are two random variables the conditional expectation is conventionally defined by $\mathrm{E}(Y \mid X = x)$, which is a real number for fixed x. One can define $\mathrm{E}(Y \mid X)$ which is a random variable taking value $\mathrm{E}(Y \mid X = x)$ when $X = x$. It is equivalent to write $\mathrm{E}(Y \mid X)$ or $\mathrm{E}(Y \mid \sigma(X))$, where $\sigma(X)$ is the sigma-algebra generated by X. The random variable $\mathrm{E}(Y \mid \sigma(X))$ is measurable for the sigma-algebra $\sigma(X)$. We can now state the Doob-Meyer decomposition for a counting process:

$$N(t) = \Lambda(t) + M(t), \quad t \ge 0, \tag{3.7}$$

where $\Lambda(t)$ is a non-decreasing predictable process called "compensator," and $M(t)$ is a martingale. For a given probability law and filtration, this decomposition is unique. When it exists, the differential representation of this decomposition is:

$$\mathrm{d}N(t) = \lambda(t)\mathrm{d}t + \mathrm{d}M(t), \quad t \ge 0,$$

where $\lambda(t)$ is the intensity of the process; $\Lambda(t)$ can also be called the "cumulative intensity" of the process. The link between $\lambda(t)$ and the hazard function $\alpha(t)$ is the following. Let us define the indicator $Y(t)$ which takes value 1 if the subject is at risk, and 0 otherwise. Consider the uncensored case where $Y(t) = 1$ if $T \geq t$ and $Y(t) = 0$ if $T < t$. By definition of the hazard function we have: $P(t \leq T < t + dt) \mid T \geq t) = \alpha(t)dt$. We have $E(dN(t) \mid \mathcal{F}_{t-}) = \lambda(t)dt$. We have also $E(dN(t) \mid T \geq t) = P(t \leq T < t + dt) \mid T \geq t)$ and $E(dN(t) \mid T < t) = 0$. Thus one can write:

$$\lambda(t) = Y(t)\alpha(t).$$

This multiplicative model (called "Aalen multiplicative model") also applies if $Y(t)$ is an indicator of at risk subject when there is right-censoring and if $N(t)$ represents the number of observed events of interest at time t.

This theory which includes many developments (predictable variation processes, stochastic integrals, martingale convergence theorems) can be used to find natural non-parametric estimators and to approximate their distributions.

3.7.4 Nelson-Aalen and Breslow estimators

We give here just the heuristic definition of the Nelson-Aalen estimator of the cumulative hazard function and its extension to the proportional hazards model, the Breslow estimator. Consider a sample of n possibly right-censored survival times, identically and independently distributed. The at-risk status indicator is $Y_i(t)$, which takes the value 1 if the subject is at risk, and 0 otherwise. The subject is at risk in t if he/she is neither dead nor censored before t. A counting process $N_i(t)$ may be associated with each subject and its Doob-Meyer decomposition is: $dN_i(t) = \lambda_i(t)dt + dM_i(t)$. The multiplicative model for the intensity is:

$$\lambda_i(t) = Y_i(t)\alpha(t).$$

Summing the n equations we obtain: $dN_\bullet(t) = Y_\bullet(t)\alpha(t) + dM_\bullet(t)$, where $N_\bullet(t) = \sum N_i(t)$, $Y_\bullet(t) = \sum Y_i(t)$ and $M_\bullet(t) = \sum M_i(t)$. Note that $Y_\bullet(t)$ is the size of the at-risk set at time t. If $Y_\bullet(t) > 0$, it is natural to estimate $\alpha(t)$ by $\hat{\alpha}(t) = \frac{dN_\bullet(t)}{Y_\bullet(t)}$. Let the ordered observed times of events be denoted as before by $t_{(1)} < t_{(2)} < \ldots < t_{(k)}$. Then, $\hat{\alpha}(t) = \frac{dN_\bullet(t)}{Y_\bullet(t)}$ takes value zero if there has been no event in t and the value $\frac{1}{Y_\bullet(t_{(j)})}$ at time $t_{(j)}$ when an event occurred. One does not obtain a good estimator of $\alpha(t)$ but one can obtain a good estimator of the cumulative hazard by summing these estimators of instantaneous hazards:

$$\hat{A}(t) = \sum_{j:t_{(j)} \leq t} \frac{1}{Y_\bullet(t_{(j)})}.$$

This is the Nelson-Aalen estimator. It can be shown that its variance can be estimated by

$$\sum_{j:t_{(j)} \leq t} \frac{1}{[Y.(t_{(j)})]^2}.$$

The asymptotic results allow to approximate the distribution of $\hat{A}(t)$ by a normal distribution.

Note that the Nelson-Aalen and the Kaplan-Meier estimators define the same distribution of event times. This is a distribution with probability masses only at observed event times, and a null density elsewhere. In general, the survival function can be expressed as a function of the cumulative hazard by the product-integral (Andersen et al., 1993). In the continuous case, this takes the form $S(t) = e^{-A(t)}$. In the case where the distribution has masses at $t_{(j)}$, the survival function and the hazard function are connected by the equation: $S(t) = \Pi_{0 < t_{(j)} < t}[1 - dA(t_{(j)})]$. The survival distribution function characterized by the Nelson-Aalen estimator is $\Pi_{0 < t_{(j)} < t}[1 - \frac{1}{Y.(t_{(j)})}]$, which is the Kaplan-Meier estimator. In conclusion, the Kaplan-Meier and the Nelson-Aalen estimators specify the same distribution.

In the proportional hazards model, the cumulative baseline hazard function can be estimated by the Breslow estimator which is:

$$\hat{A}_0(t) = \sum_{j:t_{(j)} \leq t} \frac{1}{\sum_{l=1}^{n} Y_l(t_{(j)}) \exp(\hat{\beta}^\top Z_l)},$$

and one retrieves the Nelson-Aalen estimator if $\hat{\beta} = 0$ (because in that case $\sum_{l=1}^{n} Y_l(t_{(j)}) \exp(\hat{\beta}^\top Z_l) = Y.(t_{(j)})$, the number of at-risk subjects in $t_{(j)}$). An estimator of the cumulative hazard for subject i is:

$$\hat{A}_i(t) = \hat{A}_0(t) \exp(\hat{\beta}^\top Z_i) = \sum_{j:t_{(j)} \leq t} \frac{\exp(\hat{\beta}^\top Z_i)}{\sum_{l=1}^{n} Y_l(t_{(j)}) \exp(\hat{\beta}^\top Z_l)}.$$

One calls *estimated martingale* $\hat{M}_i(t) = N_i(t) - \hat{A}_i(t)$, and the martingale residuals discussed in Section 3.5.8 are defined by $\hat{M}_i(\tilde{T}_i)$.

3.8 Additive risks models

The formalism of the theory of stochastic processes allows presenting the Aalen additive risk model which is another alternative to the Cox model.

3.8.1 The additive risks models: specification and inference

The Cox proportional hazards model is a multiplicative model which assumes that the hazard function is the product of a basic hazard function and a function of the explanatory variables. Aalen (1989) proposed an additive risk model, in which the hazard is the sum of a baseline hazard function and a linear function of explanatory variables. In a number of cases, the additive hazards model provides a better fit to the data than the multiplicative model (although comparison between the two is not obvious). As in the Cox model, the explanatory variables may depend on time. The simplicity of the additive hazards model allows an additional extension to a model whose coefficients depend on time, with no additional parametric assumption. The estimation of the cumulative effects is computationally simple. The hazard function for the individual i is modeled as:

$$\alpha_i(t) = \beta_0(t) + \beta_1(t)X_{1i}(t) + \ldots + \beta_p(t)X_{pi}(t), \qquad (3.8)$$

where $\beta_0(t)$ is the baseline hazard function and $\beta_j(t)$ represents the increment of the risk at time t for a one-unit increment of the explanatory variable $X_{ji}(t)$. The model is completely non-parametric and the fact that the coefficients can depend on time gives greater flexibility. Additivity facilitates the estimation and provides some robustness to the model. The weakness of the model is that it is not guaranteed that the hazard is positive (as is the case in the Cox model).

The estimation focuses mainly on the cumulative regression functions $B_j(t) = \int_0^t \beta_j(u)\, du$. The inference method uses the counting process theory and the Doob-Meyer decomposition presented in Section 3.7.1. The counting process $N_i(t) = 1_{\{T_i \geq t\}}$ has the intensity:

$$\lambda_i(t) = Y_i(t)[\beta_0(t) + \beta_1(t)X_{1i}(t) + \ldots + \beta_p(t)X_{pi}(t)], \qquad (3.9)$$

where $Y_i(t) = 1$ if the individual i is at risk at time t, $Y_i(t) = 0$ otherwise. The differential representation of the Doob-Meyer decomposition for N_i is: $dN_i(t) = d\Lambda_i(t) + dM_i(t)$. If Λ_i is differentiable, we can write $d\Lambda_i(t) = \lambda_i(t)dt$. However, in the non-parametric approach, we can only estimate the $B_j(t)$ but not their derivatives $\beta_j(t)$ and, for this reason, the following equations are written in terms of differential elements $dB_j(t)$:

$$dN_i(t) = Y_i(t)dB_0(t) + \sum_{j=1}^{p} dB_j(t)Y_i(t)X_{ji}(t) + dM_i(t). \qquad (3.10)$$

For a given time t, this equation has the form of a linear regression, where $dN_i(t)$ is the dependent variable, $Y_i(t)$ and $X_{ji}(t)$ are the explanatory variables, $dB_j(t)$ the parameters to be estimated and $dM_i(t)$ the random error.

We can write the equations using matrices. We define the following vectors: $N(t) = (N_1(t), \ldots, N_n(t))^\top$; $M(t) = (M_1(t), \ldots, M_n(t))^\top$; $B(t) = (B_1(t), \ldots, B_p(t))^\top$. We call $X(t)$ the $(n \times (p+1))$ matrix whose line i is $(Y_i(t), Y_i(t)X_{1i}(t), \ldots, Y_i(t)X_{pi}(t))$. With this notation, Equation (3.10) is written:

$$dN(t) = X(t)dB(t) + dM(t). \qquad (3.11)$$

The classical solution of the parameters estimates of a linear regression gives:

$$d\hat{B}(t) = [X(t)^\top X(t)]^{-1} X(t)^\top dN(t),$$

when the matrix $X(t)$ has full rank. We note $X^-(t) = [X(t)^\top X(t)]^{-1} X(t)^\top$, called the "left generalized inverse." To obtain an estimator of $B(t)$ one accumulates the increments $d\hat{B}(t)$ at event times $t_{(1)} < t_{(2)} < \dots$ (otherwise $d\hat{B}(t) = 0$) only for the times $t_{(k)}$ where the matrix $X(t_{(k)})$ has full rank (denoted $J(t_{(k)}) = 1$, 0 otherwise). A necessary condition for $X(t_{(k)})$ to have full rank is that there are more than p subjects at risk at time $t_{(k)}$; there are also conditions on the explanatory variables: among at risk subjects there must be more than p subjects with different values of explanatory variables. We have thus:

$$\hat{B}(t) = \sum_{t_{(k)} \leq t} J(t_{(k)}) X^-(t_{(k)}) \Delta N(t_{(k)}), \tag{3.12}$$

where $\Delta N(t_{(k)})$ contains zeros except for the individual who had the event at $t_{(k)}$. An interesting property of this estimator is that in the case of a single binary variable, the estimator of the cumulative risk for both terms of this variable is identical to the Nelson-Aalen estimator for each of the subgroups. Remember that the Nelson-Aalen estimator of the cumulative risk and the Kaplan-Meier estimator of the survival function characterize the same distribution of survival time.

By martingale methods it can be shown that an estimator of the variance of $\hat{B}(t)$ is:

$$\hat{\Sigma}(t) = \sum_{t_{(k)} \leq t} J(t_{(k)}) X^-(t_{(k)}) \Delta N(t_{(k)}) X^-(t_{(k)})^\top. \tag{3.13}$$

Moreover $\hat{B}(t)$ is consistent for $B(t)$ (if $J(u) = 1, u \leq t$) and has approximately a multivariate normal distribution centered around the true value of $B(t)$. Thus, the confidence interval $(1 - \alpha)\%$ for $B_j(t)$ is

$$[\hat{B}_j(t) - |z_{\alpha/2}| \sigma_{jj}(t), \hat{B}_j(t) + |z_{\alpha/2}| \sigma_{jj}(t)],$$

where $\sigma_{jj}^2(t)$ is the j-th diagonal element of the matrix $\hat{\Sigma}(t)$ and $z_{\alpha/2}$ the quantile $\alpha/2$ of the standard normal distribution.

Statistical tests for a null effect of a variable on the risk can be constructed. The null hypothesis is defined by $H_0 : B_j(t) = 0, t > 0$. Aalen (1989) proposed a test of this hypothesis against alternative hypotheses of the form $\beta_j(t) > 0$ or $\beta_j(t) < 0$ for any $t < t_0$, i.e., alternatives where there is no crossover of the hazards. The test statistic is a weighted sum of $\Delta \hat{B}_j(t_{(k)})$:

$$Z_j = \sum_{t_{(k)} \leq t_0} L_j(t_{(k)}) \Delta \hat{B}_j(t_{(k)}).$$

The variance of Z_j can be estimated by:

$$V_j = \sum_{t_{(k)} \leq t_0} L_j^2(t_{(k)}) \Delta \hat{\sigma}_{jj}^2(t_{(k)}),$$

where $\Delta \hat{\sigma}_{jj}^2(t_{(k)})$ is the increment of the j-th diagonal element of $\hat{\Sigma}(t)$. So the test statistic is $Z_j/\sqrt{V_j}$. Aalen proposed to choose the weight $L_j(t)$ as the inverse of the j-th diagonal element of the matrix $[X(t)^\top X(t)]^{-1}$, i.e., weights that consider the inverse of the variance of $\Delta \hat{B}_j(t_{(k)})$. This test, called TST, has the advantage of being identical to the log-rank test in case where the effect of a binary variable is tested (in the absence of other variables).

Other developments include the hypothesis test for several covariates, the test for a constant effect of a covariate, tests or graphical methods to evaluate the fit of the model. We refer the reader to the books of Martinussen and Scheike (2006) and Aalen et al. (2008).

3.8.2   Application to mortality in institution

We take the example of the survival of subjects living in institution. We are interested in the effect of age at entry in institution, sex and educational level.

We take as basic time-scale the time in years since institutionalization (called *time*). The age at entry into institution was centered around 85 years, the average entry age. The educational level is represented here by a binary variable called *education*: 0 for "no education," 1 for "at least primary school diploma." Sex is coded 0 for men, 1 for women. This model can be fitted using the R package survival and the function aareg, or with the R package timereg and the function aalen.

Table 3.2 shows the results of the tests of the null hypotheses of no effect $B_j(t) = 0$ for the age at entry in institution, sex and educational level. All these hypotheses are rejected.

TABLE 3.2
Results of the statistical tests for the effect of the explanatory variables in the additive hazards model applied to the survival analysis in institution.

Variable	Test statistic	p-value
Intercept	10.56	< 0.001
Age at entry	4.79	< 0.001
Education	-2.27	0.027
Sex	-4.76	< 0.001

The estimated cumulative regression curves $\hat{B}_j(t)$ are presented in Figure 3.2 together with 95% point-by-point confidence intervals. First, have a look at the intercept. If the baseline hazard was constant, the baseline cumulative hazard would be a line whose slope would be the baseline hazard. It is not far from being so. This result is not completely obvious epidemiologically because the subjects are ageing and one would expect an increase of the baseline hazard with time. But we have very strong selection effects in this population, which may explain this result, in agreement with the result found by Commenges et al. (2007). The effect of age at entry into institution is positive and appears to increase with time (a test, not detailed here confirms this increase). The effect of education is negative, indicating that subjects with high educational level have a lower risk of mortality than subjects without an educational level. However, this effect is not constant: it seems low for the first two years and seems to disappear after about six years. We observe the same kind of evolution for sex. Women have a lower risk than men, but this effect seems to disappear after about 7 years.

3.9 Degradation models

The class of *degradation models* is obtained by considering that the event of interest is the result of a continuous degradation. This process can be either a wear process or a process of accumulation. It is not surprising that this approach is widely used in industrial reliability applications where the failure of a machine part occurs with a high probability if a certain degree of wear has been reached. This point of view is also interesting in epidemiology. For example, myocardial infarction (MI) is the consequence of atherosclerotic deposits in the arteries: these deposits build up gradually and at some stage a heart attack occurs. Here, it is more an accumulation process than a wear process. The degradation process $U(t)$ is usually modelled by a Brownian motion with drift:

$$U(t) = \lambda_U t + B(t),$$

where B is a Brownian motion (or Brownian process) and λ_U is the drift. The Brownian process is a Gaussian process with independent increments and continuous path that takes a central role in the theory of stochastic processes; see Klebaner (2005) for a gentle introduction.

The event occurs when the process $U(t)$ exceeds a certain threshold η. Figure 3.3 illustrates the trajectory of a Brownian motion with drift representing the atherosclerotic process that is supposed to start from zero at the age of 20 years; the threshold η is equal to 17.5, a value that has been estimated in Commenges and Hejblum (2013). This path crosses the threshold at 68 years.

The event time T then follows an inverse Gaussian distribution whose density is:

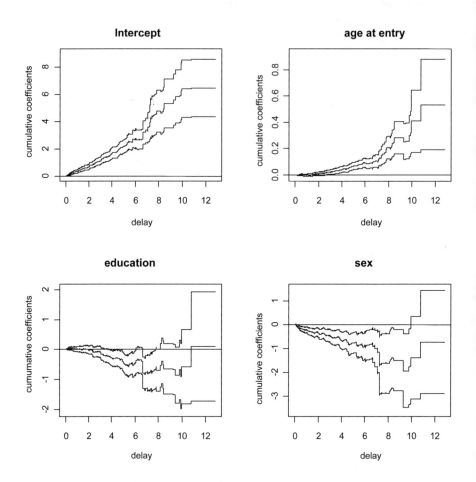

FIGURE 3.2
Cumulative regression curves: intercept and cumulative effect of the age at entry into institution, the educational level and sex on mortality in institution.

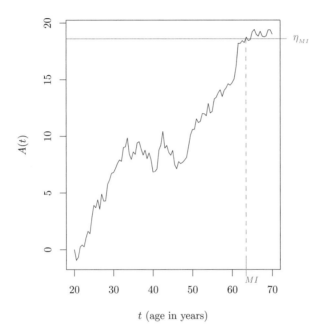

t (age in years)

FIGURE 3.3
Example of path of the atheromatous process $U(t)$; η is the threshold of appearance of a myocardial infarction which is reached in this example at 68 years.

$$f^{(\lambda_U,\eta)}(t) = \left[\frac{\eta^2}{2\pi t^3}\right]^{1/2} \exp\left(\frac{-\lambda_U^2\left(t - \frac{\eta}{\lambda_U}\right)^2}{2t}\right).$$

Both drift and threshold may depend on covariates. Drift for the individual i can be modelled by $\lambda_{Ui} = \beta X^i$, where X^i is a vector of explanatory variables. This approach provides a family of parametric models that may be well adapted in some contexts. The application to myocardial infarction has been developed by Commenges and Hejblum (2013). Aalen et al. (2008, Section 10.3.8) provide an example of data analysis on the carcinoma of the oropharynx.

4

Models for longitudinal data

This chapter is devoted to models for the analysis of longitudinal data defined as time-dependent repeated data. The dependent variable Y of interest is measured repeatedly at different times on the same subjects. Such longitudinal data are frequent in epidemiology. For example, in observational cohort studies and clinical trials of HIV infected patients, the concentration of CD4 + T lymphocytes (CD4) (CD4 counts) and the plasma viral load are measured repeatedly during the follow-up. The analysis of the time course of these two markers that are predictors of the clinical progression of the disease enables the natural history of the disease to be described, and the effectiveness of treatments to be evaluated. In many other diseases, repeated measures of biomarkers are used to track the progression of a patient's condition and anticipate the occurrence of clinical events. For instance, in prostate cancer, an increase of the prostate specific antigen (PSA) is a predictor of prostate cancer relapse after an initial treatment. The study of normal and pathological cognitive aging in the elderly is also based on repeated measures of cognitive tests. In the three above examples, the variables of interest are quantitative variables either continuous (CD4 counts, viral load, PSA) or discrete (cognitive tests). There are also numerous examples of longitudinal binary data, such as daily measures of truancy among children or of asthma attacks in asthmatic patients.

In a longitudinal study on a sample of N subjects, N series of measures of the same variable at different times are collected. Data therefore consist in a large number (N) of series generally including a small number of repeated measures (n_i measures for subject i denoted Y_{ij} for $j = 1, \ldots, n_i$). This is in contrast with time series that consist in one or two series of measures of larger sizes. Furthermore, in longitudinal studies, the number of measurements n_i and the dates of measurements can be different from one subject to the other and not equally spaced.

In most cases, the purpose of longitudinal data analysis is to describe the time course of the variable of interest and to identify factors that influence this time course. These analyses cannot be performed with standard regression models since repeated measures of a subject at different times are not independent. The repeated measurements induce a within-subject correlation, whereas standard regression models assume that observations are independent. To get rid of the within-subject correlation, it is sometimes proposed to summarize the repeated data of each subject by a single variable, for example the difference (crude or relative) between the final and initial values. Although sometimes useful for simple problems, the limitations of this approach are fairly obvious: a major loss of information (n_i measures summarized by one) and extreme sensitivity to missing data (the summarized variable cannot be calculated if the last measure is missing). In addition it is not possible to study the impact of time-dependent predictors on the change of Y with this approach.

In this chapter, we focus on the models for the analysis of longitudinal data that use all the available data. We first describe the mixed models (linear models, generalized linear models and non-linear models) which are the most commonly used models for longitudinal data analysis and have been extended in various directions. Marginal models estimated by generalized estimating equations are then presented briefly, mainly to contrast them with mixed models. The last two sections are respectively devoted to the treatment of incomplete longitudinal data and to a discussion of modeling strategies. The next chapter presents several extensions of mixed models.

4.1 Linear mixed models

4.1.1 Genesis

In this section, the outcome variable Y is supposed to be quantitative Gaussian. Let us denote Y_{ij} the observation of Y for subject i, $i = 1, \ldots, N$ at time t_{ij}, $j = 1, \ldots, n_i$ and X_{ij} a vector of explanatory variables of size p that may include fixed or time-dependent variables as well as time or any function of time.

The standard linear model that assumes an independence between repeated measures of a subject is defined by:

$$Y_{ij} = X_{ij}^{\top}\beta + \epsilon_{ij} \text{ with } \epsilon_{ij} \sim \mathcal{N}(0, \sigma^2) \text{ and } \epsilon_{ij} \perp \epsilon_{ij'} \forall j \neq j'. \tag{4.1}$$

The symbol $\perp$ means independence.

The parameters (β, σ) of this model can be estimated by maximum likelihood under the assumption of independence between the observations, and the variance estimator of the parameters is obtained by the inverse of the Hessian matrix (see Section 2.2.2). However when the data are correlated, the variance estimator is biased as well as the associated tests (Wald test for instance). In particular, the variances of the regression parameters that correspond to time-constant explanatory variables are underestimated under the independence assumption and the associated tests are anti-conservative.

A naive solution to account for within-subject correlation while remaining under ordinary regression models could be the inclusion of a subject-specific intercept in model (4.1):

$$Y_{ij} = \alpha_i + X_{ij}^\top \beta + \epsilon_{ij} \text{ with } \epsilon_{ij} \sim \mathcal{N}(0, \sigma^2) \text{ and } \epsilon_{ij} \perp \epsilon_{ij'} \forall j \neq j'. \quad (4.2)$$

However, the estimation of this model leads to three major problems that make this approach unusable:

- The total number of model parameters is $N + p + 1$ (N subject-specific parameters + p regression parameters + the residual variance) or $N - 1 + p + 1 = N + p$ because if β includes an intercept, only $N - 1$ subject-specific parameters are added. The asymptotic theory of the maximum likelihood thus fails since the number of parameters increases with the sample size (see Section 2.2.2). Moreover, the large number of parameters may cause convergence problems of numerical algorithms.

- If the vector X_{ij} includes at least one time-constant explanatory variable X_{ki} (a variable with fixed value whatever time), the associated regression coefficient β_k is not identifiable; only the sum $b_i + X_{ki}\beta_k$ is identifiable.

- The findings of the analysis are not generalizable to other subjects because the identifier of the subject is an explanatory variable, and it is not recommended to extrapolate results of a statistical analysis to values of explanatory variables that are not observed in the sample.

To overcome these problems, the fixed subject-specific effects may be replaced by a random variable: the subject-specific intercept in Equation (4.2) is not a parameter anymore but a random variable that is usually assumed Gaussian with zero mean and variance σ_b^2. The subject effect is thus taken into account by adding a single parameter in the model: the variance σ_b^2 of the random effect. The total number of parameters is reduced to $p + 2$ and independent of N. It is possible to introduce other subject-specific random effects such as a random slope (in association with time, for example). These models are called "random-effect models" or "mixed-effect models" because they contain both random and fixed effects. Most frequently, they are called "mixed models" for brevity.

4.1.2 Definition of the linear mixed model

The standard linear mixed model is defined by Laird and Ware (1982):

$$Y_{ij} = X_{ij}^\top \beta + Z_{ij}^\top b_i + \epsilon_{ij} \text{ with } \epsilon_{ij} \sim \mathcal{N}(0, \sigma^2) \text{ and } b_i \sim \mathcal{N}(0, B), \quad (4.3)$$

where X_{ij} is a p-vector of explanatory variables for the observation j of subject i, β is a p-vector of fixed effects (usually including the global intercept); Z_{ij} is a sub-vector of X_{ij} of size q ($q \leq p$). The vectors b_i of size q are vectors of random effects identically and independently distributed according to a Gaussian distribution with mean 0 and variance matrix B. This distribution is called *a priori* distribution or prior. In most cases, the matrix B is left unstructured which means that all the random effects can be correlated and B includes $q \times (q+1)/2$ parameters. To limit the number of parameters in the presence of multiple random effects, it is sometimes assumed that the random effects are independent of each other, i.e., matrix B is diagonal. The residual errors ϵ_{ij} are assumed independent of each other and independent of b_i. Thus, *given b_i, the variables Y_{ij} are independent.*

Let us denote $Y_i = (Y_{i1}, Y_{i2}, \ldots, Y_{in_i})^\top$ the vector of responses for subject i, $\epsilon_i = (\epsilon_{i1}, \epsilon_{i2}, \ldots, \epsilon_{in_i})^\top$ the vector of errors, and X_i ($n_i \times p$) and Z_i ($n_i \times q$), the matrices of explanatory variables for all the observation times of subject i. Row vectors j ($j = 1, \ldots, n_i$) of X_i and Z_i are $X_{ij}^\top$ and $Z_{ij}^\top$. The model may be written in vector form as:

$$Y_i = X_i\beta + Z_i b_i + \epsilon_i \text{ with } \epsilon_i \sim \mathcal{N}(0, \sigma^2 I_{n_i}). \tag{4.4}$$

Formulas (4.3) and (4.4) define the linear mixed model conditionally on the random effects. As all the variables are Gaussian, by defining $\varepsilon_i = Z_i b_i + \epsilon_i$, the marginal formulation of the model is obtained as:

$$Y_i = X_i\beta + \varepsilon_i \text{ with } \varepsilon_i \sim \mathcal{N}(0, V_i = Z_i B Z_i^\top + \sigma^2 I_{n_i}). \tag{4.5}$$

Thus, the linear mixed model (4.3) implies that the response vector for a subject is a multivariate Gaussian variable, $Y_i \sim \mathcal{N}(X_i\beta, V_i)$, with a covariance matrix whose structure is determined by the choice of the random effects. We distinguish the marginal expectation:

$$\mathrm{E}(Y_i) = X_i\beta,$$

that is the expectation of Y_i for the entire population sharing features X_i and the expectation of Y_i given the random effects

$$\mathrm{E}(Y_i \mid b_i) = X_i\beta + Z_i b_i.$$

that is the specific expectation for subject i.

Throughout this chapter, independence of responses between individuals is assumed: $Y_i \perp Y_{i'}$. However, when individuals are grouped, e.g., within hospitals or families, this assumption of independence between subjects can be violated. The intra-group correlation may sometimes disappear after adjustment for explanatory variables or may be handled by including a fixed group-effect if the number of groups is small. In other cases, the intra-group correlation is taken into account by including a group-specific random effect in addition to the subject-specific random effects. This hierarchical model therefore includes nested random effects (subject effect nested within group effect). Such models with more than two levels will not be described further in the remaining of the chapter but the methodology is similar given that the groups are independent.

Example 7 *(Random intercept model)*

The simplest linear mixed model is the random intercept model also called "uniform correlation model." It includes only one random effect ($q = 1$ and $Z_{ij} = 1$ for all i and j) and therefore assumes that only the mean level of Y varies between subjects:

$$Y_{ij} = X_{ij}^\top \beta + b_{0i} + \epsilon_{ij} \text{ with } \epsilon_{ij} \sim \mathcal{N}(0, \sigma_\epsilon^2) \text{ , } b_{0i} \sim \mathcal{N}(0, \sigma_0^2)$$

where ϵ_{ij} and b_{0i} are independent.

The marginal expectation and variance are $\mathrm{E}(Y_{ij}) = X_{ij}^\top \beta$ and $\mathrm{var}(Y_{ij}) = \sigma_\epsilon^2 + \sigma_0^2$, while the conditional expectations and variances are $\mathrm{E}(Y_{ij} \mid b_{0i}) = X_{ij}^\top \beta + b_{0i}$ and $\mathrm{var}(Y_{ij} \mid b_{0i}) = \sigma_\epsilon^2$. This model therefore assumes that the variance is constant in time as well as the covariance between two measures of the same subject:

$$\mathrm{cov}(Y_{ij}, Y_{ik}) = \mathrm{E}\{(b_{0i} + \epsilon_{ij})(b_{0i} + \epsilon_{ik})\} = \sigma_0^2 \ \forall i, j, k$$

The variance of the random intercept represents the covariance between any couple of measures of a subject. The correlation between two measures is also constant $\mathrm{corr}(Y_{ij}, Y_{ik}) = \frac{\sigma_0^2}{\sigma_0^2 + \sigma_\epsilon^2}$ and is called "intra-class correlation." This explains why the random intercept model is sometimes named "uniform correlation model." Because of these properties, the random intercept model is often considered as too rigid to model longitudinal data. It is indeed common that the variance increases with time and that the correlation between two measurements depends on the time interval between these measurements.

Example 8 *(Model with random intercept and slope)*

The model with random intercept and slope is often better suited for longitudinal data. Here, both initial level and slope vary from one subject to the other:

$$Y_{ij} = X_{ij}^\top \beta + b_{0i} + b_{1i} t_{ij} + \epsilon_{ij} \text{ with } \epsilon_{ij} \sim \mathcal{N}(0, \sigma_\epsilon^2)$$
$$\text{and } b_i = (b_{0i}, b_{1i})^\top \sim \mathcal{N}\left(0, B = \begin{bmatrix} \sigma_0^2 & \sigma_{01} \\ \sigma_{01} & \sigma_1^2 \end{bmatrix}\right).$$

It is reminded that t_{ij} is the time at which Y_{ij} is observed. This model assumes that the variance and covariance between two measures depend on the time of measurements:

$$\mathrm{var}(Y_i) = V_i = Z_i B Z_i^\top + \sigma^2 I_{n_i}$$

where Z_i is a $n_i \times 2$ matrix consisting of row vectors $Z_{ij}^\top = (1 \ t_{ij})$. As Z_{ij} was defined as a sub-vector of X_{ij}, the average intercept and slope must be included in the vector β. Otherwise, as the random effects have a zero expectation, the expectation of Y at $t = 0$ and the mean slope would be constrained to be null. Specifically, the covariance between two observations of subject i is

$$\mathrm{cov}(Y_{ij}, Y_{ik}) = \sigma_0^2 + \sigma_1^2 t_{ij} t_{ik} + \sigma_{01}(t_{ij} + t_{ik})$$

and the variance is

$$\text{var}(Y_{ij}) = \sigma_0^2 + \sigma_1^2 t_{ij}^2 + 2\sigma_{01} t_{ij}.$$

Whenever independence is assumed between the random effects (i.e., $\sigma_{01} = 0$), the variance and the covariance are imposed to be increasing with time.

Generalization:

In some cases, the independence assumption between the responses Y_{ij} given the random effects may be considered as too strict leading to an unrealistic correlation structure between Y_{ij}. The most general formulation of the linear mixed-effect model therefore admits correlated residual errors in addition to the random effects. Conditional on the random effects, the model can be written as in Jones and Boadi-Boateng (1991):

$$Y_i = X_i\beta + Z_i b_i + \epsilon_i \text{ with } \epsilon_i \sim \mathcal{N}(0, \Sigma_i) \text{ and } b_i \sim \mathcal{N}(0, B), \qquad (4.6)$$

and the marginal form is:

$$Y_i = X_i\beta + \varepsilon_i \text{ with } \varepsilon_i \sim \mathcal{N}(0, V_i = Z_i B Z_i^\top + \Sigma_i). \qquad (4.7)$$

For example, the error ϵ_{ij} may be the sum of two terms, a Gaussian autoregressive process capturing the residual correlation between successive measurements of Y and an independent measurement error:

$$\epsilon_{ij} = w_i(t_{ij}) + e_{ij} \qquad (4.8)$$

where e_{ij} are independent with distribution $\mathcal{N}(0, \sigma_e^2)$ and $w_i(t_{ij})$ follows a Gaussian distribution with expectation 0, variance σ_w^2 and correlation

$$\text{corr}(w_i(t_{ij}), w_i(t_{ik})) = \exp(-\gamma|t_{ij} - t_{ik}|) \text{ with } \gamma > 0.$$

The random effects b_i, the autoregressive error $w_i(t_{ij})$ and the independent error e_{ij} are mutually independent for all i and j. The variance matrix of vector ϵ_i is therefore the sum of two terms:

$$\Sigma_i = \Sigma_{wi} + \sigma_e^2 I_{n_i}$$

with Σ_{wi} the variance matrix of the autoregressive process.

In this model, $X_i\beta$ represents the mean profile of the subjects with covariate values X_i, the random effects stand for the individual long-term trend, the autoregressive error accounts for the short-term individual variations and e_{ij} represents the independent residual error often associated with measurement instruments. This independent residual error is almost always necessary because measurement tools generally induce a random measurement error and the correlation between two measurements taken almost at the same time is not equal to 1. Other correlation structures are possible to account for the time-dependent correlation (for example $w_i(t_{ij})$ may be a Brownian motion). One can also define directly the covariance matrix V_i without including random effects in the model.

4.1.3 Estimation

Parameters of a linear mixed model are estimated by maximizing the log-likelihood or the restricted (or residual) log-likelihood.

4.1.3.1 Maximum likelihood estimation

The likelihood of a linear mixed model (or more generally a multivariate Gaussian model) can be obtained from the marginal model formulation

$$Y_i = X_i\beta + \varepsilon_i \text{ with } \varepsilon_i \sim \mathcal{N}(0, V_i).$$

Let us denote ϕ the vector of covariance parameters in V_i. For instance, in the model defined by (4.8), $\phi = (\sigma_e^2, \gamma, \sigma_w^2, \sigma_\varepsilon^2)$. The log-likelihood is:

$$
\begin{aligned}
L(\beta, \phi) &= \sum_{i=1}^{N} \log(f_{Y_i}(Y_i)) \qquad\qquad (4.9)\\
&= -\frac{1}{2}\sum_{i=1}^{N}\left\{ n_i \log(2\pi) + \log|V_i| + (Y_i - X_i\beta)^\top V_i^{-1}(Y_i - X_i\beta) \right\}
\end{aligned}
$$

where $|V_i|$ is the determinant of V_i. The score equation for parameters β is:

$$\frac{\partial L(\beta, \phi)}{\partial \beta} = \sum_{i=1}^{N} X_i^\top V_i^{-1}(Y_i - X_i\beta) = 0.$$

When ϕ is known, β is estimated by:

$$\hat{\beta} = (\sum_{i=1}^{N} X_i^\top V_i^{-1} X_i)^{-1}(\sum_{i=1}^{N} X_i^\top V_i^{-1} Y_i). \qquad (4.10)$$

In practice, the variance parameters must be estimated. The maximum likelihood estimator of ϕ may be obtained by replacing β by (4.10) in (4.9) and maximizing the resulting log-likelihood on ϕ by an iterative procedure (most often a Newton-Raphson or Quasi-Newton algorithm, see Section 2.5.2). An alternative is to directly maximize (4.9) according to β and ϕ using an iterative procedure.

4.1.3.2 Restricted or Residual Maximum Likelihood (REML)

In a standard linear model (where Y_i is of dimension 1 and X_i is a p-vector), it is well known that the maximum likelihood estimator of the residual variance $\sum_i^N (Y_i - X_i\hat{\beta})^2 / N$ is biased because it does not take into account the estimation of β. For samples of small size (relative to the number of parameters), the unbiased estimator $\sum_i^N (Y_i - X_i\hat{\beta})^2 / (N - p)$ (where p is the size of β) is recommended. The same problem arises for mixed models on small samples:

the maximum likelihood estimator of ϕ is biased because it does not take into account the loss of degrees of freedom induced by the fixed effects estimation. To correct this bias, ϕ can be estimated by maximizing the restricted or residual likelihood (REML). The restricted likelihood is the likelihood of $\sum_{i=1}^{N} n_i - p$ variables

$$U = A^\top Y,$$

where A is a full rank matrix of size $\sum_{i=1}^{N} n_i \times (\sum_{i=1}^{N} n_i - p)$ whose columns are orthogonal to the columns of the matrix of explanatory variables X (i.e., $A^\top X = 0$). The vector U has thus a Gaussian distribution with expectation zero ($E(U) = A^\top X\beta = 0$) and variance $A^\top \text{var}(Y)A$ that does not depend on β. Harville (1974) showed that the restricted log-likelihood is, up to a constant and whatever the matrix A, equal to:

$$L_{\text{REML}}(\phi) = L(\hat{\beta}, \phi) - \frac{1}{2} \log | \sum_{i=1}^{N} X_i^\top V_i^{-1} X_i| \qquad (4.11)$$

Note that *the restricted likelihood cannot be used to compare models that do not contain the same fixed effects.* Indeed, if the matrices of explanatory variables X are different in two models, the matrices A change and the REML of the two models are thus calculated for different outcome variables U.

The estimates obtained by ML and REML are usually very close when the sample size is large. REML estimator is preferred when the sample is small and/or the number of fixed effects is large, particularly when the focus is on the variance parameters.

4.1.4   Inference for fixed effects

According to the maximum likelihood theory, the estimators $\hat{\beta}$ have an asymptotic multivariate normal distribution centered on the true value of β and variance:

$$\text{var}(\hat{\beta}) = \left\{ -E\left(\frac{\partial^2 L(\beta, \phi)}{\partial\beta\partial\beta^\top} \right) \right\}^{-1} = \left(\sum_{i=1}^{N} X_i^\top V_i^{-1} X_i \right)^{-1}. \qquad (4.12)$$

An estimator of $\text{var}(\hat{\beta})$ is obtained by replacing ϕ in V_i by their ML or REML estimates. This allows the computation of confidence intervals and Wald test statistics for the regression parameters. The likelihood ratio test and the score test (rarely available in software) can also be used to test hypotheses about fixed effects.

For small sample sizes, the variance estimator of $\hat{\beta}$ (4.12) underestimates the variance of $\hat{\beta}$ because it does not take into account the estimation of ϕ. This problem could be solved by computing by finite difference the observed

Fisher information matrix for all parameters $\theta = (\beta^\top, \phi^\top)^\top$ to obtain the asymptotic variance of $\hat{\theta}$ by:

$$\text{var}(\hat{\theta}) = \left\{ -\frac{\partial^2 L(\theta)}{\partial \theta \partial \theta^\top} \right\}^{-1}. \tag{4.13}$$

The asymptotic variance of $\hat{\beta}$ is a sub-matrix of $\text{var}(\hat{\theta})$. However, this calculation is rarely available in software because the likelihood is most often maximized iteratively on ϕ replacing β by (4.10) in (4.9). Thus, the test for fixed effects are corrected by approximating the distribution of the Wald test statistic under the null hypothesis by an F distribution instead of a χ^2 distribution. The degree of freedom of the numerator of the statistic is equal to the number of tested constraints on the parameters and several methods of calculation have been proposed for the degree of freedom of the denominator, such as the Satterthwaite approximation (see Verbeke and Molenberghs, 2009, Chapter 6).

4.1.5 Choice of the covariance structure

To select the best covariance structure (i.e., the matrix V_i) for the data, models including different covariance structures may be compared. The models (nested or not) may be compared with the Akaike criterion:

$$\text{AIC} = -2 \times \text{ Log-Likelihood } + 2 \times \text{ number of parameters.}$$

The model with the minimum AIC provides the best fit. Using AIC, it is possible for instance to compare a model that includes random intercept and slope with a model that includes an autoregressive process instead.

If the correlation is accounted for by random effects, it may be useful to test whether the addition of a random effect improves the model fit, that is whether the variance of additional random effect σ_b^2 is different from zero. The variances of the random effects cannot be tested at 0 with standard tests (Wald or likelihood ratio) because the null hypothesis $H_0 : \sigma_b^2 = 0$ is on the boundary of the parameter space (because $\sigma_b^2 \geq 0$) and the standard results on the asymptotic distribution of the test statistic under H_0 are not valid. However, Stram and Lee (1994) proposed an approximation of the distribution of the likelihood ratio statistic for the test of q correlated random effects *vs.* $q + 1$:

$$H_0 : B = \begin{bmatrix} B_{qq} & \mathbf{0} \\ \mathbf{0}^\top & 0 \end{bmatrix} \text{ vs. } H_1 : B = \begin{bmatrix} B_{qq} & \mathbf{C} \\ \mathbf{C}^\top & \sigma_{q+1}^2 \end{bmatrix}$$

where B_{qq} is the variance matrix of the first q random effects, σ_{q+1}^2 is the variance of the random effect $q + 1$ and $\mathbf{C}$ is the vector of the q covariances between the new random effect and the first q ones. Thus the test focuses on

$q + 1$ parameters since it does not require independence between the random effects. The likelihood ratio statistic (ML or REML) is:

$$\text{LR} = -2 \log \frac{\mathcal{L}(H_0)}{\mathcal{L}(H_1)} = \text{Dev}(H_0) - \text{Dev}(H_1)$$

where $\text{Dev}(H_0)$ is the deviance $(-2 \times L$ or $-2 \times L_{\text{REML}})$ of the model with q random effects and $\text{Dev}(H_1)$ is the deviance of the model with $q + 1$ random effects. Under H_0, the asymptotic distribution of the statistic LR is a mixture of a χ^2 distribution with $q + 1$ degrees of freedom (denoted χ^2_{q+1}) and a χ^2 distribution with q degrees of freedom (denoted χ^2_q) with equal probabilities 0.5. This mixture distribution is denoted $\chi^2_{q+1:q}$. The p-value is computed as:

$$p = \text{P}(\chi^2_{q+1:q} > \text{LR}) = 0.5 \times \text{P}(\chi^2_{q+1} > \text{LR}) + 0.5 \times \text{P}(\chi^2_q > \text{LR})$$

Example 9 *Let us consider a linear random intercept model:*

$$Y_{ij} = X_{ij}^\top \beta + b_{0i} + \epsilon_{ij} \text{ with } \epsilon_{ij} \sim \mathcal{N}(0, \sigma^2) \text{ , } b_{0i} \sim \mathcal{N}(0, \sigma_0^2)$$

where ϵ_{ij} and b_{0i} are independent. The hypothesis of homogeneity between the N subjects or of independence within each subject is defined by:
$H_0 : \sigma_0^2 = 0$ *vs.* $H_1 : \sigma_0^2 > 0$.

The test statistic is $\text{LR} = \text{Dev}(H_0) - \text{Dev}(H_1)$, *where* $\text{Dev}(H_0)$ *is the deviance of the model for independent data and* $\text{Dev}(H_1)$ *is the deviance of the random intercept model. Under H_0, LR follows a mixture distribution $\chi^2_{1:0}$ where χ^2_0 is the distribution defined by $\text{P}(\chi^2_0 = 0) = 1$. The p-value is given by:*

$$p = \text{P}(\chi^2_{1:0} > \text{LR}) = 0.5 \times \text{P}(\chi^2_1 > \text{LR}) + 0.5 \times \text{P}(\chi^2_0 > \text{LR}) = 0.5 \times \text{P}(\chi^2_1 > \text{LR})$$

Example 10 *Let us consider a linear model with random intercept and slope:*

$$Y_{ij} = X_{ij}^\top \beta + b_{0i} + b_{1i} t_{ij} + \epsilon_{ij} \text{ with } \epsilon_{ij} \sim \mathcal{N}(0, \sigma_\epsilon^2)$$

and $b_i = (b_{0i}, b_{1i})^\top \sim \mathcal{N} \left(0, B = \begin{bmatrix} \sigma_0^2 & \sigma_{01} \\ \sigma_{01} & \sigma_1^2 \end{bmatrix} \right)$.

To assess whether the random slope is necessary, this model is compared to the random intercept model of example 9 using a likelihood ratio test. The null and alternative hypotheses are defined by:

$$H_0 : B = \begin{bmatrix} \sigma_0^2 & 0 \\ 0 & 0 \end{bmatrix} \text{ vs. } H_1 : B = \begin{bmatrix} \sigma_0^2 & \sigma_{01} \\ \sigma_{01} & \sigma_1^2 \end{bmatrix}.$$

The test statistic is $\text{LR} = \text{Dev}(H_0) - \text{Dev}(H_1)$, *where* $\text{Dev}(H_0)$ *is the deviance of the random intercept model and* $\text{Dev}(H_1)$ *is the deviance of the model with correlated random intercept and slope. Under H_0, LR follows a mixture distribution $\chi^2_{2:1}$. The p-value is:*

$$p = \text{P}(\chi^2_{2:1} > \text{LR}) = 0.5 \times \text{P}(\chi^2_2 > \text{LR}) + 0.5 \times \text{P}(\chi^2_1 > \text{LR})$$

Stram and Lee (1994) have also given the approximate distribution of the likelihood ratio statistic under the null hypothesis for testing simultaneously several independent random effects (a mixture of several χ^2 distributions), but the assumption of independence between random effects is rarely realistic. Molenberghs and Verbeke (2007) have also proposed a correction for the Wald test of the random effects but they recommend the corrected likelihood ratio test as its use is simpler. Let us note that the conventional test ignoring the constraint of the parameter space is conservative (the null hypothesis is less often rejected). Thus it leads to overly parsimonious models.

4.1.6 Estimation of random effects

Although the main goal of the analysis is usually the estimation of the regression parameters (β), the estimation of the random effects may be useful, especially for individual predictions. The random effects are estimated by the expectation of their *posterior* distribution $E(b_i \mid Y_i = y_i)$, that is the distribution given the observed data. Given that the vector $[Y_i^\top, b_i^\top]^\top$ has a multivariate Gaussian distribution of dimension $n_i + q$,

$$\begin{bmatrix} Y_i \\ b_i \end{bmatrix} \sim \mathcal{N} \left(\begin{bmatrix} X_i\beta \\ 0 \end{bmatrix}, \begin{bmatrix} V_i & Z_iB \\ BZ_i^\top & B \end{bmatrix} \right).$$

By using properties of the multivariate Gaussian distribution, we obtain:

$$\begin{aligned} E(b_i \mid Y_i) &= E(b_i) + \text{cov}(b_i, Y_i)\text{var}(Y_i)^{-1}[Y_i - E(Y_i)] \\ &= BZ_i^\top V_i^{-1}(Y_i - X_i\beta) \end{aligned} \tag{4.14}$$

The parameters β and ϕ are replaced by their maximum likelihood estimators (or REML estimator for ϕ) in (4.14) to obtain the *empirical Bayes estimator* of b_i, denoted $\hat{b}_i$ (also called BLUP for Best Linear Unbiased Prediction).

Further:

$$\widehat{\text{var}}(\hat{b}_i) = \hat{B}Z_i^\top \hat{V}_i^{-1} \left\{ \hat{V}_i - X_i \left(\sum_{i=1}^{N} X_i^\top \hat{V}_i^{-1} X_i \right)^{-1} X_i^\top \right\} \hat{V}_i^{-1} Z_i \hat{B}.$$

Note that the histogram of the empirical Bayes estimators of the random effects gives little information on the validity of the Gaussian assumption for the random effects because it is strongly influenced by the prior distribution, and especially when the residual variance is large (an illustration is given in Chapter 7.8 of Verbeke and Molenberghs (2009)).

4.1.7 Predictions

In this section, prediction means estimation of values of Y, often at the time of observations. These predictions are not necessarily estimates of future values of Y. Let us consider the mixed model:

$$Y_i = X_i\beta + Z_i b_i + \epsilon_i \text{ with } \epsilon_i \sim \mathcal{N}(0, \Sigma_i) \text{ and } b_i \sim \mathcal{N}(0, B).$$

The variance is defined as $\text{var}(Y_i) = V_i = Z_i B Z_i^\top + \Sigma_i$. From this model, at least two types of predictions can be defined: the estimate of the marginal expectation,

$$\text{E}(Y_i) = X_i\beta$$

or the estimate of the conditional expectation given the random effects

$$\text{E}(Y_i \mid b_i) = X_i\beta + Z_i b_i.$$

The first one is the expectation of Y_i for all the subjects who share the same characteristics X_i as subject i, while the second is the expectation specific to subject i, including individual trend accounted for by the random effects.

The marginal prediction is obtained by $\hat{E}(Y_i) = X_i\hat{\beta}$ and the conditional prediction given the random effects is computed from the empirical Bayes estimators:

$$\hat{Y}_i = \hat{E}(Y_i \mid b_i) = X_i\hat{\beta} + Z_i\hat{b}_i.$$

Replacing $\hat{b}_i$ by its estimator (4.14) computed with $\hat{\beta}$ and $\hat{\phi}$, this leads to:

$$
\begin{aligned}
\hat{Y}_i &= X_i\hat{\beta} + Z_i B Z_i^\top V_i^{-1}(Y_i - X_i\hat{\beta}) \\
&= (I_{n_i} - Z_i B Z_i^\top V_i^{-1}) X_i\hat{\beta} + Z_i B Z_i^\top V_i^{-1} Y_i \\
&= \Sigma_i V_i^{-1} X_i\hat{\beta} + (I_{n_i} - \Sigma_i V_i^{-1}) Y_i
\end{aligned}
$$

The individual prediction including the random effects is therefore the weighted average of the marginal prediction $X_i\hat{\beta}$ and the observed value Y_i. The weights depend on the ratio between the within-subject variance Σ_i and the total variance V_i. When the within-subject variance increases compared to the between-subject variance (variance of the random effects), the individual prediction gets closer to the average profile. This is the phenomenon of "shrinkage."

If the model includes an autoregressive component (defined by (4.6) and (4.8)), it may also be useful to estimate the conditional expectation including individual short-term variations

$$\text{E}(Y_i \mid b_i, W_i) = X_i\beta + Z_i b_i + W_i$$

with $W_i = (w_i(t_{i1}), \ldots, w_i(t_{in_i}))^\top$. It is again obtained by using the properties of the multivariate normal distribution.

4.1.8   Residuals

As several different predictions may be computed from the mixed model, several types of residuals may also be defined: marginal residuals

$$Y_i - X_i\hat{\beta}$$

of variance

$$V_i^{res} = V_i - X_i \left(\sum_{i=1}^{N} X_i^\top V_i^{-1} X_i \right)^{-1} X_i^\top$$

and subject-specific residuals

$$\hat{\epsilon}_i = Y_i - X_i \hat{\beta} - Z_i \hat{b}_i.$$

Replacing $\hat{b}_i$ by its empirical Bayes estimator, this leads to

$$\hat{\epsilon}_i = \Sigma_i V_i^{-1} (Y_i - X_i \hat{\beta})$$

and thus

$$\text{var}(\hat{\epsilon}_i) = \Sigma_i V_i^{-1} V_i^{res} V_i^{-1} \Sigma_i.$$

Let us remark that, even when the mixed model has independent errors, i.e., $\Sigma_i = \sigma^2 I_{n_i}$, subject-specific residuals are correlated. In particular, their distribution depends on the choice of V_i and on the *prior* for the random effects.

Standardized residuals are the residuals divided by their standard deviations while Cholesky residuals are uncorrelated residuals. They are obtained by the following formula:

$$R_i = U_i (Y_i - X_i \hat{\beta}).$$

where U_i is the upper triangular matrix obtained by Cholesky transformation of the inverse of the variance matrix $V_i^{res}{}^{-1}$, according to the relationship $V_i^{res}{}^{-1} = U_i^\top U_i$. Cholesky residuals therefore follow a standard Gaussian distribution, $R_i \sim \mathcal{N}(0, I_{n_i})$, if the model is well specified. Cholesky transformation of conditional residuals is identical to Cholesky transformation of marginal residuals.

4.1.9 Goodness of fit analyses

The evaluation of the fit of a linear mixed model is complicated by the non-independence of residuals (Grégoire et al., 1995; Jacqmin-Gadda et al., 2007). However, the following graphs and analyses make the assessment of some model assumptions possible:

- Displaying the predicted values (marginal or conditional) *vs.* the observed values is useful but the differences between predictions and observations are difficult to interpret if the data are incomplete. They may reflect either model misspecification or the impact of missing data if they are not completely at random (see Section 4.5). When the data are incomplete, it may be better to use the predicted values given the random effects that should fit the observed data under the less restrictive assumption of missing at random data.

- The graph of standardized residuals (residuals divided by the standard deviation) *vs.* time or *vs.* a quantitative explanatory variable can be used to assess whether the effect of this variable is correctly specified or to identify outliers.

- The Quantile-Quantile plot of uncorrelated residuals (Cholesky residuals) assess the fit of the residuals to the standard Gaussian distribution $\mathcal{N}(0, I)$.

- To detect extreme individuals or incorrect specification of the impact of subject-specific explanatory variables, Park and Lee (2004) proposed a summarized statistic for the subject-specific residuals, that is

$$(Y_i - X_i\hat{\beta})V_i(\hat{\phi})^{-1}(Y_i - X_i\hat{\beta})$$

  that has a χ^2 distribution with n_i degrees of freedom when the model is well specified.

- Assessing the assumption of constant variance of the residual error ϵ_{ij} is difficult since the conditional residuals $\hat{\epsilon}_{ij}$ do not have a constant variance and are correlated. Especially, $\text{var}(\hat{\epsilon}_{ij})$ depends on time if the model includes a random slope. However, whether $\hat{\sigma}_1^2 t_{ij}^2$ is small compared to the variances of the random intercept σ_0^2 and the error σ_e^2, $\text{var}(\hat{\epsilon}_{ij})$ may be considered as approximately time-constant and the homoscedasticity assumption may be assessed by drawing $\hat{\epsilon}_{ij}$ *vs.* $\text{E}(Y_{ij} \mid \hat{b}_i)$ or t_{ij}.

Furthermore, various simulation studies have shown that the fixed effects estimators and their variances were quite robust to misspecification of the distribution of the errors or of the random effects and, under some conditions, to a violation of the homoscedasticity assumption (Jacqmin-Gadda et al., 2007; Neuhaus et al., 1991). Nevertheless, when heteroscedasticity is obvious, it can be taken into account through a model for the residual variance (Foulley et al., 1992).

4.1.10   Application

The purpose of this application is to compare three antiretroviral treatment strategies on the change in T CD4+ lymphocytes concentration (denoted CD4) over time in the clinical trial ALBI ANRS 070. The treatment strategies are: (1) patients treated with zidovudine and lamivudine (AZT + 3TC) for 24 weeks, (2) patients treated with stavudine and didanosine (ddI + d4T) for 12 weeks followed by AZT + 3TC for 12 weeks, and (3) patients treated with d4T + ddI for 24 weeks. The first treatment strategy is considered as the reference. An indicator variable was built for the two other treatment strategies (X_{2i} and X_{3i}, respectively).

Following treatment initiation, the increase in CD4 evokes a certain effectiveness of treatments (Figure 4.1). The observed average change in CD4

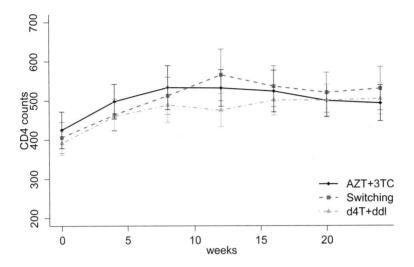

FIGURE 4.1
Mean trajectory of T CD4+ lymphocytes (CD4) (and 95% confidence bands) in the three antiretroviral treatments regimens in HIV-1 infected patients from the clinical trial ALBI ANRS 070

suggests a non-linear trend with time (e.g., quadratic) but we use a linear model for educational purposes. Similarly, the model is presented with a quite simple covariance structure.

Let us assume a linear model with random intercept and slope:

$$Y_{ij} = \beta_0 + \beta_1 t_{ij} + \beta_2 X_{2i} + \beta_3 X_{3i} + \beta_4 X_{2i} t_{ij} + \beta_5 X_{3i} t_{ij} + b_{0i} + b_{1i} t_{ij} + \epsilon_{ij} \quad (4.15)$$

with

$$(b_{0i}, b_{1i})^\top \sim \mathcal{N}\left(0, B = \begin{bmatrix} \sigma_0^2 & \sigma_{01} \\ \sigma_{01} & \sigma_1^2 \end{bmatrix}\right)$$

and

$$\epsilon_{ij} \sim \mathcal{N}(0, \sigma_\epsilon^2).$$

Y_{ij} is the measure j of $\sqrt[4]{\text{CD4}}$ for subject i collected at time t_{ij} where t_{ij} is the time since subject i inclusion in the ALBI trial. The time in days is divided by 100 to avoid very small variance estimates for the random slope (σ_1^2). Such rescaling of time or explanatory variables is often useful to limit convergence issues of optimization algorithms. The fourth root of CD4 is used to ensure normal and homoscedastic distribution of residuals (see the last paragraph of the application).

The meaning of parameter estimates is the following: β_0 is the fixed intercept representing the average value of $\sqrt[4]{\text{CD4}}$ at inclusion (t=0) for treatment group 1 (AZT+3TC, reference); β_1 is the mean change (slope) of $\sqrt[4]{\mathrm{CD4}}$ by time unit (here for 100 days) for treatment group 1 (AZT+3TC); β_2 and β_3 are the mean differences of $\sqrt[4]{\mathrm{CD4}}$ at inclusion between group 1 and groups 2 and 3, respectively; β_4 and β_5 are the mean differences in the slopes of $\sqrt[4]{\mathrm{CD4}}$ between strategy 1 and strategies 2 and 3, respectively.

This model can be estimated by using the MIXED procedure of SAS, or `lme` and `lmer` functions of R. Scripts associated with this application are given in the appendix. Estimates of model parameters are presented in Tables 4.1 and 4.2.

TABLE 4.1
Estimates of fixed effects of the linear model with correlated random intercept and slope. ALBI ANRS 070.

Variable	Param.	Estimate	S.E.	Wald statistic	p-value
(intercept)	β_0	4.62	0.046	100.06	<0.0001
Time	β_1	0.072	0.022	3.31	0.001
Treatment 2	β_2	-0.068	0.066	-1.03	0.30
Treatment 3	β_3	-0.10	0.065	-1.56	0.12
Treatment 2 × time	β_4	0.067	0.031	2.17	0.030
Treatment 3 × time	β_5	0.066	0.031	-2.14	0.033

TABLE 4.2
Estimates of variance parameters of the linear model with correlated random intercept and slope. ALBI ANRS 070.

Parameter	Estimates	Standard-Error
σ_0^2	0.084	0.124
σ_1^2	0.0039	0.0028
σ_{01}	0.0035	0.0044
σ_ϵ^2	0.044	0.0024

The fixed intercept estimate shows that the mean initial level of $\sqrt[4]{\mathrm{CD4}}$ was 4.62 for patients of group 1. The slope ($\hat{\beta}_1$) shows that the mean $\sqrt[4]{\mathrm{CD4}}$ increased by 0.072 every 100 days among patients of group 1. The test for the difference of means of $\sqrt[4]{\mathrm{CD4}}$ at inclusion between treatment groups, may be performed using a multivariate Wald test or a likelihood ratio test with null hypothesis $H_0: \beta_2 = \beta_3 = 0$. The likelihood ratio test is built by comparing the full model defined by (4.15) and the model without the terms $\beta_2 X_{2i} + \beta_3 X_{3i}$.

The result shows that the initial difference between the means of the three groups is not significant (LR $=2.52$, p$=0.28$). This was expected given that the treatment groups were randomized. However, the likelihood ratio test for the effect of the treatment strategy on the slope (H_0: $\beta_4 = \beta_5 = 0$) is significant (LR $=6.12$, p$=0.047$). The slopes for the 2nd ($\hat{\beta}_1 + \hat{\beta}_4 = 0.140$ $\sqrt[4]{CD4}/100$ days) and the 3rd groups ($\hat{\beta}_1 + \hat{\beta}_5 = 0.138$ $\sqrt[4]{CD4}/100$ days) are significantly larger than that of the first group (0.072 $\sqrt[4]{CD4}/100$ days) as evidenced by the interaction terms significantly different from 0 (p$=0.030$ and 0.033, respectively, for β_4 and β_5).

The variance parameters for the random effects are displayed in Table 4.2: σ_0^2 is the between-subject variance of the initial level of $\sqrt[4]{CD4}$, σ_1^2 is the between-subject variance of the slope, σ_{01} is the covariance between individual initial level and slope.

The likelihood ratio test between a model with correlated random intercept and slope ($L_1 = -70.4$) and a model with only a random intercept ($L_0 = -73.1$) shows that the variance of the random slope is significantly different from 0 ($p = 0.044$) although its value is very low ($\sigma_1^2 = 0.0039$). Under H_0, the test statistic follows a mixture of χ^2 with 1 and 2 degrees of freedom. The p-value is thus

$$p \simeq 0.5\mathrm{P}(\chi_1^2 > 5.4) + 0.5\mathrm{P}(\chi_2^2 > 5.4) = (0.020 + 0.067)/2 = 0.044$$

The covariance between the random intercept and the random slope was not significantly different from 0: $\sigma_{01} = 0.0035, Z = 0.0035/0.0044 = 0.79, p = 0.21$. In fact, estimates and tests of fixed effects were very close when using a random intercept model.

The transformation of CD4 was validated with the analysis of standardized residuals of the model with a random intercept. This indicated heteroscedasticity when the CD4 count was modeled in its natural scale (left part of Figure 4.2). Heteroscedasticity disappeared when using $\sqrt[4]{CD4}$ (right part of Figure 4.2).

4.2 Generalized mixed linear models

The linear mixed model is used to analyze the change over time of a continuous Gaussian dependent variable. When the dependent variable is binary or discrete quantitative, it is not suitable anymore. Discrete data are typically analyzed using generalized linear models such as the logistic model or the log-linear Poisson model. The analysis of longitudinal discrete data can be achieved through generalized linear models with random effects (or with mixed effects named more briefly generalized linear mixed models) that are built on the same principle as the linear mixed models. Conditional on the

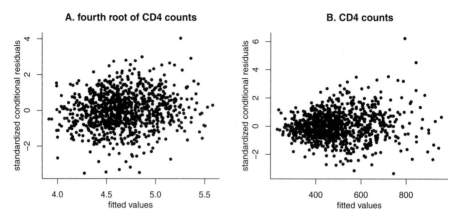

FIGURE 4.2
Standardized conditional residuals *vs.* predicted values of the random-intercept model when the dependent variable CD4 count is transformed in $\sqrt[4]{\text{CD4}}$ (left) and when it is in its natural scale (right).

random effects, the response variable follows a generalized linear model and the random effects are introduced into the linear predictor.

4.2.1 Model specification

A generalized linear model is defined by:

- the distribution of the response variable that belongs to the exponential family including in particular the Gaussian, Bernoulli, Binomial and Poisson distributions,

- a linear predictor (linear combination of explanatory variables and parameters), and

- a link function connecting $E(Y)$ to the linear predictor.

Let Y_{ij} be the outcome variable for observation j $(j = 1, \ldots, n_i)$ of subject i $(i = 1, \ldots, N)$. Generalized linear mixed models are defined by specifying first the distribution of Y_{ij} in the exponential family (4.16) and second a model for the expectation of Y_{ij} (4.18). The distribution of Y_{ij} belongs to the exponential family defined by:

$$f_{Y_{ij}}(y; \theta_{ij}, \psi) = \exp\left\{\psi^{-1}\left[\theta_{ij}y - g(\theta_{ij})\right] + C(y, \psi)\right\}, \qquad (4.16)$$

where θ_{ij} is the canonical parameter which is equal to the linear predictor

$$\theta_{ij} = X_{ij}^{\top}\beta + Z_{ij}^{\top}b_i, \qquad (4.17)$$

where X_{ij} is a vector of explanatory variables of size p and β is the associated p-vector of fixed effects; Z_{ij} is a sub-vector of X_{ij} of size q $(q \leq p)$ and b_i is a q-vector of random effects identically and independently distributed with mean 0 and variance matrix B. Let us denote $f_{b_i}(b)$ the density of this distribution *a priori* which is most often Gaussian.

With this formulation, the link function between $E(Y_{ij} \mid b_i)$ and the linear predictor is the inverse of the derivative of the function g, that is:

$$E(Y_{ij} \mid b_i) = g'(\theta_{ij}) = g'(X_{ij}^\top \beta + Z_{ij}^\top b_i). \tag{4.18}$$

Furthermore, according to the properties of generalized linear models, we have:

$$\text{var}(Y_{ij} \mid b_i) = g''(\theta_{ij})\psi.$$

4.2.2 The mixed-effect logistic model

For binary data, Stiratelli et al. (1984) introduced the mixed effects logistic model by assuming a Gaussian distribution for the random effects. This model may be defined by:

$$\text{logit}(P(Y_{ij} = 1 \mid b_i)) = X_{ij}^\top \beta + Z_{ij}^\top b_i \text{ with } b_i \sim \mathcal{N}(0, B). \tag{4.19}$$

and thus

$$P(Y_{ij} = 1 \mid b_i) = \frac{\exp(X_{ij}^\top \beta + Z_{ij}^\top b_i)}{1 + \exp(X_{ij}^\top \beta + Z_{ij}^\top b_i)}. \tag{4.20}$$

When $q = 1$ and $Z_{ij} = 1 \; \forall i, j$, we obtain the random intercept logistic model sometimes called "normal logistic model."

4.2.3 The mixed proportional-odds and cumulative probit models

The mixed effects proportional odds logistic model generalizes the mixed effects logistic model for ordinal response variables (i.e., variables with values in $\{0, 1, \ldots, M\}$) taking into account the order of these values. It may be written as:

$$\text{logit}(P(Y_{ij} \leq m \mid b_i)) = \log\left(\frac{P(Y_{ij} \leq m \mid b_i)}{P(Y_{ij} > m \mid b_i)}\right)$$
$$= \alpha_{m+1} - X_{ij}^\top \beta - Z_{ij}^\top b_i \text{ for } m \in \{0, ..., M-1\}. \tag{4.21}$$

X_{ij}, β, Z_{ij} and b_i are defined as previously and the parameters $(\alpha_m)_{m \in \{1,...,M\}}$ are the intercepts specific to each level of the outcome. These parameters are ordered and a constraint must be imposed to ensure identifiability of the model. For instance with the constraint $\alpha_1 = 0$, we obtain the standard formula for the logistic model in the binary case ($M = 1$). Another option is to remove the intercept of the vector of fixed effects β.

The logit link may be replaced by the probit link, that is the inverse of the cumulative distribution function of a standard Gaussian variable Φ^{-1}:

$$\text{probit}(P(Y_{ij} \leq m \mid b_i)) = \Phi^{-1}(P(Y_{ij} \leq m \mid b_i))$$
$$= \alpha_{m+1} - X_{ij}^\top\beta - Z_{ij}^\top b_i \text{ for } m \in \{0, ..., M - 1\}.$$
$$(4.22)$$

These two models are very close. They differ by the distribution of the errors. For a better understanding, we can introduce a continuous latent process underlying the observed ordinal variable. Indeed, the ordinal outcome Y_i may be considered as an ordinal measure of a continuous latent process $(\Lambda_i(t))_{t \in \mathbb{R}}$. This latent process represents the true quantity of interest measured by Y, such as pain measured by an ordinal subjective scale (no pain /mild pain/moderate pain/intense pain) or physical dependence measured by a scale (autonomy, mild dependence, moderate dependence, severe dependence). The latent process is modeled by a linear mixed model,

$$\Lambda_i(t_{ij}) = X_{ij}^\top\beta + Z_{ij}^\top b_i + \epsilon_{ij},$$

and the relationship between the observed outcome and the underlying process is defined by

$$Y_{ij} = m \Leftrightarrow \alpha_m < \Lambda_i(t_{ij}) \leq \alpha_{m+1} \text{ for } m \in \{0, \ldots, M\}$$

with $\alpha_0 = -\infty$ and $\alpha_{M+1} = +\infty$. In other words, the observed variable takes the value m when the true quantity of interest lies in the interval $]\alpha_m, \alpha_{m+1}]$. Assuming a logistic distribution for the error ϵ_{ij}, the proportional odds logistic model is obtained whereas the probit model is defined by assuming a unit Gaussian distribution for the error.

It has been shown that these two models had a very similar behavior except for extreme probabilities. The parameters β and $(\alpha_m)_{m \in \{1,...,M\}}$ from the two models are equivalent except for a multiplicative coefficient $\pi/\sqrt{3}$ that is the ratio of the standard-errors of a logistic variable and a Gaussian variable. Similarly, the parameters of the variance matrix B of the random effects are equivalent for the two models except for the multiplicative coefficient $\pi^2/3$.

4.2.4 The mixed Poisson model

For count data, the Poisson model with mixed effects is defined by:

$$P(Y_{ij} = k) = \frac{\lambda_{ij}^k \exp(-\lambda_{ij})}{k!}$$

and

$$\log(\lambda_{ij}) = X_{ij}^\top\beta + Z_{ij}^\top b_i$$

where b_i is either $\mathcal{N}(0, B)$ or Gamma distributed. For the log-linear Poisson model, the chosen prior for the random effects is often a Gamma distribution because this leads to a closed form for the likelihood. However, most software only offers the Gaussian distribution (proc `NLMIXED` and `GLIMMIX` in `SAS` and function `glmer` in `lme4` `R` package for example). The choice of the prior usually has little impact on the estimated regression parameters.

4.2.5 Estimation

By denoting ϕ the vector of variance parameters (ψ and the elements of the matrix B), the individual contribution to the log-likelihood of generalized linear mixed model is:

$$L_i(\beta, \phi) = \log \int \prod_{j=1}^{n_i} f_{Y_{ij}|b_i}(Y_{ij} \mid b) f_{b_i}(b) db.$$

Given the independence assumption between the individuals, the total log-likelihood is:

$$L(\beta, \phi) = \sum_{i=1}^{N} L_i(\beta, \phi). \tag{4.23}$$

The functional form for f_{b_i} is chosen *a priori*, and the parameters β and ϕ can be estimated by maximizing the log-likelihood (4.23). However, the calculation of the log-likelihood involves an integral over b_i whose multiplicity is equal to the dimension of the vector of random effects b_i, that is q. In most cases, this integral has no analytic solution. The log-linear Poisson model is an exception when the gamma distribution is chosen as *prior* for the random effects. In the other cases, the most commonly used distribution for the random effects is the Gaussian one, and the integral is computed numerically.

Numerical computation of the integral over the random effects makes the computation of the likelihood quite complicated so that the maximum likelihood estimation of generalized linear mixed models is much more cumbersome than that of linear mixed model. Several algorithms have been proposed for solving this problem. For numerical integration, three methods are used: adaptive Gaussian quadrature, Monte-Carlo and Laplace approximation. Gaussian quadrature is the most common approach when the number of random effects is not too large because it gives a good compromise between accuracy and speed of calculation. This method approximates the integral by a sum of the integrand computed at predefined points (or abscissas) and weighted by tabulated weights according to the type of integral (Abramowitz and Stegun, 1972). When the random effects are Gaussian, the abscissas and weights of the Gauss-Hermite quadrature (a_l, w_l) are used and the approximate formula for an integral of size 1 is:

$$\int \prod_{j=1}^{n_i} f(Y_{ij} \mid b) f(b) db \approx \sum_{l=1}^{n_{GH}} \prod_{j=1}^{n_i} f(Y_{ij} \mid b = \sqrt{2}\sigma_0 a_l) \frac{w_l}{\sqrt{\pi}}.$$

where n_{GH} is the number of quadrature points that determines the accuracy of the approximation. The adaptive quadrature that centers the quadrature points around the predicted values of b_i at each iteration is recommended because it results in a more accurate approximation of the integral (Lesaffre and Spiessens, 2001).

The Monte Carlo approach approximates the integral by

$$\int \prod_{j=1}^{n_i} f(Y_{ij} \mid b) f(b) db \approx \sum_{k=1}^{K} \prod_{j=1}^{n_i} f(Y_{ij} \mid b_{ik}).$$

where b_{ik} are generated according to the prior distribution of the random effects f_{b_i}. With a large number of simulations K (for instance $K \geq 1000$), the accuracy can be good but the computation time quickly becomes prohibitive.

When the number of random effects is large, the Laplace approximation is a useful alternative to reduce the computation time although the accuracy of the estimates deteriorates. In this approach, the integrand is approached by a Taylor expansion around its maximum $\hat{b}_i$ allowing an analytical calculation of the integral (Wolfinger, 1993).

To maximize the likelihood, the main software uses Newton-like algorithms (Newton-Raphson, Quasi-Newton or Fisher Scoring) most often combined with adaptive Gaussian quadrature (default method with SAS proc `NLMIXED` and available with SAS proc `GLIMMIX` and R function `glmer`) or Laplace approximation (default method with R `glmer` and available with SAS proc `GLIMMIX` and SAS proc `NLMIXED`).

The EM algorithm (Dempster et al., 1977) can also be used to estimate mixed-effect models by considering b_i like missing data. The advantage of this algorithm is that the maximization step does not require integration. On the other side, each iteration includes an optimization process. As the EM algorithm converges slowly, it was supplanted by the combination Quasi-Newton/Quadrature for the estimation of generalized linear mixed-effect models. It remains useful for more complex models, particularly thanks to stochastic extensions of the EM algorithm that include Monte Carlo simulations in step E (Celeux et al., 1996). For instance, the SAEM algorithm is implemented in the software `monolix` (Kuhn and Lavielle, 2005).

In all cases, it is recommended to take the estimates from the fixed effects model as initial parameter values of the optimization procedure.

4.2.6 Confidence intervals and tests

Confidence intervals and tests for the fixed effects are obtained from the theory of maximum likelihood. The estimators are asymptotically Gaussian, their variances are estimated by the inverse of the Hessian matrix and the three classical tests (Wald, likelihood ratio test and score test) are valid. They are also valid for testing parameters variance if the null hypothesis is not on the boundary of the definition space of the parameters (test of covariance to 0 for example). On the other side, they cannot be used to test the nullity of a variance and thus to compare two different models including unequal numbers of random effects. However, the corrected likelihood ratio test described in Section 4.1.5 is also valid for generalized linear mixed models.

4.2.7 Estimation of random effects

As for linear mixed-effect models, the random effects may be estimated by the *posterior* mean $E(b_i \mid Y_i, \hat{\beta}, \hat{\phi})$. However, when the model is not linear in the parameters or not Gaussian, the conditional distribution $f(b_i \mid Y_i)$ has no closed form. Using the following relationship:

$$f_{b_i \mid Y_i}(b_i \mid Y_i) = \frac{f_{Y_i \mid b_i}(Y_i \mid b_i) f_{b_i}(b_i)}{f_{Y_i}(Y_i)} \propto f_{Y_i \mid b_i}(Y_i \mid b_i) f_{b_i}(b_i)$$

the expectation $E(b_i \mid Y_i)$ is approximated by the mode of $f_{Y_i \mid b_i}(Y_i \mid b_i) f_{b_i}(b_i)$ that does not require the computation of integrals but requires an optimization procedure to find the maximum of the function $f_{Y_i \mid b_i}(Y_i \mid b_i) f_{b_i}(b_i)$.

4.2.8 Application

The objective of this analysis is to describe the change over time of depressive symptomatology in the elderly and to evaluate the impact of sex on this trajectory.

In the general population, depressive symptomatology is measured by the CES-D (Center of Epidemiological Studies of Depression), a self-administered questionnaire of 20 items providing a score between 0 and 60, 0 being no symptoms. Figure 4.3 displays the CES-D distribution in a sample of 500 subjects randomly drawn from the Paquid cohort described in Section 1.4.1. This distribution is highly skewed with more than 20% of values equal to 0. The change over time of the CES-D can therefore not be analyzed with a conventional linear mixed model. As CES-D scores are ordinal, a proportional odds model or a probit model could be considered but, with 61 possible different levels and 51 levels observed in the Paquid sample of 500 subjects, such approaches would be very difficult to implement (this aspect will be reviewed in Section 5.1).

An alternative is to choose a clinically meaningful threshold, such as a threshold beyond which it is assumed that depressive symptoms become

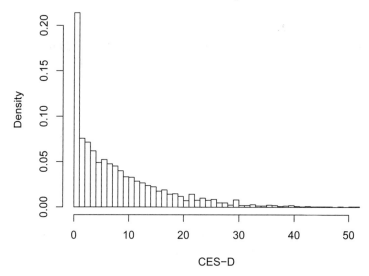

FIGURE 4.3
Distribution of CES-D scores in a sample of 500 subjects of Paquid cohort.

pathological. The outcome variable thus becomes binary, and its change over time can be described by a mixed-effect logistic model. In this illustration, we model the probability of having a CES-D score greater than or equal to 16, 16 being a clinically recognized threshold. The outcome variable (`cesd16`) is described as a function of age and sex.

The age variable (`age`) is centered at 65 years, so that the intercept of the model has a meaning and it is divided by 10 to avoid numerical issues due to very small estimated parameters (the random-slope variance mainly): `age65=(age-65)/10`. The binary variable for sex is denoted `male`.

Assuming a linear trajectory with age and including only a random intercept to account for the inter-individual variability, the mixed-effect logistic model is written for subject i at measurement j:

$$\text{logit}(\text{P}(\texttt{cesd16}_{ij} = 1)) = \beta_0 + \beta_1 \, \texttt{age65}_{ij} + \beta_2 \, \texttt{male}_i + \beta_3 \, \texttt{male}_i \times \texttt{age65}_{ij} + b_{0i} \tag{4.24}$$

with $b_{0i} \sim \mathcal{N}\left(0, \sigma_0^2\right)$. This model can be estimated by the SAS procedures NLMIXED or GLIMMIX and several R functions, including `glmer` of `lme4` package. The scripts for this application are given in the appendix.

4.2.8.1 Interpretation of the fixed effects

Table 4.3 gives the estimates of the fixed effects. The probability of having depressive symptomatology over 16 increases significantly with age with an estimated odds ratio for women of $\exp(0.436) = 1.55$ $(p = 0.0037)$ by decade. The interaction age65$\times$male being not significant $(p = 0.406)$, the increase with age is not different for the men. In contrast, men have a significantly lower risk to have a high depressive symptomatology at age 65 compared to women: the odds ratio for men *vs.* women at age 65 is $\exp(-1.475) = 0.23$ $(p = 0.0072)$.

TABLE 4.3

Estimated fixed effects of mixed-effects logistic model for the outcome variable cesd16 in the Paquid sample of 500 subjects.

Variable	Parameter	Estimate	Standard Error	Wald statistic	p-value
(intercept)	β_0	-2.684	0.292	-9.20	<0.0001
age65	β_1	0.436	0.150	2.90	0.0037
male	β_2	-1.475	0.549	-2.69	0.0072
age65$\times$male	β_3	0.259	0.313	0.83	0.406

Note that these odds ratios are calculated by conditioning on the random effects. In other words, they correspond to an increased risk for two subjects that differ only by the explanatory variable of interest (male) or (age65) and share the same random deviation from the intercept b_{0i}. If a random slope was added to the model (addition of $b_{1i} \times$ age65 in Equation 4.2.8), the interpretation of the regression coefficient for age65 would be less easy. Indeed, the odds-ratio for a 1 year increase of age65 would be $OR(\text{age65} \mid b_{0i}, b_{1i}, \text{male}) = \exp(\beta_1 + \beta_3\text{male} + b_{1i})$ and should therefore be given for a specific value of male and b_{1i}. In practice, the odds ratio is given for $b_{1i} = 0$.

4.2.8.2 Covariance structure for the random effects

The variance of the random intercept is estimated at $\hat{\sigma}_0^2 = 4.1$. As in the linear mixed models, the null hypothesis $H_0 : \sigma_0^2 = 0$ can be tested by the likelihood ratio test that follows a mixture distribution $\chi_{1:0}^2$ under H_0 (see Section 4.1.5). The log-likelihood for the random intercept model is $L = -842.7$ (AIC= 1695.4) and the one for the model without random effect (standard logistic model) is $L = -951.4$ (AIC= 1902.8). The likelihood ratio statistic is thus equal to 217.4 and the variance of the random intercept is significantly different from 0 $(p < 0.0001)$. This shows a large inter-individual variability in the probability of having depressive symptomatology over 16. In other words, individuals who had a higher probability of being depressed at the entry in the study continued to have a higher probability of being depressed afterwards. When adding a random slope correlated with the random intercept, the likelihood of the model becomes $L = -840.9$ (AIC= 1695.8). The likelihood ratio statistic which follows a $\chi^2_{2:1}$ distribution under the null hypothesis is equal to 3.6 with a p-value of 0.11. Thus, as soon as the variability of the intercept is taken into account, there was no significant inter-individual variability at the 5% level on the change over time of the probability of having high depressive symptomatology. The inclusion of a random slope was not necessary.

4.3   Non-linear mixed models

In the previous two sections, we detailed linear mixed models and generalized linear mixed models. In fact, most statistical models can be generalized by including random effects. For example, survival models with random effects are called "frailty models" and will be presented in Chapter 6. To finish this inventory of mixed-effects models for repeated longitudinal data, we give a brief presentation of non-linear mixed-effects models for Gaussian repeated data. Other examples of non-linear mixed models based on differential equations will be given in Chapter 9 about causality. The term "linear" in linear mixed models comes from the fact that the model is linear in the parameters (fixed and random). In contrast, a non-linear mixed model includes also non-linear functions of the fixed and random effects.

Let us denote Y_i the n_i-vector of outcome measures for subject i, $i = 1, \ldots, N$, a non-linear model may be defined by:

$$Y_i = g(X_i, \beta, b_i) + \epsilon_i \text{ with } \epsilon_i \sim \mathcal{N}(0, \Sigma_i) \text{ and } b_i \sim \mathcal{N}(0, B). \qquad (4.25)$$

where X_i is a matrix of explanatory variables, β a vector of fixed effects and b_i a vector of random effects, most often Gaussian. The function $g(X_i, \beta, b_i)$ is any parametric function which is *a priori* specified.

Example 11 *The evolution of the plasma viral load in HIV patients is commonly described by the following biexponential model with four random effects (Wu and Ding, 1999):*

$$Y_{ij} = \log_{10}\left[(\beta_1 + b_{1i})\exp\{-(\beta_2 + b_{2i})t_{ij}\}\right] + (\beta_3 + b_{3i})\exp\{-(\beta_4 + b_{4i})t_{ij}\} + \epsilon_{ij} \qquad (4.26)$$

where Y_{ij} is the $\log_{10}$ of the viral load, $\epsilon_i \sim \mathcal{N}(0, \Sigma_i)$ and $b_i = (b_{1i}, b_{2i}, b_{3i}, b_{4i})^\top \sim \mathcal{N}(0, B)$.

These models can be estimated by the maximum likelihood. As the model is non-linear in b_i, the likelihood has usually no closed form. By denoting ϕ the vector of variance parameters and given the independence between individuals, the marginal log-likelihood is:

$$L(\beta, \phi) = \sum_{i=1}^{N} \log \int f_{Y_i|b_i}(Y_i \mid b) f_{b_i}(b) db. \qquad (4.27)$$

The evaluation of the log-likelihood requires a numerical integration over the random effects distribution which is computed similarly as described for the generalized linear mixed models in Section 4.2.5. Standard optimization algorithms may be used. Sometimes, the model is linearized by a first-order Taylor approximation around the expectation of the random effect, i.e., 0 (Beal and Sheiner (1982); method FIRO with SAS NLMIXED) or around the current empirical Bayesian prediction of the random effect $(\hat{b}_i)$ (Lindstrom and Bates, 1990) but these approaches are less efficient than direct maximization of the likelihood when possible.

4.4 Marginal models and generalized estimating equations (GEE)

Mixed models are extensions of standard regression models that define the joint distribution of a vector of variables, including the correlation between these variables. These models are estimated by applying the standard results of the maximum likelihood theory. Liang and Zeger (1986) introduced another approach for the analysis of longitudinal data using generalized linear models. Instead of changing the model, they proposed to modify the estimation procedure to obtain robust estimates of the parameters of standard regression models and their variances when the data were correlated. To do this, they replaced the score equations whose solution gives the maximum likelihood estimators under the assumption of independence, by generalized estimating equations (GEE). These equations involve a *working covariance matrix* that usually depends on a vector of parameters δ to estimate. In addition, Liang and Zeger (1986) proposed a new estimator of the variance of the estimated regression parameters, $\hat{\beta}$, said robust estimator or "sandwich" estimator, and they proved that these estimators of β and of their variances were consistent even when the working covariance matrix was misspecified. The next section describes the GEE method whose merits will be contrasted with those of mixed models in Section 4.4.2.

4.4.1　The GEE approach

The marginal distribution of the variable Y_{ij} is described by a generalized
linear model:

$$f_{Y_{ij}}(y; \theta_{ij}, \psi) = \exp\left\{\psi^{-1}[\theta_{ij}y - g(\theta_{ij})] + C(y, \psi)\right\}$$

where θ_{ij} is the canonical parameter, $\theta_{ij} = X_{ij}^\top \beta$, and β is a p-vector of fixed
parameters. Under the independence assumption, the log-likelihood is:

$$L(\beta, \psi) = \sum_{i=1}^{N} \sum_{j=1}^{n_i} \left\{\psi^{-1}[\theta_{ij}Y_{ij} - g(\theta_{ij})] + C(Y_{ij}, \psi)\right\},$$

and the score equations that must be solved to obtain the maximum likelihood
estimators under the independence assumption are:

$$\frac{\partial L}{\partial \beta}(\beta, \psi) = \sum_{i=1}^{N} \psi^{-1} X_i^\top (Y_i - \mu_i) = 0, \tag{4.28}$$

where Y_i is the n_i-vector of outcome variables for subject i, $Y_i = (Y_{i1}, \ldots, Y_{in_i})^\top$, μ_i is the n_i-vector of expectations, $\mu_i = (\mu_{i1}, \ldots, \mu_{in_i})^\top$ with
$\mu_{ij} = g'(\theta_{ij})$, and $X_i = (X_{i1}, \ldots, X_{in_i})^\top$ is the $n_i \times p$ matrix of explanatory
variables for subject i.

Liang and Zeger (1986) generalized this equation to take account of the
within-subject correlation of the data. Let $V_i(\delta, \psi)$ (denoted V_i in the following) be a symmetric working covariance matrix $n_i \times n_i$ between repeated
measures of Y_{ij} that depends on ψ and on a vector of parameters δ of size q.
The generalized estimating equation is defined by:

$$\sum_{i=1}^{N} D_i^\top V_i^{-1}(Y_i - \mu_i) = 0 \tag{4.29}$$

where $D_i = \partial \mu_i / \partial \beta = A_i X_i$ and $A_i = \text{diag}\{g''(\theta_{ij})\}$. This equation reduces
to the score equation (4.28) when the diagonal matrix $V_i = \psi A_i$ is chosen as
a working covariance matrix (independence working hypothesis).

Regression parameters β are estimated by solving Equation (4.29) after
replacing ψ and δ by consistent estimates. Under these conditions, Liang and
Zeger proved that $\hat{\beta}$ was asymptotically multivariate Gaussian with expectation equal to the true value of β and variance matrix given by:

$$V_R(\hat{\beta}) = \left\{\sum_{i=1}^{N} D_i^\top V_i^{-1} D_i\right\}^{-1} \left\{\sum_{i=1}^{N} D_i^\top V_i^{-1} \text{var}(Y_i) V_i^{-1} D_i\right\} \left\{\sum_{i=1}^{N} D_i^\top V_i^{-1} D_i\right\}^{-1} \tag{4.30}$$

Replacing $\text{var}(Y_i)$ by $(Y_i - \hat{\mu}_i)(Y_i - \hat{\mu}_i)^\top$, and β, ψ and δ by their expectations, we obtain $\hat{V}_R(\hat{\beta})$, the robust (or sandwich) estimator of the variance of $\hat{\beta}$. Without time-dependent explanatory variables, the convergence of $\hat{\beta}$ and $\hat{V}_R$ relies only on a correct modeling of the expectation of Y_{ij} and not on the choice of V_i. Therefore $\hat{\beta}$ and $\hat{V}_R$ are asymptotically unbiased even when the working covariance matrix does not correspond to the actual covariance structure of the data. With time-dependent explanatory variables, this result is valid only for a diagonal working covariance matrix or if the following condition is valid (Pepe and Anderson, 1994):

$$E(Y_{it} \mid X_{it}) = E(Y_{it} \mid X_{it}; X_{ij}, j \neq t)$$

Pepe and Anderson (1994) shown that this condition failed when response at time t directly influences the subsequent responses.

When V_i is the true covariance matrix of the data, V_R reduces to the classical formula (variance assuming that the model is correctly specified and called "naive" or "model-based variance"):

$$V_M(\hat{\beta}) = \left\{ \sum_{i=1}^{N} D_i^\top V_i^{-1} D_i \right\}^{-1}. \tag{4.31}$$

In practice, it is recommended to use the robust variance whose value varies little when the working covariance matrix is changed (at least when the data are complete, see Section 4.5). When the working matrix is close to the true covariance matrix, values of the robust and model-based variances are close.

It can be emphasized that Liang and Zeger's results prove that GEE estimates obtained under the working independence assumption are convergent (Liang and Zeger, 1986). As for generalized linear models, GEE with the independence working covariance matrix are identical to the score equations for the MLE, these estimates may be obtained using softwares dedicated to maximum likelihood estimation of generalized linear models assuming independence of the data. However, variance of these estimates has to be estimated by the robust estimator (4.30), as it is possible with many softwares for estimating GLM.

Liang and Zeger suggested to estimate ψ by a moments estimator:

$$\hat{\psi} = \sum_{i=1}^{N} \sum_{j=1}^{n_i} \frac{(Y_{ij} - \mu_{ij})^2}{g''(\theta_{ij})(N-p)}.$$

The moments estimator of δ depends on the chosen correlation structure. One of the simplest, said exchangeable correlation structure (or compound symmetry), assumes that $\mathrm{corr}(Y_{ij}, Y_{ij'}) = \delta \; \forall j \neq j'$ where δ is a scalar; δ is therefore estimated by:

$$\hat{\delta} = \left\{ \sum_{i=1}^{N} \frac{n_i(n_i - 1)}{2} - p \right\}^{-1} \left\{ \sum_{i=1}^{N} \sum_{j=1}^{n_i} \sum_{j'>j}^{n_i} \frac{(Y_{ij} - \mu_{ij})(Y_{ij'} - \mu_{ij'})}{\psi \sqrt{g''(\theta_{ij})g''(\theta_{ij'})}} \right\}.$$

Software offers a wide choice of working correlation structures. Outside the exchangeable and independence structures, here are some working correlation matrices commonly used for balanced design:

- Unstructured: $\text{corr}(Y_{ij}, Y_{ij'}) = \delta_{jj'}\ \forall j \neq j'\ (n_i(n_i - 1)/2$ parameters)

- Autoregressive: $\text{corr}(Y_{ij}, Y_{ij'}) = \delta^{|j-j'|}\ \forall j \neq j'\ (1$ parameter)

- Banded diagonal by: $\text{corr}(Y_{ij}, Y_{ij+h}) = \delta_h\ (n_i - 1$ parameters)

4.4.2 Mixed models and maximum likelihood *vs.* marginal models and GEE

4.4.2.1 Required assumptions

The maximum likelihood estimation of a mixed model requires to specify the complete joint distribution of the response variable. Indeed, by defining both the conditional distribution $f(Y_{ij} \mid b_i)$ and the *a priori* law of the random effects $f(b_i)$, the joint distribution of the vector Y_i, denoted $f(Y_i)$, is entirely defined, even if this distribution has usually no closed form for non-linear mixed models.

The maximum likelihood theory ensures that the estimators are asymptotically unbiased when the model is well specified. In particular, the covariance structure of the data (number of random effects and structures of matrices B and Σ_i) and the random effects distribution must, theoretically, be well specified in order to have a consistent $\hat{\beta}$. Conversely, the convergence of GEE estimators of regression parameters only requires that the marginal expectation of Y_{ij} is correct. Theoretical results prove consistency of the estimators when the working covariance matrix is misspecified (for example, when the working matrix assumes independency while data are correlated) (Liang and Zeger, 1986). According to the theory, GEE estimators are significantly more robust.

In practice, these results must be qualified. Indeed, on one hand, several simulation studies showed that the estimators of the regression parameters of mixed models were robust when the covariance structure (Jacqmin-Gadda et al., 2007) or the random effects distribution were misspecified (Neuhaus et al., 1991). On the other hand, when the working covariance matrix is very poorly specified, GEE estimators are asymptotically unbiased but they can have poor efficiency. In addition, the consistency of GEE estimators is guaranteed only when the missing data are completely at random, while the maximum likelihood estimators are consistent under the less restrictive missing at random assumption (see Section 4.5).

Finally, it should be noted that the sandwich variance estimator, originally proposed by White (1982) may be applied to obtain a robust estimator of the variance of MLE of mixed models. This estimator is robust when the within-subject covariance assumed in the mixed model is poorly specified, leading to robust confidence intervals and tests.

4.4.2.2 Parameter interpretation

Because of their different meanings, the mixed-effect models are also called "cluster-specific models" and the marginal models are called "population-averaged models" (Neuhaus et al., 1991). In this section, β and β^* denote the parameters from mixed models and marginal models, respectively.

In mixed-effects models, the expectation of the response variable is defined conditional on the random effects. To simplify the presentation, we present the case of a random intercept model:

$$E(Y_{ij} \mid b_{0i}) = g'(X_{ij}^\top \beta + b_{0i}).$$

In contrast, in the marginal approach, we define the marginal expectation of Y_{ij}:

$$E(Y_{ij}) = g'(X_{ij}^\top \beta^*).$$

In the case of homogeneity between subjects, that is when the variance of the random effect and thus the within-subject correlation is zero, the parameters β and β^* are equal. In the other cases, if $g'()$ is not a linear function of b_{0i}, β and β^* are different because:

$$E(Y_{ij}) = E\{E(Y_{ij} \mid b_{0i})\} = E\{g'(X_{ij}^\top \beta + b_{0i})\} \neq g'(X_{ij}^\top \beta).$$

Each element of the vector β measures the effect of an explanatory variable, the others and the value of the random effect being constant. The random intercept can be considered as representing the set of subject-specific explanatory variables that were omitted so that it has a similar status as the explanatory variables. This makes natural the interpretation of β conditional on the values of these variables and the random effect.

An element of the vector β^* measures the mean effect of an explanatory variable on the whole population. The value of β^* depends on both the strength of the association between the explanatory variables and the response variable and on the degree of heterogeneity in the population. For the logistic model, it was shown that $|\beta^*| < |\beta|$, unless one of the two is zero, in which case the other is also null (Neuhaus et al., 1991) .

Due to the different interpretations of the parameters, the use of mixed-effects models is rather advised in an explanatory perspective (to assess the specific effect of each explanatory variable on the response variable), while the marginal models are more suitable in a pragmatic approach (to assess the apparent effect of a change in X on the mean of Y for the whole population).

Nevertheless the parameters β and β^* are identical when the function $g'()$ is linear:

$$E(Y_{ij}) = E\{E(Y_{ij} \mid b_{0i})\} = E\{X_{ij}^\top \beta + b_{0i}\} = X_{ij}^\top \beta.$$

They have therefore the two interpretations: "population-averaged" and "cluster-specific."

4.4.3 Application

We take the example of Section 4.2.8 on generalized linear models that aims at describing the evolution of depressive symptoms in the elderly population and evaluating the effect of sex on this trajectory. In Section 4.2.8, the change over time of the probability of having a CES-D score above 16 was described by a mixed-effects logistic model in a sample of 500 subjects from the Paquid cohort.

Using the same variables (age65 and male) and still assuming a linear trajectory with age, and an effect of sex on the initial level and on the slope with age, the marginal logistic model is written:

$$\text{logit}(\text{P}(\texttt{cesd16}_{ij} = 1)) = \beta_0 + \beta_1 \ \texttt{age65}_{ij} + \beta_2 \ \texttt{male}_i + \beta_3 \ \texttt{male}_i \times \texttt{age65}_{ij}$$
(4.32)

This model can be estimated by the SAS procedure GENMOD or the R function gee of the package gee. Scripts associated with this application are given in the appendix.

4.4.3.1 Estimated parameter interpretation

Table 4.4 displays the estimated parameters using an unstructured (the least constrained) working covariance matrix X. The table shows both the naive and robust estimators of the standard deviation of each parameter. We see that the naive standard deviations tend to underestimate the variability of the estimates even if the difference is quite small in this example.

TABLE 4.4
Estimated parameters from the marginal logistic model for the outcome variable CES-D$\geq$16 *vs.* CES-D$<$16 in the sample of 500 subjects from Paquid with an unstructured working covariance matrix (GEE method).

Variable	Parameter	Estimate	Standard-Error		Wald statistic (robust)	p-value
			Naive	Robust		
(intercept)	β_0	-1.600	0.200	0.208	-7.688	<0.0001
age65	β_1	0.224	0.106	0.112	2.009	0.045
male	β_2	-0.865	0.380	0.398	-2.174	0.030
age65×male	β_3	0.054	0.218	0.228	0.238	0.812

As in the mixed-effects logistic model, the probability of having high depressive symptoms (greater than 16) increased significantly with age in women (OR= $\exp(0.224) = 1.251$ for 10 years, $p = 0.045$) as well as in men since

TABLE 4.5
Estimated parameters from the marginal logistic model for the outcome variable CES-D$\geq$16 *vs.* CES-D$<$16 in the sample of 500 subjects from Paquid with an exchangeable working covariance matrix (GEE method).

Variable	Parameter	Estimate	Standard-Error Naive	Robust	Wald statistic (robust)	p-value
(intercept)	β_0	-1.602	0.185	0.197	-8.121	<0.0001
age65	β_1	0.254	0.095	0.100	2.550	0.011
male	β_2	-0.963	0.345	0.373	-2.581	0.010
age65$\times$male	β_3	0.190	0.187	0.198	0.959	0.338

the interaction age65$\times$male is not significant ($p = 0.81$). As previously, the probability of having high depressive symptoms at age 65 is lower in men (OR$= \exp(-0.865) = 0.421$, $p = 0.030$) than in women. Thus, whatever the age, women have an increased risk of depressive symptomatology than men but this excess risk among women does not change with age.

In comparison, Table 4.5 presents the parameter estimates of the same model estimated with an exchangeable working covariance matrix. The conclusions are basically the same but the estimates are slightly larger in absolute value and variance estimates are lower leading to greater significance levels. Contrary to what was expected, the robust standard deviations in this application are as sensitive to changes of working covariance matrix as naive standard deviations. This can be explained by the frequency of missing data in the Paquid cohort. Indeed, we will see in next section that GEE estimators are not robust when the data are incomplete, which raises a problem in population-based cohort studies, like Paquid, that often exhibit large dropout rates.

As explained in Section 4.4.2.2, parameter estimates obtained by GEE (Table 4.4) are smaller in absolute value than the maximum likelihood estimates of the mixed model including the same explanatory variables (Table 4.3). The ORs from the mixed model are approximations of the OR adjusted for variables that might explain inter-individual variability and are not necessarily included in the model, while the ORs estimated by GEE are interpreted as averaged over these factors.

4.5 Incomplete longitudinal data

In longitudinal studies, the whole set of data planned in the protocol is rarely collected. Participants can leave the study prematurely (own decision, moving, ...), refuse to participate in certain visits or complete only a part of the questionnaire. Missing data always lead to a loss of information and thus a decrease of the power of the study. In addition, depending on the relation between the observation process and the outcome and explanatory variables, they might induce biases. Note that the issues of follow-up truncated by death will be discussed in Section 9.4.

Little and Rubin (1987) proposed a classification of missing data to identify cases leading to biases. In this chapter, we focus on the missing data on the response variable in the analysis of longitudinal data. When the explanatory variables are incomplete, various approaches are possible, but multiple imputation is often recommended (Van Buuren and Groothuis-Oudshoorn, 2011) as it is easy to implement and avoids underestimation of variance of estimated parameters that arises with simple imputation.

4.5.1 Terminology

We use the standard and intuitive notation introduced by Little and Rubin (1987) for missing data (see the remark in Section 4.5.2 about more rigorous notation). Let Y be the vector of responses partitioned in $Y = (Y^o, Y^m)$, where Y^o are actually observed responses and Y^m are the unobserved responses. Let R be the indicator variable of observation: $R(t) = 1$ if $Y(t)$ is observed, $R(t) = 0$ if not. Missing data are *monotone* if $P(R(t) = 0 \mid R(s) = 0, s < t) = 1$, they are *intermittent* if not. Monotone missing data correspond to *dropouts* of study; in this case, the vector of observation indicators $R_i^{\top} = (R_{i1}, R_{i2}, \ldots, R_{in_i})$ can be summarized by the follow-up time and a binary variable indicating whether the subject dropped out prematurely or at the scheduled end of the study.

Little and Rubin's classification of missing data includes three categories (Little and Rubin, 1987). When R does not depend on Y, responses are called *missing completely at random (MCAR)*. In longitudinal studies, this case may include situations where the probability of response depends on observed explanatory variables:

$$P(R \mid Y^o, Y^m, X) = P(R \mid X).$$

When R depends on observed responses Y^o but not on missing responses Y^m, data are called *missing at random (MAR)*:

$$P(R \mid Y^o, Y^m, X) = P(R \mid Y^o, X).$$

Finally, the missing data are *informative* or *not at random (MNAR)* when R depends on unobserved responses Y^m.

Example 12 *In the study of the change over time of depressive symptoms in the Paquid cohort described in Sections 4.2.8 and 4.4.3, the data are missing completely at random if the probability of completing the CES-D scale is independent of the past and present CES-D values. Under this assumption, the probability of response may depend on age, sex, education or any other variable whose value is known even when CES-D score is missing. The data are missing at random if, after adjustment for explanatory variables, the probability of completing the CES-D scale at time t depends on the CES-D values observed at previous visits but not on the CES-D value at time t: for example, if depressed subjects at a visit tend to refuse participation in the next visit. Finally, the data are missing not at random, and are thus informative if, after adjustment for explanatory variables and the scores observed at previous visits, the probability of completing the CES-D at time t depends on the CES-D at time t (that is not observed if the subject does not respond). This is the case if the depressed subjects at t tend to refuse the visit of the investigator at that time.*

4.5.2 Analysis under the MAR assumption

When the data are missing at random and the parameters θ of the model for the expectation of Y are distinct from parameters ψ of the observation process R, missing data are called *ignorable* and the estimators obtained by the maximum likelihood method using the observed data Y^o are not biased.

Indeed, the likelihood of the observed data, Y^o and R, is:

$$f(Y^o, R \mid \theta, \psi) = \int f(Y^o, Y^m \mid \theta) f(R \mid Y^o, Y^m, \psi) dY^m.$$

If the data are MAR, this leads to:

$$
\begin{aligned}
f(Y^o, R \mid \theta, \psi) &= f(R \mid Y^o, \psi) \int f(Y^o, Y^m \mid \theta) dY^m \\
&= f(R \mid Y^o, \psi) f(Y^o \mid \theta).
\end{aligned}
$$

and the log-likelihood can be written as the sum of two terms

$$L(\theta, \psi \mid Y^o, R) = L(\theta \mid Y^o) + L(\psi \mid R, Y^o).$$

When parameters ψ and θ are distinct, θ can be estimated without bias (asymptotically) by maximizing the log-likelihood computed on the available data, that is $L(\theta \mid Y^o)$. The missing data are said *ignorable*. In contrast, if the model is estimated by GEE, the parameters are biased if the MCAR assumption is not valid. Estimating equations weighted by the probability of observation have been proposed to correct the GEE estimators under the MAR assumption (Robins et al., 1995).

Remark: In the above definitions of missingness mechanisms and in the demonstration of *ignorability*, we chose to use the standard notations Y^o, Y^m and R because they are very intuitive. However, these notations are ambiguous because Y^o is itself a function of R. For instance, the length of Y_i^o is $\sum_j R_{ij}$. Seaman et al. (2013) propose more rigorous definitions of missingness mechanisms. They denote $o(Y, R)$ the subvector of Y consisting of elements of Y whose associated elements in R are 1 ($o(Y, R)$ is equivalent to Y^o). With this notation, they define data as *everywhere missing at random* (everywhere MAR) if $\forall \psi$,

$$P(R = r \mid Y = y) = P(R = r \mid Y = y^*) \forall r, y, y^* \text{ such that } o(y, r) = o(y^*, r)$$

This means that the probability of any missingness pattern does not depend on missing values of Y given the observed values of Y. This is the condition required for unbiased frequentist likelihood inference.

Example 13 *Estimates from mixed models for the change over time of the CES-D in Paquid estimated by maximum likelihood are unbiased if the probability of completing the CES-D scale depends on the observed values at the previous visit (MAR assumption) but not on the current value (MNAR). In contrast, GEE estimates are unbiased only under the MCAR assumption, i.e., if the probability of completing the CES-D does not depend on the observed values (past) or missing values (current or future) of the CES-D.*

4.5.3   Analysis in the MNAR case

When the observation probability may depend on unobserved responses Y^m (e.g., when it depends on the current response: $P(R(t) = 1) = g(Y(t))$), missing data are MNAR. In this case, no standard estimation method is unbiased. The joint log-likelihood $L(Y^o, R)$ must be maximized on the whole set of observed data of the two processes Y and R. Several methods corresponding to different decompositions of this likelihood have been proposed. In those, it is usually assumed that Y follows a mixed-effects model.

With *Pattern Mixture Models* (Little, 1993; Michiels et al., 2002), the distribution of Y_i, $f(Y_i \mid R_i)$, is defined conditionally on the observation pattern R_i and constraints must be specified so that all parameters are identifiable for all observation patterns R_i. For example, a slope cannot be estimated from subjects having only one measure. An advantage of this approach is that the constraints needed to estimate these models are clearly identified and the estimates obtained under different assumptions can be compared in a sensitivity analysis. In addition, these mixture models can usually be estimated using software devoted to the estimation of standard mixed-effect models by adjusting or stratifying on the follow-up duration or other variables defining the observation pattern. Nevertheless, the target distribution $f(Y \mid X)$ is not directly estimated; its parameters are estimated in a second step as the average of the estimates of the conditional distributions $f(Y \mid X, R)$ weighted by the proportion of each observation pattern: $f(Y \mid X) = \Sigma_r f(Y \mid X, R = r)P(R = r)$.

On the other hand, the approach by *selection models* allows the direct estimation of the distribution of interest $f(Y \mid X)$. Indeed, in models, the distribution of R_i is defined conditionally on Y_i^o and Y_i^m (outcome-dependent selection models) or conditionally on the random effects b_i (random-effects dependent selection models or shared random-effects model) and the joint likelihood is computed using one of the following two decompositions:

$$f(Y_i^o, R_i \mid X_i) = \int f(Y_i^o, Y_i^m \mid X_i)f(R \mid Y_i^o, Y_i^m, X_i)dY_i^m$$

or

$$f(Y_i^o, R_i \mid X_i) = \int f(Y_i^o \mid X_i, b_i)f(R_i \mid X_i, b_i)f(b_i)db_i.$$

Modelling the observation process R as a function of Y may seem more natural than modelling Y given R which is generally not useful in itself, except when the dropouts are caused by an identified event. When the missing data are monotone, the most common selection models are joint models for longitudinal data and time-to-events that are detailed in Chapter 8.

Although these approaches initially aroused much enthusiasm, it has quickly become clear that the estimates from pattern mixture models and selection models were very sensitive to unverifiable parametric assumptions about the relationship between R and Y^m. Selection models are also sensitive to the distribution of the response variable. Currently, it is recommended to perform the primary analysis under the assumption of random missing data (MAR) and use pattern mixture or selection models to assess the robustness of the findings of the main analysis to assumptions about missing data in the framework of a sensitivity analysis (Verbeke et al., 2001; Thijs et al., 2002).

4.5.4   Censored longitudinal data

When a measuring instrument has one or several detection limits, the measured variable is censored. The measure is left-censored (respectively right-censored) when the value is lower (respectively higher) than the low (respectively high) detection limit. For instance, measurement tools for the viral load in HIV-infected patients generally have a lower detection limit (from 10 000 copies/mL in the mid-1990s to 20 copies/mL and less today). Among patients under highly active antiretroviral treatment, the value of the viral load frequently goes below this threshold. Thus, in clinical trials and other longitudinal studies of changes in viral load among HIV infected patients, a large proportion of the measures of the response variable is left censored. Some analyses were performed by replacing the censored values by the threshold value or half of this value. This strategy generally induces a bias and a systematic underestimation of the variances of the model parameters since, like any method of single imputation, the imputed data are treated as observed data (Jacqmin-Gadda et al., 2000).

In fact, these censored data are a special case of non-random missing data for which the observation mechanism is known: the probability that a value is missing equals the probability that the same value is below the detection limit (for left-censoring). The longitudinal data analysis when the response variable is censored by a lower detection limit can be conducted with a mixed model by modifying the likelihood. The contribution to the likelihood of censored measures equals the probability to be below the threshold, while the contribution of observed measures is the density. Let us denote Y_i^o the vector of response variables completely observed for subject i, Y_i^c the vector of censored responses and C_i the vector of detection thresholds (which may vary over time and across subjects). At each measurement time t_{ij}, the observations are $\max(C_{ij}, Y_{ij})$. With these notations, the global likelihood is:

$$\mathcal{L}(\theta) = \prod_{i=1}^{N} f_{Y_i^o}^{\theta}(Y_i^o) F_{Y_i^c|Y_i^o}^{\theta}(C_i \mid Y_i^o) \tag{4.33}$$

If the model is a mixed Gaussian linear model, f and F are respectively the density and the cumulative distribution functions of multivariate normal distributions. The computation of the distribution function requires a numerical integration whose dimension is the number of censored measures for the subject (Jacqmin-Gadda et al., 2000). When the number of censored measures is large, the computation time can be reduced by using an alternative formulation of the likelihood conditional on the random effects (Lyles et al., 2000):

$$\mathcal{L}(\theta) = \prod_{i=1}^{N} \int_{\mathbb{R}^q} \prod_{j=1}^{n_{oi}} f_{Y_{ij}^o|b_i}^{\theta}(Y_{ij}^o \mid b) \prod_{j=1}^{n_{ci}} F_{Y_{ij}^c|b_i}^{\theta}(C_{ij} \mid b) f_{b_i}(b) db, \tag{4.34}$$

with n_{oi} and n_{ci} the numbers of observed and censored measures for subject i. In this formulation, the dimension of the integral is the number of random effects while the computation of $F_{Y_{ij}^c|b_i}^{\theta}(C_{ij} \mid b)$ requires only univariate integration of Gaussian density for which very efficient algorithms exist. Nevertheless, the function to be integrated in 4.34 is quite complex and, with this method, the mixed model cannot include correlated errors. A Fortran program is available on the Web (http://www.isped.u-bordeaux.fr/BIOSTAT) for the estimation of the model with the formulation (4.33). Thiébaut and Jacqmin-Gadda (2004) give the SAS code for maximizing the likelihood (4.34) and compare the two approaches.

4.6 Modeling strategies

4.6.1 Description of the data

In all cases, the first step of a longitudinal data analysis must be a comprehensive description of the data including:

- the available data (sample size, number of measures, duration of follow-up, measured variables),

- graphs illustrating both the mean and individual profiles of change of the marker,

- graphs of non-parametric predictions (e.g., LOESS), especially in the case of highly imbalanced data where the description by measurement time is not easy,

- an empirical semi-variogram (Diggle, 1988) representing the difference $d^2_{jk} = 0.5[y(t_j) - y(t_k)]^2$ *vs.* $u_{jk} = t_j - t_k$ can be useful if there is no *a priori* available information for modeling the covariance.

4.6.2 Choice of the fixed effects

The choice of fixed effects should be guided by the objectives of the analysis and the data description. It is recommended to test only the interactions that have a clinical meaning because the model can become quite complex with multiple parameters and it reduces false positive results. Indeed, the simple study of the effect of a variable on the change over time of the marker generates a first-order interaction with time. Seeking a modification of this effect by another explanatory variable produces a second-order interaction. As the study of the change over time of the marker according to the explanatory variables is often the main objective in longitudinal data analyses, the interactions with time (first order) are readily enforced, i.e., they are kept in the model although they are not significant. If one opts for a step-by-step selection of fixed effects, simple effects and interactions with time will be tested separately. Non-significant interactions can be removed by keeping the simple effect if its interpretation is relevant. In fact, the withdrawal of the interaction with time changes the interpretation of the simple effect. Without the interaction with time, the coefficient of an explanatory variable measures the mean effect at all times. With interaction with time, the coefficient for the simple effect accounts for the effect of the explanatory variable at time 0.

Non-significant simple effects are rarely removed from the model when the interaction is significant but this is not a strict rule. When the change over time is accounted for by several terms (e.g., t and t^2 for a quadratic trend), testing the effect of a factor on changes involves testing several interactions simultaneously ($X \times t$ and $X \times t^2$ for a quadratic trend).

4.6.3   Choice of the covariance matrix

In mixed-effects models, the definition of the covariance matrix influences fixed effects and vice versa. The most useful criteria for choosing the covariance structure are:

- The objective of the analysis: if the goal is the estimation of fixed effects, parsimonious covariance structures are used. On the contrary, if the aim is to make individual predictions, more flexible covariance structures may be selected (including several random effects and/or an autoregressive process).

- The number of measurements per subject and the frequency of measurements: the larger the number of measurements per subject, the larger the number of covariance parameters. When the number of measurements per subject is large, an autocorrelated process is often necessary to take into account individual variations over time and variability of the correlation between the measures according to the time interval between them.

Covariance structure involving both random effects and autocorrelated error is possible but requires rich enough data to be able to distinguish between intra- and inter-individual variability. In addition to the arguments above, the choice can be guided by significance tests or model choice criteria such as AIC.

Different strategies have been suggested to choose the fixed effects and the variance matrix. The first, mainly recommended for clinical trials, is to define a full model for fixed effects and then to define the covariance matrix (Diggle, 1988). In this case, time is often included as a discrete variable (a dummy variable for measurement times). This strategy therefore applies mainly to study designs in which all patients are assumed to be seen at the same times and the number of explanatory variables is small (such as in clinical trials). When the number of visiting times is low, an unstructured variance matrix V_i is often more suitable than random effects.

For cohort studies with varying measurement times between subjects, different strategies are possible. For (almost) complete data, the fixed effects may be selected by using a marginal model estimated by GEE and Wald tests in a first step; then some random effects and/or autocorrelated error (plus an independent residual error) may be included, and the best mixed-effects model selected using for instance AIC. An alternative approach is to choose a covariance structure from a mixed model including the main explanatory variables. Then the selection of fixed effects can be proceeded by a conventional strategy (step-by-step for instance). On the final selected model, the choice of the covariance structure is checked and, if necessary, refined. Whatever the strategy, it is essential to perform the selection of fixed effects taking into account the within-subject correlation. Note that the number of parameters to be estimated can be large, especially when the variance matrix B for the random effects is unstructured, that is when all the covariances between the random effects are estimated (the number of variance parameters to be estimated is $\frac{q(q+1)}{2}$ for q random effects).

4.6.4 Goodness of fit

It is recommended to check some model assumptions early in the analysis procedure because the transformation of the response variable (e.g., the logarithm or square root as in Section 4.1.10) or corrections of outliers, would require to perform again all the analyses. Heteroscedasticity can also be modeled by relaxing the variance structure of the measurement error. Residuals analysis is very useful for detecting outlying individuals or observations compared to model predictions.

Missing data may also alter the modeling strategy. Indeed, either the missingness process is clearly informative and it is necessary to implement an appropriate model (e.g., a joint model), or the missingness process may be assumed at random (MAR) and robustness analyses will be performed in a second step after the primary analysis based on a mixed model with maximum likelihood estimation.

Part II

Advanced Biostatistical Models

5

Extensions of mixed models

The mixed model theory has been extended to take into account various problems encountered in practice. This chapter will focus on some of them with mixed models for curvilinear outcomes, mixed models for multivariate longitudinal data, and mixed models involving also latent classes.

5.1 Mixed models for curvilinear outcomes

The linear mixed model provides a framework to analyze changes in a quantitative Gaussian dependent variable and the generalized linear mixed model extends the approach to the analysis of binary, ordinal or count variables. In practice, some variables of interest do not enter these frameworks and are thus difficult to analyze. Examples include subjective measures of health such as scales of quality of life, dependency or pain, and psychometric scales such as neuropsychological tests used to assess cognitive functioning.

Subjective measures are usually ordinal bounded variables with a number of different levels that varies a lot but may reach 40 or even 100. When the number of levels is large, it is natural to consider such variables as quantitative variables, and to analyze their change over time through linear mixed models. However, their distributions may greatly deviate from the normal distribution which is assumed in the linear mixed model. Indeed, subjective measures may have a ceiling (or a floor) effect corresponding to the fact that the maximum (or the minimum) of the scale is reached for a non-negligible part of the sample. They also usually present an unequal interval scaling also called *curvilinearity* reflecting the fact that the difference between two successive levels of the scale does not have a constant meaning. For example, on a 100-point quality-of-life scale, a difference of 1 point between scores 10 and 11, and a 1-point difference between 90 and 91 do not necessarily have the same meaning in terms of intensity of change in quality of life: a change from 10 to 11 could correspond to a significant increase in quality of life, whereas the same increase between 90 and 91 could translate into a minor increase (or vice versa). Yet the linear mixed model implicitly assumes that a difference between two values has the same meaning throughout the whole range of the variable of interest by assuming constant effects of predictors.

An alternative is to use a model for ordinal data (the actual nature of most measurement scales), namely a proportional odds logistic model or a cumulative probit model which involve a link function between the observed data and the linear predictor variable (see Section 4.2.3). Thanks to the specific intercept for each level of the variable, the curvilinearity problem is properly taken into account. However, first, the estimation of a proportional odds logistic mixed model or of a cumulative probit mixed model requires that each level of the dependent variable is observed, which is not necessarily the case when the variable has a large number of different levels. Second, these models are quite complicated to estimate due to the numerical integration over the random effects and the number of parameters involved (regression parameters plus as many thresholds as there are different levels of the variable).

To overcome this problem, it is possible to define a curvilinear mixed model that can be seen either as an extension of the linear mixed model to analyze quantitative data that are subject to curvilinearity and/or ceiling/floor effects, or as an approximation (numerically simpler) of the cumulative probit mixed model.

5.1.1 Model specification

Following the notations of Chapter 4, the curvilinear mixed model is defined for subject i $(i = 1, ..., N)$ at occasion j $(j = 1, ...n_i)$ by:

$$H(Y_{ij}; \eta) = X_{ij}^\top \beta + Z_{ij}^\top b_i + \epsilon_{ij} \text{ with } b_i \sim \mathcal{N}(0, B)$$
$$\text{and } \epsilon_i = (\epsilon_{i1}, ..., \epsilon_{in_i})^\top \sim \mathcal{N}(0, \Sigma_i) \tag{5.1}$$

The vector of responses for subject i is denoted $Y_i = (Y_{i1}, Y_{i2}, \ldots, Y_{in_i})^\top$. The errors ϵ_i can be divided into a Gaussian process w_i with variance-covariance matrix R_i and independent Gaussian measurement errors e_i with variance $\sigma^2 I_{n_i}$ so that $\epsilon_i = w_i + e_i$ and $\Sigma_i = R_i + \sigma^2 I_{n_i}$.

The link function H is a monotonous increasing function parameterized with vector η of size p_η. When H is a linear function, the model reduces to the standard linear mixed model (apart from an identifiability constraint - see Section 5.1.2).

To obtain a large flexibility in the shape of the relationship between the observed variable and its "normalized" version $\tilde{Y}_{ij} = X_{ij}^\top \beta + Z_{ij}^\top b_i + \epsilon_{ij}$, the link function H is chosen inside a family of flexible monotonous increasing functions. One example of flexible and parsimonious family is the family of cumulative Beta distribution functions recentered and standardized. They are defined as:

$$H(Y_{ij}; \eta) = \frac{1}{\eta_4} \left(\int_0^{Y_{ij}^*} \frac{x^{\eta_1-1}(1-x)^{\eta_2-1}}{B(\eta_1, \eta_2)} dx - \eta_3 \right), \tag{5.2}$$

where $B(\eta_1, \eta_2)$ is the complete Beta function and Y_{ij} is rescaled in $(0, 1)$ using $Y_{ij}^* = \frac{Y_{ij} - \min(Y) + \epsilon_Y}{\max(Y) - \min(Y) + 2\epsilon_Y}$ and a constant $\epsilon_Y > 0$.

With only four parameters, this transformation can capture concave, convex and sigmoïd relationships. Any other simple family of parameterized monotonous increasing functions could be used instead, such as the cumulative distribution functions of Weibull or logistic variables (see Proust et al., 2006, for more details) also rescaled. In order to overcome limits of classical parametric functions, the link function H can also be approximated by a basis of I-splines $(B_m^I)_{m=1, p_\eta - 1}$, the integrated version of M-splines (Proust-Lima et al., 2013). The link function is then defined as:

$$H(Y_{ij}; \eta) = \eta_0 + \sum_{m=1}^{p_\eta - 1} \eta_m B_m^I(Y_{ij}). \tag{5.3}$$

By choosing a relatively small number of knots and quadratic splines, the I-splines link function provides a family of extremely flexible link functions with a reasonable number of parameters.

5.1.2 Identifiability

It is essential to note that the curvilinear mixed model as defined by Equation (5.1) with a parameterized link function H (for example the ones given in (5.3) or in (5.2)) is not identifiable. Most often, identifiability is met by removing the intercept of the vector of parameters β ($\beta_0 = 0$) and fixing the variance of the independent Gaussian errors σ^2 to 1.

Indeed, in the case of a link function approximated by I-splines (5.3), β_0 is absorbed by η_0 and σ is absorbed by $\sum_{m=1}^{p_\eta - 1} \eta_m$. In the case of a linear link function, $H(y; \eta) = \frac{y - \eta_0}{\eta_1}$ so that η_0 and η_1 replace, respectively, the intercept β_0 and the standard error σ of the standard linear mixed model.

5.1.3 Maximum likelihood estimation

As the link function is a continuous monotonous increasing function, the Jacobian formula can be used to link the density of the vector Y with the density of its normalized version, vector $\tilde{Y}$, defined by elements $\tilde{Y}_l = H(Y_l; \eta)$:

$$f_Y(y) = f_{\tilde{Y}}(\tilde{y}) \mid J_H \mid$$

where J_H is the Jacobian diagonal matrix with l^{th} element $H'(y_l)$ the first derivative of transformation H, and $\mid J_H \mid$ is the determinant of J_H.

The vector $\tilde{Y}_i$ is multivariate normal with expectation $X_i \beta$ and variance-covariance matrix $V_i = Z_i B Z_i^\top + \Sigma_i$ (X_i and Z_i are the matrices with $X_{ij}^\top$

and $Z_{ij}^{\top}$ as row vector j). So by denoting ϕ the parameters of variance and covariance in V_i, the log-likelihood of the model can be written:

$$L(\beta, \phi, \eta) = -\frac{1}{2} \sum_{i=1}^{N} \left\{ n_i \log(2\pi) + \log |V_i| + \right.$$

$$\left. (H(Y_i; \eta) - X_i\beta)^{\top} V_i^{-1} (H(Y_i; \eta) - X_i\beta) \right\} + \sum_{i=1}^{N} \sum_{j=1}^{n_i} \log(H'(Y_{ij}; \eta)) \quad (5.4)$$

with $H(Y_i)$ the n_i-vector with j^{th} element $H(Y_{ij})$.

The maximum likelihood estimators of β, ϕ and η are obtained simultaneously by maximizing the log-likelihood (5.4) using an iterative procedure (a Newton-Raphson algorithm for instance). This model is implemented in the function `lcmm` of `lcmm` R package (Proust-Lima et al., 2015).

5.1.4 Difference with the generalized linear mixed model

Although both approaches introduce the concept of link function, the curvilinear mixed model differs from generalized linear models. Indeed, in both cases the idea is to use a transformation (or link function) to reduce the regression to a linear mixed model. However, curvilinear mixed models apply directly this transformation to the observations of the variable of interest, and therefore include measurement errors in the linear regression with mixed effects. In contrast, generalized linear models apply the transformation to the expectation of the variable of interest so that no error is added to the linear regression with mixed effects.

A second difference is that in generalized linear models, the link function is determined (logit, logarithm, etc.), while in curvilinear mixed models, the transformation involves parameters to be estimated. Nevertheless, the two approaches are very close, and the linear mixed model is a special case of both the generalized linear mixed model and the curvilinear mixed model.

5.1.5 Concept of underlying latent process

Just as the proportional odds logistic mixed model or the cumulative probit mixed model, the curvilinear mixed model can be seen as a mixed model involving an underlying latent process. Indeed, the "normalized version" of the variable of interest is a latent process whose change over time is described with a linear mixed model. This latent process is the actual quantity of interest for which the observed dependent variable constitutes an imperfect measure. This is the case for instance with psychometric tests which are imperfect measures of the cognitive level, or perceived pain scales that aim to measure the intensity of pain, or also questionnaires assessing quality of life. The concept of underlying latent process actually applies to any subjective measure, i.e., measurements collected using a scale, a questionnaire or a test.

Using this definition, one can easily link the curvilinear models that assume a continuous parameterized transformation between the underlying latent process and the observed variable with models for ordinal data (described in Section 4.2.3) that define a discrete relationship between these two quantities. Indeed, by rewriting the curvilinear mixed model formula (5.1) as $Y_{ij} = F(\tilde{Y}_{ij}; \eta)$ with $F(.; \eta) = H^{-1}(.; \eta)$ since H are invertible functions, the cumulative probit mixed model may enter the same family of models with the surjective link function F defined for a discrete variable y in $(\min, \max)$ by:

$$\forall k \in \{\min, \max\}, \quad F(y; \eta) = k \mathbb{1}_{\eta_k < y \leq \eta_{k+1}} \text{ and } \eta_{\min} = -\infty \; ; \; \eta_{\max+1} = +\infty \tag{5.5}$$

This model will be further called "latent process mixed model" with a thresholds link function or cumulative probit mixed model. Using this alternative definition $Y_{ij} = F(\tilde{Y}_{ij}; \eta)$, the curvilinear mixed model can be seen as a continuous approximation of the cumulative probit mixed model for ordinal data with a large number of values or an extension of this model to the non-Gaussian quantitative data.

A difficulty with the curvilinear mixed model is that the regression parameters are interpreted in the scale of the latent process (or transformed variable $\tilde{Y}$). To interpret the estimates, it is thus often useful to plot the trajectory of the variable Y in its natural scale according to the explanatory variables values, that is $\mathrm{E}(Y \mid X, \hat{\beta}, \hat{\phi}, \hat{\eta})$. However, when the transformation $H(Y; \eta)$ is not linear, $\mathrm{E}(Y \mid X, \hat{\beta}, \hat{\phi}, \hat{\eta}) \neq H^{-1}(\mathrm{E}(\tilde{Y} \mid X, \hat{\beta}, \hat{\phi}); \hat{\eta})$ and the computation of $\mathrm{E}(Y \mid X, \hat{\beta}, \hat{\phi}, \hat{\eta})$ may not be straightforward. The Monte-Carlo method can be used to calculate easily this expectation. It consists in generating a large number of values $\tilde{y}_s$ from the Gaussian distribution of $\tilde{Y}$ conditional to the explanatory variables and the estimated parameters, and calculating the mean (or median) of $H^{-1}(\tilde{y}_s)$. The 2.5^{th} and 97.5^{th} percentiles of the distribution of $H^{-1}(\tilde{y}_s)$ also provide the 95% confidence bands.

5.1.6 Application

In studies of cognitive aging such as the Paquid cohort, various measurement scales are collected, with sometimes distributions very far from the Gaussian distribution, and potential problems of curvilinearity. This is the case for psychometric tests (Proust-Lima et al., 2011, 2013) but also for scales of dependency or depressive symptoms.

We illustrate here the use of the curvilinear mixed models with the analysis of repeated measures of depressive symptoms according to gender. In Sections 4.2 and 4.4, the probability of having high depressive symptoms, defined by a CES-D above 16, was described as a function of age and gender in a logistic mixed effects model and a marginal logistic model. This model is interesting to accurately describe the passage above a clinically relevant threshold of the CES-D scale. However, it leads to a significant loss of information since the CES-D measures depressive symptomatology quantitatively on a scale ranging from 0 to 60 and subtle changes above or below the clinically meaningful threshold may be of interest.

To take into account all available information and precisely describe the change over time of this measurement scale, the ordinal nature of the CES-D would lead to consider a proportional odds mixed model or a cumulative probit mixed model. However, with 61 different levels in theory and 51 different levels in the sample of 500 subjects from Paquid cohort, this approach is very difficult to implement in practice. An alternative is to apply the latent process mixed model for curvilinear data that is numerically simpler, and which takes into account the deviation from the normality of the variable (as shown in Figure 4.3 of Chapter 4) as opposed to the linear mixed model.

For this illustration, as in Chapter 4, we chose to describe the change over time of CES-D (`cesd`) according to gender (using the binary variable `male`) and age using the variable `age65 = (age-65) / 10` which is centered at 65 and described in decades to avoid numerical problems.

For subject i at occasion j, the latent process linear mixed model is defined as:

$$H(\texttt{cesd}_{ij}; \eta) = \beta_1 \, \texttt{age65}_{ij} + \beta_2 \, \texttt{male}_i + \beta_3 \, \texttt{male}_i \times \texttt{age65}_{ij} + b_{0i} + b_{1i} \, \texttt{age65}_{ij} + \epsilon_{ij} \tag{5.6}$$

where $b_i = \begin{pmatrix} b_{0i} \\ b_{1i} \end{pmatrix} \sim \mathcal{N}\left(\begin{pmatrix} 0 \\ 0 \end{pmatrix}, \begin{pmatrix} \sigma_0^2 & \sigma_{01} \\ \sigma_{01} & \sigma_1^2 \end{pmatrix} \right)$ and $\epsilon_{ij} \sim \mathcal{N}(0, 1)$.

Two continuous link functions H were considered: a linear function which defines a standard linear mixed model, and a linear combination of I-splines as defined in (5.3) with 5 knots at the quantiles. We also estimated this latent process mixed model with a thresholds link function as discussed in Section 5.1.5 and Equation (5.5). These three models were estimated with `lcmm` function of `lcmm` R package. Calls for this application are detailed in the appendix.

The three different estimated functions that link the underlying latent process to the observed CES-D are shown in Figure 5.1. The thresholds link function defined in the cumulative probit mixed model is more flexible since it models non-parametrically the relationship between the observed variable and its "normalized" version that is the underlying latent process. The linear function considered in the standard linear mixed model is very far from this thresholds link function, which results in a much worse fit to the data with an *AIC for discrete data* (Proust-Lima et al., 2013) of 460 points higher than the one of the cumulative probit mixed model. In contrast, the estimated splines link function is very close to the estimated thresholds link function, and the discrete AIC even favors the more parsimonious I-splines link function by 8.3

points. This shows that the latent process mixed model with continuous transformations can very well approximate the cumulative probit mixed model and provides a numerically attractive alternative for ordinal variables of interest with a relatively large number of values.

We note here that models were compared in terms of *AIC for discrete data* rather than naive (or standard) AIC for each model. Indeed, in the model with a thresholds link, the data are considered as discrete and the densities are computed with respect to the counting measure. In the models with continuous link functions, the same data are considered as continuous and the densities are computed with respect to the Lebesgues measure. AIC derived from likelihoods computed with Lebesgues and counting measures cannot be compared, so a unified *AIC for discrete data* was proposed (Proust-Lima et al., 2013) and further validated (Commenges et al., 2015) in which the densities are computed *a posteriori* according to the counting measure whatever the model, and are thus comparable in terms of AIC.

The estimated transformations displayed in Figure 5.1 also highlight the property of curvilinearity of CES-D scale: a change of one point of CES-D in very low values of the CES-D (between 0 and 5) represents a much more dramatic change in the scale of the latent process than a one-point change in the highest values (between 20 and 30).

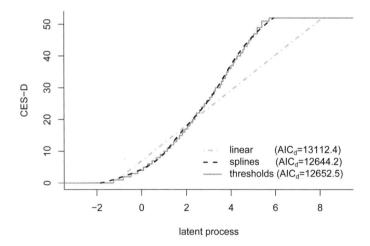

FIGURE 5.1
Estimated linear, I-splines (with 5 knots at the quantiles) and thresholds link functions to link the observed CES-D scores with its underlying latent process representing the normalized depressive symptoms.

The fixed effects estimates of the model are given in Table 5.1. The interpretation of these parameters is the same as in any conventional linear mixed model. The only difference is that they are expressed in the scale of the latent process underlying the CES-D, i.e., the normalized or ("actual") depressive symptoms rather than on the CES-D scale directly. According to Table 5.1, men have in mean a significantly lower depressive symptomatology than women at age 65 (β_2 = - 0.831, p<0.0001); depressive symptomatology increases significantly with age (β_1 = 0.424, p <0.0001), and this increase is higher in men than in women (β_3 = 0.234, p = 0.023). These interpretations cannot be directly translated in a quantitative way in the natural scale of the CES-D. Indeed, the effects, that are linear in the scale of the latent process, are no longer linear in the original CES-D scale because of the curvilinearity captured by the non-linear link function. One way to interpret the results in the scale of the CES-D is to depict the marginal predictions of the model according to each level of the covariate of interest as evoked in Section 5.1.5. This is shown in Figure 5.2. Because of the curvilinearity (or in other words the non-linearity of the relationship with the underlying latent process), although the regression model assumes linear trajectories by sex in the scale of latent process, the trajectories are non-linear in the scale of the CES-D.

The results of this analysis differ from those of the logistic model with mixed effects described in Section 4.2.2. Indeed, with the logistic model no interaction between gender and age had been found ($p = 0.406$) on the probability of having high depressive symptoms (i.e., CES-D greater than 16 *vs.* lower) while in this model, depressive symptoms increase significantly more with age in men than in women ($p = 0.026$) although men remain at a lower level than women (see Figure 5.2). It should be noted that the information used in these two approaches is different. Here, the depressive symptomatology spectrum is assessed in a more subtle way compared to the previous analysis that focused solely on the passing above a clinically meaningful threshold.

TABLE 5.1

Fixed effects estimated in the latent process mixed model with a I-splines link function (5 knots at the quantiles) for the CES-D in the 500-subject PAQUID sample.

Parameter	Estimated value	Standard-error	Wald statistic	p-value
intercept (not estimated)	0			
age65	0.424	0.063	6.76	<0.0001
male	-0.831	0.197	-4.21	<0.0001
age65×male	0.234	0.103	2.23	0.023

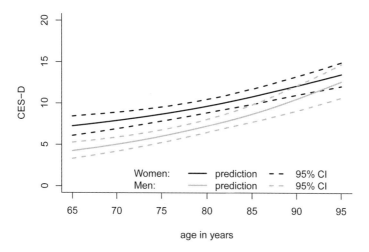

FIGURE 5.2
Predicted trajectories of CES-D according to gender obtained by a Monte-Carlo method. The solid line corresponds to the median prediction and the dashed lines correspond to the 2.5% and 97.5% predictions of the trajectories obtained from 2000 random draws.

5.2 Mixed models for multivariate longitudinal data

In cohort studies and clinical trials, different variables are usually measured at each visit. When these variables are correlated, it may be useful to study them together in order to increase the power of the analysis and to assess the association between the different processes. For example, the monitoring of HIV+ patients is based on two main correlated and complementary markers: plasma viral load and CD4 count. The joint analysis of their trajectories enables a better understanding of their interrelationships. Another example is the study of cognitive decline in the elderly which is usually based on repeated measurements of a battery of neuropsychological tests. Although these tests evaluate different aspects of cognition, they are highly correlated and mostly measure the same underlying quantity: cognition.

In this section, we present two extensions of the mixed model for the analysis of multivariate longitudinal data. When the number of markers is small (2 or 3) and one wants to make the fewest assumptions as possible about the markers interrelations, a direct extension of the univariate mixed model (for one marker) to the multivariate setting is envisaged. In contrast, when the number of markers is larger and it is reasonable to consider that they all essentially measure the same underlying process, a multivariate mixed model involving a common latent process for all the markers may be favored. This approach is more parsimonious than conventional multivariate mixed models and may increase the power of the analysis when the main interest is in the change over time of the common process underlying the change of various markers and in the assessment of factors associated with this process.

We note that in these two approaches, the number and the times of measurement can vary from one subject to another, and from one marker to another.

5.2.1 Multivariate linear mixed model

To make the notation clearer, we only present here the bivariate linear mixed model. However, the extension to more than two markers is straightforward. In addition, we detail the principle of the multivariate mixed model in the linear framework only but the same extension applies to generalized linear mixed models and non-linear mixed models.

5.2.1.1 Model specification

Let us denote Y_{ki} the vector of size n_{ki} of observations for marker k ($k = 1, 2$) and subject i ($i = 1, ..., N$) collected at measurement times $t_{ki} = (t_{ki1}, ..., t_{kin_{ki}})^\top$. The trajectory of each marker can be described with a linear mixed model:

$$Y_{1i} = X_{1i}\beta_1 + Z_{1i}b_{1i} + \epsilon_{1i}, \tag{5.7}$$

and

$$Y_{2i} = X_{2i}\beta_2 + Z_{2i}b_{2i} + \epsilon_{2i}, \tag{5.8}$$

where the vectors of random effects b_{ki} and the measurement errors ϵ_{ki} are Gaussian with zero expectations and variance-covariance matrices B_k and Σ_{ki}, respectively. To take into account the correlation between the markers, the two models can be combined by assuming a correlation between the random effects b_{1i} and b_{2i}, and possibly between the measurement errors ϵ_{1i} and ϵ_{2i}. The multivariate mixed model is then written:

$$Y_i = X_i\beta + Z_ib_i + \epsilon_i, \tag{5.9}$$

with $Y_i = [Y_{1i}^\top \; Y_{2i}^\top]^\top$, $\beta = [\beta_1^\top \; \beta_2^\top]^\top$,

$$X_i = \begin{bmatrix} X_{1i} & \mathbf{0} \\ \mathbf{0}^\top & X_{2i} \end{bmatrix}, Z_i = \begin{bmatrix} Z_{1i} & \mathbf{0} \\ \mathbf{0}^\top & Z_{2i} \end{bmatrix}.$$

The vectors $b_i = [b_{1i}^\top \; b_{2i}^\top]^\top$ and $\epsilon_i = [\epsilon_{1i}^\top \; \epsilon_{2i}^\top]^\top$ follow multivariate normal distributions with zero expectations and variance-covariance matrices

$$B = \begin{bmatrix} B_1 & B_{12} \\ B_{12}^\top & B_2 \end{bmatrix} \text{ and } \Sigma_i = \begin{bmatrix} \Sigma_{1i} & \Sigma_{12i} \\ \Sigma_{12i}^\top & \Sigma_{2i} \end{bmatrix}, \text{ respectively.}$$

The submatrix B_{12} defines the covariance between the random effects of the two markers, while Σ_{12i} defines the covariance between the measurement errors of the two markers. The latter can be constrained to 0 when the measurement errors are supposed to be independent between the markers.

This model has exactly the same structure as the standard linear mixed model and it can be estimated with standard SAS or R linear mixed model estimation procedures when the structure of Σ_i remains simple (for example when $\Sigma_i = \sigma^2 I_{n_i}$). The principle is to set the repeated measures of the two markers in a unique response vector Y of length $n_{1i} + n_{2i}$, and specify an indicator variable of each marker to distinguish the repeated data of each one (see Thiébaut et al., 2002).

This approach is limited to a small number of correlated markers. Indeed the number of random effects and thus the number of variance-covariance parameters increases proportionally with the number of markers. Other more parsimonious parametric (Sy et al., 1997) or non-parametric (Brown et al., 2001) models have been proposed. When the number of markers increases, Fieuws and Verbeke (2006) have proposed a pairwise approach using pseudo-likelihood to avoid computational issues due to the size of the covariance matrix.

5.2.1.2 Application

The bivariate linear mixed model is illustrated through an application in HIV infection. The objective consists in assessing the viro-immunological response, characterized by the plasma viral load and the CD4 count (concentration of CD4+ T cells in the blood), after the initiation of an antiretroviral therapy in the cohort ANRS EP11 APROCO. This French multicenter observational cohort included 1281 patients who initiated an antiretroviral triple therapy including a protease inhibitor. Patients had a measurement of the two markers every 4 months. Further information on the data and several types of bivariate mixed models are detailed in the following publications (Thiébaut et al., 2002, 2003).

Plasma viral load and CD4 count are fundamentally correlated since CD4 cells are the main target of HIV and the virus is produced by infected CD4 cells. The study of the effect of the treatment on these two markers leads to the modelling of two correlated markers repeatedly collected over time. The dynamics of the markers over time does not appear to be linear, especially that of viral load. So, in order to characterize at best the dynamics of the markers over time, a piecewise linear model is used. It consists in defining a first time variable $(\min(t_{ij}, t_1))$ that represents time until time t_1 and a second time variable $((t_{ij} - t_1)\mathbb{1}_{t_{ij}>t_1})$ that represents the time elapsed since t_1. This second time variable is defined in a way that ensures continuity in t_1. Time t_1

was set at four months, that is the date of the first monitoring.

Each univariate mixed model therefore includes potentially three fixed effects and three random effects (intercept, first slope and second slope), and a bivariate model taking into account the correlation between these parameters would therefore include nine additional variance-covariance parameters. This illustrates the rapid inflation of the number of parameters with this type of approach.

In this example, it was proposed to work on the difference with time 0:

$$\check{Y}_{kij} = Y_{kij} - Y_{ki0}$$

for $t_{ij} > 0$. Working on the difference removes the fixed intercepts and the random intercepts since the initial value of the difference is 0 for all the individuals by definition. These initial values of the difference are naturally excluded from the analysis. The model can be written for each marker k ($k = 1$ for the CD4 count and $k = 2$ for viral load for example):

$$\check{Y}_{kij} = \beta_{1k} \min(t_{ij}, t_1) + \beta_{2k}(t_{ij} - t_1)\mathbb{1}_{t_{ij}>t_1} + b_{1ik} \min(t_{ij}, t_1) + \\ b_{2ik}(t_{ij} - t_1)\mathbb{1}_{t_{ij}>t_1} + \epsilon_{kij}. \tag{5.10}$$

The variance-covariance matrix of the marker-specific random effects associated with the slopes is left unstructured. Thus it includes all the covariances between the subject-specific slopes for the two markers. The distribution of the random effects can be written:

$$(b_{1i1}, b_{2i1}, b_{1i2}, b_{2i2})^{\top} \sim \mathcal{N} \left(0, B = \begin{bmatrix} \sigma_1^2 & \sigma_{12} & \sigma_{13} & \sigma_{14} \\ \sigma_{12} & \sigma_2^2 & \sigma_{23} & \sigma_{24} \\ \sigma_{13} & \sigma_{23} & \sigma_3^2 & \sigma_{34} \\ \sigma_{14} & \sigma_{24} & \sigma_{34} & \sigma_4^2 \end{bmatrix} \right)$$

and

$$\epsilon_{kij} \sim \mathcal{N}(0, \sigma_{\epsilon_k}^2).$$

The variance-covariance matrix B of the random effects includes the variances of the random effects (first and second slopes of CD4 count and first and second slopes of viral load) in its diagonal, and covariances within and between the markers in the non-diagonal terms. For example, σ_{12} is the covariance between the first slope and the second slope of the CD4; σ_{24} denotes the covariance between the second slope of the CD4 and the second slope of viral load. Both residual errors are assumed to be independent. However, the variance-covariance matrix of the errors could be further enhanced to take into account the fact that each dependent variable is a difference in marker values rather than directly the value of the marker.

A total of 16 parameters were estimated in this model. Viral load was transformed using the logarithmic function in base 10 to meet the assumptions of the model (homoscedastic Gaussian errors). This transformation is common for the viral load that may range from a few copies/mL to several millions of copies/mL in primary infection. CD4 counts were divided by 10 for numerical reasons. Examples of scripts in R and SAS are given in the appendix.

We note that viral load may be potentially left-censored by lower detection threshold. In the context of this application of multivariate mixed models, a simple imputation of half the value of the detection limit was done for data below the detection limit. However, it is possible to take into account this left-censoring of the marker in the context of a multivariate mixed model as described for the univariate mixed model in Section 4.5.4 (Thiébaut et al., 2003).

The multivariate mixed model resulted in a better fit than the two univariate mixed models and their total of 12 parameters (AIC=50420 *vs.* AIC=50638). Estimates of the fixed parameters showed a rapid change in the first four months (first slopes exhibited an increase of 25 CD4 cells per mm^3 per month and a fall of viral load of 0.5 $\log_{10}$ per month) and a slower dynamics for both markers after four months (seconds slopes) as reported in Table 5.2.

The covariance matrix of the random effects displayed in Table 5.3 showed significant associations between the slopes of the same marker (especially for the CD4) and the slopes of the two markers. The correlation matrix of the individual slopes of the markers given in Table 5.4 further exhibited strong negative correlations among individual first or second slopes of the two markers (-0.60 before 4 months, and -0.41 after 4 months) reflecting the association between the dynamics of the immune response and the virological response that the bivariate mixed model can take into account.

The mean predicted subject-specific trajectories plotted in Figure 5.3 along with the observed mean trajectories underline the good fit of the model to the data and the biphasic trajectories of CD4 count and viral load.

5.2.2 Multivariate mixed model with latent process

In some applications, several measures may be simultaneously collected to describe the same phenomenon of interest. For example, several growth indicators (head circumference, femur length, etc.) are measured to describe the growth of a fetus in utero. Similarly, a series of psychometric tests assessing memory, language, attention, etc. is usually collected to assess the cognitive level of a person. Finally, questionnaires involving a large number of different items is most often used to quantify the quality of life.

In these examples, the interest is not in the analysis of one or the other markers taken separately but in the analysis of the underlying quantity that

TABLE 5.2
Fixed effect estimates from the bivariate linear mixed model (with time in months). APROCO ANRS EP11 cohort (CD4 for CD4+ T cells, VL for Viral Load).

Covariate	Parameter	Estimated value	Standard-error	Wald Statistic	p-value
1st slope CD4	β_{11}	2.54	0.10	25.03	<0.0001
2nd slope CD4	β_{21}	0.59	0.03	19.77	<0.0001
1st slope VL	β_{12}	-0.49	0.0096	-51.34	<0.0001
2nd slope VL	β_{22}	-0.0047	0.0021	-2.25	0.025

TABLE 5.3
Estimated covariance of the random effects from the bivariate linear mixed model. APROCO ANRS EP11 cohort (CD4 for CD4+ T cells, VL for Viral Load).

Covariance	Parameter	Estimated value	Standard-error	Wald Statistic	p-value
1st slope CD4, 2nd slope CD4	σ_{12}	0.53	0.10	5.31	<0.0001
1st slope CD4, 1st slope VL	σ_{13}	-0.30	0.032	-9.24	<0.0001
1st slope CD4, 2nd slope VL	σ_{14}	0.015	0.0067	2.30	0.021
2nd slope CD4, 1st slope VL	σ_{23}	-0.025	0.0092	-2.74	0.0062
2nd slope CD4, 2nd slope VL	σ_{24}	-0.016	0.0020	-8.13	<0.0001
1st slope VL, 2nd slope VL	σ_{34}	-0.0014	0.00065	-2.13	0.033

the set of markers is supposed to measure. One possibility is to use a multivariate linear mixed model to account for the correlation between the markers. However, a more astute and parsimonious way to simultaneously model these markers is to actually assume that there is a common latent process underlying all the dependent variables, to describe this latent process over time using a standard linear mixed model, and to simultaneously link each marker with the latent process through an equation which is specific to it, and called *equation of observation* or *measurement model*.

Whether in the presence of repeated data or not, the introduction of latent

TABLE 5.4

Estimated correlation matrix of the random effects from the bivariate linear mixed model. APROCO ANRS EP11 cohort (CD4 for CD4+ T cells, VL for Viral Load).

Parameter	CD4		Viral load	
	1st slope	2nd slope	1st slope	2nd slope
1st slope CD4	1			
2nd slope CD4	0.37	1		
1st slope VL	-0.41	-0.16	1	
2nd slope VL	0.13	-0.60	-0.10	1

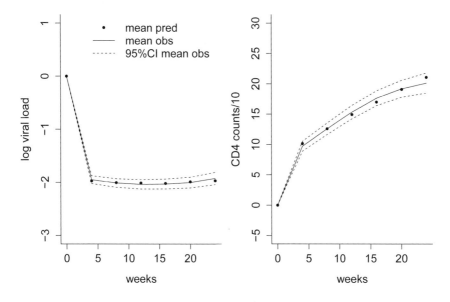

FIGURE 5.3

Mean observed trajectories (95% confidence interval) and mean subject-specific predictions for plasma viral load and CD4+ T cells in APROCO ANRS EP11 cohort.

variables is classic in psychology, a field in which most of the phenomena of interest are latent concepts (cognition, satisfaction, mood, etc.) that are measured using indicators or questionnaires. These models involving continuous latent variables are often called "structural equation models," the term *structural equation* referring to the part of the model that describes the structure of the latent phenomenon (Muthén, 2002).

5.2.2.1 Model specification

Let us denote $\Lambda_i(t)_{t \in \mathbb{R}}$ the latent process defined in continuous time and representing the common underlying component of a set of K observed longitudinal dependent variables Y_{ki} ($k = 1, ..., K$ and $i = 1, ..., N$). Change over time of the latent process is modelled in a *structural equation* with a standard linear mixed model:

$$\Lambda_i(t) = X_i(t)^\top \beta + Z_i(t)^\top b_i + w_i(t) \quad \forall t \in \mathbb{R} \tag{5.11}$$

$X_i(t)$ et $Z_i(t)$ are vectors of covariates respectively associated with the vector of fixed effects β and the vector of random effects b_i that are identically and independently distributed according to a Gaussian distribution with mean 0 and variance-covariance matrix B. An autocorrelated Gaussian process $(w_i(t))$ with zero expectation and parameterized structure of variance-covariance can be also included. One example is the Brownian process with the covariance structure $\mathrm{cov}(w_i(t), w_i(u)) = \sigma_w^2 \min(t, u) \ \forall (t, u) \in \mathbb{R}^{+2}$. We note that the linear mixed model defined in (5.11) does not involve any independent measurement error since the latent process is not observed, and is thus not subject to measurement error.

Each observed variable is linked to the latent process in a specific *equation of observation*. Linear equations of observation are most often defined for continuous Gaussian variables. By denoting Y_{kij} the response variable k ($k = 1, ..., K$) of subject i ($i = 1, ..., N$) at occasion j ($j = 1, ..., n_{ik}$) and t_{kij} the corresponding time of measurement, the equation of observation can be written:

$$Y_{kij} = \eta_{0k} + \eta_{1k} \Lambda_i(t_{kij}) + \epsilon_{kij}. \tag{5.12}$$

The vector of parameters that links the variable Y_{kij} to the latent process is $\eta_k = (\eta_{0k}, \eta_{1k})$. The measurement errors specific to variable k are ϵ_{kij}, and they have a Gaussian distribution with mean zero and variance $\sigma_{\epsilon_k}^2$.

In the case of binary or ordinal markers, the linear equation of observation defined in (5.12) can be replaced by an equation of observation that involves thresholds parameters:

$$Y_{kij} = m \Leftrightarrow \eta_m < \Lambda_i(t_{kij}) + \sigma_{\epsilon_k} \epsilon_{kij} \leq \eta_{m+1} \quad \forall m \in \{0, M\} \tag{5.13}$$

This equation reduces to a proportional odds model when the errors ϵ_{kij} are logistic, or a cumulative probit model when the errors ϵ_{kij} are normal (see Section 4.2.3 for further details). In this case, the autocorrelated Gaussian process $(w_i(t))$ is not included in the structural Equation (5.11) for numerical reasons.

When all the dependent variables are binary or ordinal and equations of observation such as (5.13) are assumed, the model constitutes a longitudinal version of the 2-parameter model for graded responses, well known in the *Item Response Theory* (IRT) literature.

In general, one can consider any type of equation of observation that is appropriate for the dependent variable. In particular, *curvilinear* equations of observation as introduced in Section 5.1 can be considered:

$$H_k(Y_{kij}; \eta_k) = \Lambda_i(t_{kij}) + \sigma_{\epsilon_k} \epsilon_{kij} \qquad (5.14)$$

where $(H_k)_{k=1,K}$ are K parameterized continuous monotonous link functions.

It is also possible to mix different types of equations of observation within the same multivariate mixed model by combining equations of observation with thresholds (5.13) for some ordinal markers with curvilinear ones (5.14) for curvilinear markers, etc.

The equations of observation can also be defined in a more sophisticated way by including covariates with effects that are specific to each observed marker (in contrast with the common effects that are supposed in the structural equation for the latent process) and/or random effects that are specific to each observed marker (and take into account a marker-specific additional variability) (Proust et al., 2006; Proust-Lima et al., 2013).

5.2.2.2 Identifiability

The multivariate latent process mixed model as defined by the structural Equation (5.11) and the equations of observation (5.12) and/or (5.13) and/or (5.14) is not identifiable. To reach identifiability, constraints on the dimension of the latent process are necessary. One way consists in eliminating the fixed intercept in $X_i(t)^\top \beta$, and constraining the variance of the random intercept in b_i to one. This second constraint on the variance of the random-intercept replaces the one on the variance of the errors in the univariate latent process mixed models described in Section 5.1. With these constraints,

- the latent process is centered around the mean level of the underlying quantity among subjects of the reference category for covariates $X_i(t) = 0$ at time $t = 0$;

- one unit of the latent process represents the inter-individual variability of this quantity at time $t = 0$ (when $Z_i(t)$ only includes functions of time).

5.2.2.3 Estimation

The parameters of the multivariate latent process mixed model are estimated by maximum likelihood. The form of the likelihood depends on the nature of the equations of observation considered for each marker of interest k. When all the equations of observation are linear or curvilinear, the marginal distribution can be used to write the likelihood of the data (as in the univariate case, see Section 4.1.3.1). When at least one equation of observation is not curvilinear or linear (as with binary or ordinal data for example), then the likelihood usually does not have an analytical solution. The likelihood is decomposed using the conditional distribution given the random effects and the integral over the random effects is computed by numerical integration.

In both cases, an iterative maximization algorithm is used to obtain the maximum likelihood estimators. With curvilinear and linear link functions, these models can be estimated with the `multlcmm` function of the R package `lcmm` (Proust-Lima et al., 2015). In the case of linear equations of observation, the SAS proc MIXED may also be used. In other cases, specific programs exist (see for instance Proust-Lima et al. (2013) for longitudinal IRT models).

5.2.2.4 Application

To illustrate the multivariate latent process mixed model, we describe cognitive change over time measured in the Paquid sample with three psychometric tests:

- the Mini Mental State Examination (MMSE), a score ranging in 0-30 and evaluating the overall cognitive level;

- the Benton Visual Retention Test (BVRT), a score ranging in 0-15 and measuring the visual and spatial memory;

- the Isaacs Set Test (IST) truncated to 15 seconds, a score ranging in 0-40 and measuring verbal fluency and semantic memory.

For these three tests, higher scores indicate better cognitive level. Histograms of the repeated measures in these three tests in the sample of 500 subjects from Paquid are given in Figure 5.4. The distribution of MMSE is very asymmetric and the maximum is reached for about 10% of the data, indicating the strong ceiling effect of this test. The distributions of other tests are far less asymmetrical with a lower ceiling effect for BVRT and almost no one for IST.

We assume that these three psychometric tests are measures with error of the same underlying latent process, that is global cognitive functioning. Change over time of this global cognitive functioning is described according to education (binary covariate CEP which equals 1 when the subject obtained the diploma from primary school, and 0 otherwise). We chose to study the cognitive trajectory according to the time since the entry in the cohort (variable time in years) and to assume a quadratic trajectory with correlated random effects on the intercept, slope and quadratic slope. No autocorrelated process was added.

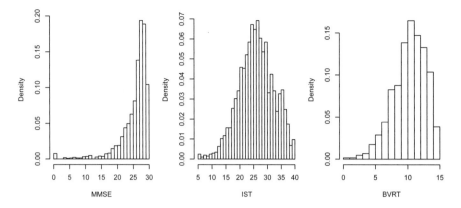

FIGURE 5.4
Distribution of the repeated measures of MMSE, IST and BVRT in the sample
of 500 subjects from Paquid cohort.

The multivariate latent process mixed model is defined in two steps. First,
the trajectory of the underlying global cognitive functioning is described according to time and education in the linear mixed model without measurement
errors, that is for subject i at time t ($t \in \mathbb{R}$):

$$\Lambda_i(t) = \beta_1\, t + \beta_2\, t^2 + \beta_3\, \text{CEP}_i + \beta_4\, \text{CEP}_i \times t + \beta_5\, \text{CEP}_i \times t^2 + b_{0i} + b_{1i}\, t + b_{2i}\, t^2 \quad (5.15)$$

Each repeated measure of each score is linked to the latent process at the
exact time of measurement by a score-specific equation of observation, that is
for subject i ($i = 1, ..., N$) and occasion j ($j = 1, ..., n_{ik}$, $k \in 1, 2, 3$):

$$H_1(\text{MMSE}_{ij}; \eta_1) = \Lambda_i(\text{time}_{1ij}) + \sigma_{\epsilon_1} \epsilon_{1ij}$$
$$H_2(\text{IST}_{ij}; \eta_2) = \Lambda_i(\text{time}_{2ij}) + \sigma_{\epsilon_2} \epsilon_{2ij} \quad (5.16)$$
$$H_3(\text{BVRT}_{ij}; \eta_3) = \Lambda_i(\text{time}_{3ij}) + \sigma_{\epsilon_3} \epsilon_{3ij}$$

The random effects $b_i = (b_{0i}, b_{1i}, b_{2i})$ follow a multivariate normal distribution with zero mean and an unstructured variance-covariance matrix (except the constraint that $\text{var}(b_{0i}) = 1$). The test-specific measurement errors
ϵ_{kij} ($k \in 1, 2, 3$) are independent and follow a standard Gaussian distribution. The three link functions H_1, H_2 and H_3, with vectors of parameters
η_1, η_2 and η_3 respectively, are defined in this example by cumulative Beta distribution functions centered and standardized. They capture the suspected
curvilinearity of the three tests with only four parameters. We note that other
families of link functions could have been chosen instead (for instance, linear
functions) and families of different types could have been assumed for each
score. The call of the model estimated with function `multlcmm` is given in the
appendix.

The estimated link functions between each test and the common latent
process are displayed in Figure 5.5. The transformation for MMSE is very

non-linear with a concave shape that illustrates the problem of ceiling effect
and curvilinearity of this test: one point lost at different levels of the test does
not represent the same loss in terms of underlying latent process. Equivalently,
a fixed loss in the scale of the latent process, for example 2 points, does not
translate into the same number of lost points in MMSE; it corresponds to a
loss of less than 1.5 points from a score of 30, a loss of 4.5 points from a score
of 27, and a loss of more than 10 points from an initial score of 20.

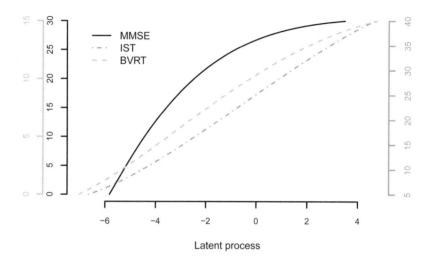

FIGURE 5.5
Estimated link functions between each test and the common underlying latent
process in the multivariate latent process mixed model and the sample of 500
subjects from Paquid cohort.

The model assumes that all the tests share the same underlying trajectory,
defined at the latent process level. In particular, it assumes that education
impacts all the tests in the exact same way through its impact on the latent
process. The estimated fixed effects of the model are reported in Table 5.5.
We do not report here the estimates of the variance-covariance of the random
effects, the estimates of the Beta link functions, nor the estimates of the
variances of the errors. We note, however, that the need for random effects
on the slope and the quadratic slopes can be tested exactly as in a standard
linear mixed model with the test described in Section 4.1.5 of Chapter 4.

The mean latent cognitive functioning is supposed to be zero in the reference category, that is in patients without the primary school diploma (CEP =
0) at baseline (time = 0). At baseline, subjects who graduated from primary
school had in mean a higher latent cognitive functioning ($\hat{\beta}_3 = 1.209$, p <

TABLE 5.5
Estimated fixed effects of the multivariate latent process mixed model. Only reported are the fixed effects at the level of the latent process underlying the three psychometric tests (MMSE, IST and BVRT) in the sample of 500 subjects from the Paquid cohort.

Variable	Parameter	Estimated value	Standard-error	Wald Statistic	p-value
(intercept)	β_0	0			
time	β_1	-0.125	0.031	-4.09	<0.0001
time^2	β_2	-0.020	0.017	-1.19	0.233
CEP	β_3	1.209	0.154	7.85	<0.0001
CEP×time	β_4	0.031	0.033	0.94	0.348
CEP×time^2	β_5	-0.014	0.018	-0.78	0.434

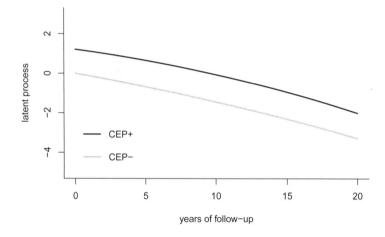

FIGURE 5.6
Predicted trajectories in the latent process scale according to the educational level (CEP+ when graduated from primary school *vs.* CEP- otherwise) in the sample of 500 subjects from the Paquid cohort. The latent process underlies MMSE, IST and BVRT psychometric tests.

0.0001) but their change over time did not differ from the change over time of those who did not obtain the diploma from primary school ($\hat{\beta}_4$ =0.031 and $\hat{\beta}_5$ = -0.014, p = 0.643). We note that testing the effect of educational level on the cognitive trajectory implies to simultaneously test the effect of CEP on variables time and time^2 using a bivariate Wald test ($\mathcal{H}_0 : \beta_4 = \beta_5 = 0$) since the change in the latent cognitive functioning is modelled by a quadratic shape.

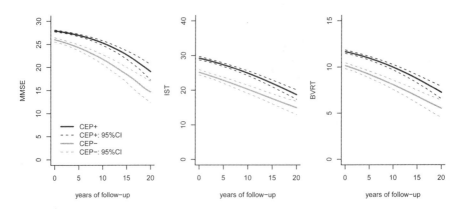

FIGURE 5.7
Predicted trajectories in the psychometric test (MMSE, IST and BVRT) scales according to the educational level (CEP+ when graduated from primary school *vs.* CEP- otherwise) in the sample of 500 subjects from the Paquid cohort.

When trajectories with time are non-linear and interactions with time are significant (note that this is not the case here), it becomes essential to plot the predicted trajectories according to the covariates to better appreciate the differences between groups and the general shape of trajectory. In the present application, the mean predicted trajectories in the scale of the latent process (the latent cognitive functioning) are plotted in Figure 5.6. Cognitive trajectories differ substantially according to the educational level. However, they remain roughly parallel throughout the follow-up underlining that the educational level does not impact the change in cognitive functioning. The same type of predictions can be computed and displayed in the natural scales of the tests, as done in Figure 5.7. However, these graphs must be interpreted with caution. Because of the important curvilinearity of MMSE, the distance between the predicted trajectories of subjects with low and high educational level increases over time. This growing difference between the trajectories is only due to the curvilinearity of the test and the large effect of educational level at baseline, not the actual impact of educational level on cognitive change.

5.3   Latent class mixed models

The linear mixed model assumes that the population under study is homogeneous; that is, it can be described by a unique mean profile of trajectory $X_i\beta$ and Gaussian individual deviations $Z_i b_i$ centered around this mean profile. In practice, it is not rare to suspect a certain heterogeneity in the population. For example, it is known that a population of old subjects *a priori* without dementia includes at least two profiles of cognitive aging: the so-called "normal" cognitive aging which is linked to the natural aging process with age, and a "pathological" cognitive aging that can lead later to a dementia like Alzheimer's disease. It is not *a priori* possible to identify these two types of trajectory using observed explanatory covariates. They consist in two latent groups or latent classes of subjects. In contrast, in a randomized clinical trial, a heterogeneity in the profiles of trajectory is also suspected according to the treatment but in this case, the groups are well identified and the inclusion of the treatment variable in the vector of predictors X_i of the linear mixed model should capture this heterogeneity and provide a unique mean profile of trajectory $X_i\beta$.

5.3.1 Model specification

The latent class mixed model which extends the theory of the standard mixed models to the study of heterogeneous populations has been first introduced by Verbeke and Lesaffre (1996) and Muthén and Shedden (1999). The model assumes that it exists a finite number G of subpopulations defining G latent classes. Each subject belongs to a unique latent class which is formalized by a discrete latent variable c_i that equals g if subject i belongs to latent class g. The probability to belong to the latent classes is generally defined in a multinomial logistic model:

$$\pi_{ig} = P(c_i = g \mid X_{1i}) = \frac{e^{\xi_{0g}+X_{1i}^\top \xi_{1g}}}{\sum_{l=1}^{G} e^{\xi_{0l}+X_{1i}^\top \xi_{1l}}} \qquad (5.17)$$

where X_{1i} is a vector of time-independent covariates. To reach identifiability, one class is defined as the reference class; in the following, this will be class G with constraints $\xi_{0G} = 0$ and $\xi_{1G} = 0$. It is not rare to include no covariate in the latent class membership probability model. In this case, $\frac{e^{\xi_{0g}}}{\sum_{l=1}^{G} e^{\xi_{0l}}}$ defines the marginal probability to belong to class g.

The trajectory of the dependent variable is simultaneously defined specifically to each latent class by a mixed model. With a continuous variable, the model for the distribution $[Y_{ij} \mid c_i = g]$ of subject i conditional on his/her membership to class g is defined by:

$$Y_{ij} = X_{2ij}^\top \beta + X_{3ij}^\top \gamma_g + Z_{ij}^\top b_i + \epsilon_{ij} \text{ with } b_i \sim \mathcal{N}(\mu_g, B_g). \qquad (5.18)$$

The three vectors X_{2ij}, X_{3ij} and Z_{ij} are vectors of covariates that do not overlap in order to ensure the identifiability of the model. Vector X_{2ij} is associated with the vector of fixed effects β that are common over the classes, vector X_{3ij} is associated with the vector of fixed effects γ_g that are different from one latent class to another, and vector Z_{ij} is associated with the vector of random effects b_i that are independent and identically distributed according to a mixture of distributions. In each latent class g, b_i follows a Normal distribution with mean μ_g and variance-covariance matrix B_g. We note that in contrast with the standard definition of the linear mixed model in which the random effects are zero-centered and all the fixed effects are modelled through the vector of covariates X, the random effects here are not zero-centered; they have a mean μ_g which is different in each latent class. This is the reason why the vectors of covariates X_{2ij}, X_{3ij} and Z_{ij} cannot overlap. The class-specific variance-covariance B_g of the random effects can also differ from one class to another. Most often, the variance is assumed to be the same in all the latent classes that is $B_g = B, \forall g \in \{1, G\}$ or the variance is assumed to be proportional from one class to another: $B_g = \omega_g^2 B, \forall g \in \{1, G\}$ with $\omega_G = 1$.

As in standard linear mixed models, the error ϵ_{ij} is Gaussian ($\epsilon_i \sim \mathcal{N}(0, \Sigma_i)$) and can be divided in two terms, one process that translates the correlated error and one independent measurement error: $\epsilon_{ij} = w_i(t_{ij}) + e_{ij}$. The measurement errors e_{ij} are independent and follow a $\mathcal{N}(0, \sigma_e^2)$ distribution, and $\{w_i(t), t \geq 0\}$ is a zero-mean Gaussian process. As evoked in Chapter 4, an example is the Brownian process with covariance structure $\text{cov}(w_i(t_{ij}), w_i(t_{ij'})) = \sigma_w^2 \min(t_{ij}, t_{ij'})$. The random effects b_i, the autocorrelated error $w_i(t_{ij})$ and the measurement error e_{ij} are independent for all subject i ($i = 1, ..., N$).

The generalized linear mixed models, the non-linear mixed models, the curvilinear mixed models and the multivariate mixed models can be extended to heterogeneous populations in the exact same way. The latent class membership model in (5.17) does not change and Equation (5.18) is replaced by the mixed model which is appropriate to the type of dependent variable, but including class-specific fixed effects and class-specific distributions for the random effects.

5.3.2   Maximum likelihood estimation

The parameters of a latent class linear mixed model are estimated most of the time in the maximum likelihood framework (Verbeke and Lesaffre, 1996; Muthén and Shedden, 1999; Proust and Jacqmin-Gadda, 2005) but Bayesian approaches have also been proposed (Elliott et al., 2005; Komarek, 2009).

The maximum likelihood estimation of the parameters is performed for a fixed number of latent classes G. The vector of parameters to estimate noted θ_G includes all the parameters that intervene in Equations (5.17) and (5.18). The distribution of vector Y_i marginally to the random effects and conditionally to the latent classes is used for the estimation:

$$[Y_i \mid c_i = g] \sim \mathcal{N}\left(X_{1i}\beta + X_{2i}\gamma_g + Z_i\mu_g, Z_i B_g Z_i^\top + \Sigma_i\right)$$

where X_{1i}, X_{2i} and Z_i are the matrices with row vectors $X_{1ij}^\top$, $X_{2ij}^\top$ and $Z_{ij}^\top$ respectively for $j = 1, ..., n_i$.

The likelihood is then:

$$\mathcal{L}(\theta_G) = \prod_{i=1}^{N}\left(\sum_{g=1}^{G} P(c_i = g \mid X_{1i}; \theta_G) \times \phi_{ig}(Y_i \mid c_i = g; X_{2i}, X_{3i}, Z_i; \theta_G)\right)$$

where ϕ_{ig} is the density of a multivariate normal distribution with mean $X_{1i}\beta + X_{2i}\gamma_g + Z_i\mu_g$ and variance $Z_i B_g Z_i^\top + \Sigma_i$.

The log-likelihood $L(\theta_G) = \log(\mathcal{L}(\theta_G))$ is maximized by an iterative algorithm of type EM or Newton-Raphson. Several software can fit this type of models including Mplus (Muthén and Muthén, 2007), GLLAMM under stata (Rabe-Hesketh et al., 2004) and `hlme` function of `lcmm` package under R (Proust-Lima et al., 2015). We will focus on the latter for the illustration. In this function, the optimization algorithm is a modified Marquardt algorithm as decribed in Section 2.5.2.

When the number of latent classes G is not known, as is often the case, it needs to be determined *a posteriori* from the models estimated for different fixed numbers of latent classes. The likelihood ratio test cannot be directly used to select the number of latent classes. Indeed, the null hypothesis can be defined in different ways (same parameters in two latent classes or a null probability for the new latent class) and the asymptotic distribution of the likelihood ratio has a very complex form. Approximations of the test were proposed but they are not widely used (Muthén, 2003). The choice of the number of latent classes in a mixture model is usually based on the Bayesian Information Criterion (BIC) (Bauer and Curran, 2003). Its formula is BIC $= -2L(\theta_G) + p_G \log(N)$ where p_G is the number of estimated parameters (the dimension of θ_G). This criterion is preferred to the most well-known Akaike Information Criterion (AIC) because it penalizes more the complexity of the model (with $\log(N)$ instead of 2), and as such, it favors more parsimonious models than AIC. Other criteria were proposed, such as the BIC-ICL which takes into account the quality of the classification in addition to the goodness-of-fit when selecting the optimal number of latent classes (Han et al., 2007). Posterior classifications obtained from latent class mixed models are discussed in the next section.

It is essential to note that the likelihood of any mixture model, including the latent class mixed model, can be multimodal, so that algorithms of types Newton-Raphson or EM may converge to local maxima. In order to ensure the convergence toward the global maximum, it is highly recommended to use different sets of initial values in the estimation procedures (Hipp and Bauer, 2006).

5.3.3 Posterior classification

The latent class linear mixed model is often used to describe profiles of change over time. However, another asset is that it provides a *posterior* classification of the subjects according to the profile that best matches their data. This is accomplished by the computation of the *posterior* latent class membership probabilities given the subject observations, that is, for class g and subject i:

$$
\begin{aligned}
\hat{\pi}_{ig}^Y &= P(c_i = g \mid X_i, Y_i; \hat{\theta}_G) \\
&= \frac{P(c_i = g \mid X_{1i}; \hat{\theta}_G)\phi_{ig}(Y_i \mid c_i = g, X_{2i}, X_{3i}, Z_i; \hat{\theta}_G)}{\sum_{l=1}^{G} P(c_i = l \mid X_{1i}; \hat{\theta}_G)\phi_{il}(Y_i \mid c_i = l, X_{2i}, X_{3i}, Z_i; \hat{\theta}_G)}
\end{aligned} \tag{5.19}
$$

From these probabilities, each subject can be assigned to the latent class to which he/she has the highest *posterior* probability to belong. This classification is useful to describe *a posteriori* the latent classes according to the characteristics of the subjects, but it is also used to assess the discriminative performances of the model. Indeed, a discriminant classification is an indicator that the latent classes actually represent distinct groups of subjects.

In the case of a perfect classification, each subject should have a *posterior* probability of 1 to belong to the latent class to which he/she is *a posteriori* assigned and probabilities of 0 to belong to the others. The techniques for assessing the discriminative performances of the latent class mixed model (and mixture model in general) consist in quantifying the departure from this perfect classification. Various indicators exist (Proust-Lima et al., 2014) including:

- the proportion of subjects with a maximal *posterior* probability above a certain threshold (0.8 for instance) or conversely below a certain threshold (0.6 or 0.5 for instance) computed for each *posterior* latent class. This provides a quantification of the proportion of subjects classified in each latent class according to a degree of discrimination or conversely a degree of ambiguity.

- an entropy measure: $1 - \frac{\text{En}}{N \log G}$ with $\text{En} = -\sum_{i=1}^{N} \sum_{g=1}^{G} \hat{\pi}_{ig}^Y \log(\hat{\pi}_{ig}^Y)$. The closer to 1, the better is the classification.

- the classification table which consists in providing the matrix of the averaged *posterior* probabilities to belong to each latent class l (with $l = 1, ..., G$) inside each *posterior* latent class g (with $g = 1, ..., G$). A discriminative classification would have values close to 1 on the diagonal (for $l = g$) and values close to 0 for all $l \neq g$.

5.3.4 Application

To illustrate the latent class linear mixed model, we explore the profiles of trajectory with age of a cognitive measure among elderly people from the sample of 500 subjects from the Paquid cohort. We chose to focus on the MMSE which is the most well-known psychometric test to describe cognitive aging. To take into account the problem of curvilinearity of MMSE, we did not use the models described in Section 5.1 for this illustration although they would have applied perfectly. For the sake of simplicity, we chose to normalize the MMSE first using a pre-transformation that was specifically designed for this test (Philipps et al., 2014). As a consequence, the cognitive measure in this application is the normalized MMSE, referred to as normMMSE.

No explanatory covariate was included in the model for the class-membership probability. The class-specific linear mixed model included age and squared age in order to account for a possible acceleration of the cognitive decline among the eldest. Correlated random effects were included on the initial level and on the functions of time (age and squared age) to account for a correlation between the repeated measures of a given subject. In addition, as educational level is a well-known risk factor of cognitive deficit (previously identified in other examples), we chose to adjust the trajectories for this factor. As previously mentioned, educational level was summarized into a binary covariate CEP that equals 1 for subjects who graduated from primary school (noted CEP+) and 0 for others (noted CEP-). Educational level was considered only on the mean cognitive level rather than on the cognitive decline with age since interactions with time were not significant in previous examples as well as in this one. As before, the age variable (age) was centered at 65 and indicated in decades (age65=(age-65)/10).

The latent class linear mixed model can be written for subject i, occasion j and latent class g:

$$\text{NormMMSE}_{ij} = b_{0i} + b_{1i}\, \text{age65}_i + b_{2i}\, \text{age65}_i^2 + \beta_1\, \text{CEP}_i + \epsilon_{ij} \qquad (5.20)$$

with $b_i = (b_{0i}, b_{1i}, b_{2i})^\top \sim \mathcal{N}((\mu_{0g}, \mu_{1g}, \mu_{2g})^\top, B)$ and $\epsilon_{ij} \sim \mathcal{N}(0, \sigma^2)$.

This model was estimated with hlme function of R package lcmm. The call is detailed in the appendix.

The model was estimated for a number of latent classes varying from 1 to 4, the model with 1 latent class corresponding to the standard linear mixed model. The results are summarized in Table 5.6. We reported the global maxima as well as the local maxima found during the various runs of the procedure in order to emphasize the importance of the multiple estimation of the models with different sets of initial values. The model with two latent classes was selected by the BIC as the model with the optimal number of latent classes. The mean predicted trajectories in each latent class are depicted in Figure 5.8 according to educational level. The latent classes are described *a posteriori* according to gender, educational level, incidence of dementia and age at

TABLE 5.6
Summary of the estimated latent class linear mixed models on the Paquid sample (N=500): number of latent classes (G), number of parameters (p), log-likelihood (L), Bayesian Information Criterion (BIC) and proportion of each latent class (in %). The model with the best BIC is in bold; the local maxima are indicated with a *.

G	p	L	BIC	Frequency of the latent classes (%)			
				1	2	3	4
1	11	-8920.6	17909.6	100			
2*	15	-8912.1	17917.4	99.2	0.8		
2	**15**	**-8899.2**	**17891.7**	**87.6**	**12.4**		
3*	19	-8898.2	17914.5	56.4	30.4	13.2	
3	19	-8890.1	17898.4	87.4	11.8	0.8	
4*	23	-8890.0	17923.0	60.6	22.0	13.2	4.2
4	23	-8889.6	17922.2	86.4	12.2	0.8	0.6

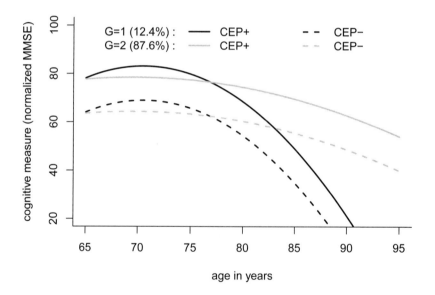

FIGURE 5.8
Mean predicted trajectories of normalized MMSE according to age in the two latent class models selected by the BIC and according to educational level (CEP- or CEP+) in the sample of 500 subjects from Paquid.

baseline in Table 5.7.

Latent class 2 is the main one. It includes 87.6% of the subjects and is

TABLE 5.7

Description of the two *posterior* latent classes according to gender (women *vs.* men), educational level (CEP+ *vs.* CEP−), incidence of dementia, and age at inclusion in years. Indicated are the counts (percentages) and the p-value of the Chi-square test for qualitative data, and the mean (standard-deviation) and the p-value of the Wilcoxon test for the quantitative variable.

| Variable | *Posterior* class: | | p-value |
| | 1 | 2 | |
	(N=62)	(N=437)	
Women	47	241	0.003
	(76.8%)	(55.0%)	
CEP+	49	306	0.180
	(79.0%)	(70.0%)	
Incident dementia	54	74	<0.0001
	(87.1%)	(16.9%)	
Age at baseline	74.5	74.2	0.444
	(5.8)	(6.5)	

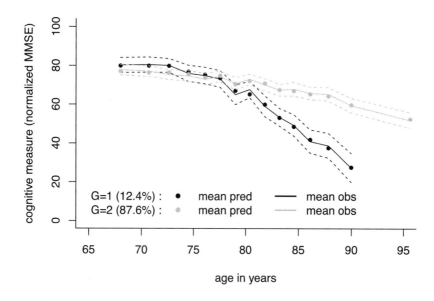

FIGURE 5.9

Weighted averaged individual predictions (mean pred) and observations (mean obs) of the normalized MMSE according to age in the two latent classes weighted by the *posterior* probabilities of belonging to each class. Dashed lines depict the 95% confidence bands for the weighted averaged observations.

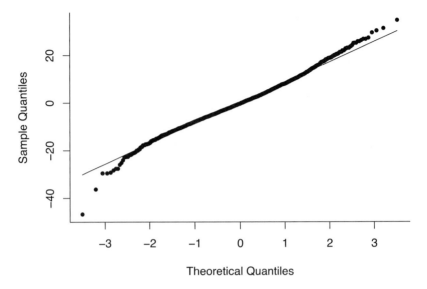

FIGURE 5.10

Q-Q plot of the conditional (or subject-specific) residuals averaged over classes.

characterized by a slight cognitive decline with age. Latent class 1 includes 12.4% of the subjects and is characterized by a largely more pronounced cognitive decline with age. We note that mean cognitive levels at 65 years old are very similar in the two latent classes. Only the slopes with age and squared age differ. According to the *posterior* description of the latent classes given in Table 5.7, the two latent classes differ significantly by the proportion of subjects that developed dementia during the follow-up of the study (87% in class 1 *vs.* 17% in class 2) and the proportion of women (76.8% in class 1 *vs.* 55% in class 2). The latent classes do not differ significantly by age at baseline nor by educational level.

From these characteristics, latent class 2 could be called "normal cognitive decline" and latent class 1 could be called "pathological cognitive decline toward dementia." Regarding educational level, subjects who graduated from primary school had in mean a significantly higher cognitive level whatever the latent class and the age ($\hat{\beta}_1 = 14.1$; p<0.0001). This effect was assumed in the model to be the same for all the latent classes and the ages since no interaction with age and common effect of educational level over classes were considered. This latter assumption could be assessed by comparing the results with those of a model that would assume a different effect of educational level in each latent class.

The goodness-of-fit of latent class linear mixed models can be evaluated in several ways. First, as in standard linear mixed models, individual predictions (either marginal or conditional on the individual random effects) can be computed and compared to the observations in order to assess the fit of the model to the data. The only difference is that these predictions are now specific to the latent classes. From these individual class-specific predictions, it is possible to compute either a unique prediction for each subject by averaging his/her predictions over the classes, or a unique prediction by latent class by computing the mean of all the measures observed (or predicted) at a given time (or in a given time interval). In both cases, the averages are weighted by the latent class membership probability (marginal probability for marginal predictions and *posterior* probabilities for conditional predictions). Thus, Figure 5.9 gives the individual predictions conditional on the random effects in a series of intervals of time; they are weighted and averaged in each latent class, and compared to the weighted averaged observations in the same intervals of time. It shows that the fit of the model is very good in the two latent classes. In addition, Figure 5.10 compares the residuals conditional to the individual random effects and averaged in each class to the theoretical normal distribution of these residuals. Again, it shows a good fit.

In addition to the predictions of the linear mixed model, most of the time it is crucial to assess the quality of the classification which is stemmed from the model using the *posterior* class membership probabilities as it was described in Section 5.3.3. We illustrate here only the classification table given in Table 5.8. If the classification was perfect, the matrix would contain only 1s in the diagonal and 0s elsewhere. In our example, the average probabilities are relatively high (>80%) showing the satisfying discrimination ability of the model. Subjects classified in latent class 1 are assigned to this class with a mean probability of 80.5% *vs.* a probability of 19.5% to belong to the second class. Conversely, subjects classified in class 2 are assigned to this class with a mean probability of 87.3% *vs.* a probability of 12.7% to belong to the first class. This quality of classification (discrimination) is essential when one wants to interpret the latent classes. Indeed, an ambiguous classification (with for instance *posterior* probabilities around 60% in a 2-class model) indicates that the latent classes cannot be really distinguished and that subjects cannot be clearly assigned to one class or the other. This is what happens especially when the latent class mixed model captures non-Gaussian random effects in a homogeneous population (Verbeke and Lesaffre, 1996). We will see in Chapter 8 about joint models an example of 4-class model in which the *posterior* classification is even clearer with average probabilities higher than 90%.

TABLE 5.8
Number (%) of subjects and mean *posterior* probabilities (given in %) of latent
class membership according to the final *posterior* classification.

Final classification	Number of subjects (%)	Mean *posterior* probability to belong to class (%)	
		1	2
1	62 (12.4%)	**80.5**	19.5
2	437 (87.6%)	12.7	**87.3**

6

Advanced survival models

In this chapter we discuss the relative survival models that compare the survival of a specific group with that in the general population. Then different extensions of survival analyses are presented: competing risks models, frailty models and cure models.

6.1 Relative survival

6.1.1 Principle

Relative survival is a way to estimate survival associated with a given pathology eliminating other causes of death. For this, the expected mortality in the population is used. We describe in this section the past (Estève et al., 1990) and recent (Perme et al., 2012) concepts and methods, and some applications of the relative survival. This approach is often used in the analysis of survival times, especially for cancer registry data where information on the cause of death is not routinely collected. We will develop primarily in this chapter the cancer data analysis, although these methods can be applied to other fields.

When we focus on death related to a specific disease (e.g., breast cancer), putting aside death from other causes (e.g., cardiovascular disease, colorectal cancer), we are interested in *net survival* (or *corrected survival*) which is the survival of patients for a given cause when all other causes have been eliminated. It can be estimated from cohort data if the exact cause of death is observed. Survival times are then censored at death times if death is not cancer-related. This approach requires one to assume that mortality rates from "other causes" and "linked to the studied disease" are not influenced by the same independent covariates (Perme et al., 2012).

Another way to estimate the net survival is the method of relative survival which does not require knowing the cause of death. In the relative survival analysis, the available data are often data from cohort of cancer patients followed for a long period of time. Time of death is recorded but information about the cause of death is difficult to get. Some deaths are related to the cancer studied, others are not, and we want to study the proportion attributable to cancer. For this, the relative survival method uses mortality tables in the general population, according to various demographic strata (age, sex, calendar year, location). These mortality tables are obtained from national statistics, e.g., the French "Institut National de la Statistique et de Études Économiques" (INSEE), or the World Health Organization (WHO). This method avoids the use of death certificates that are rarely collected, or collected with great imprecision. The assumption of "rare disease" is made, in other words the specific risk of death in the population is supposed to be small compared to that for all other causes of death. So the mortality tables are assumed to give the mortality rates without the studied disease. The net survival approach allows for comparisons between countries after eliminating other causes of mortality, often different from one country to another.

6.1.2 Specification

Two formulations are possible to describe the relative survival approach: a model based on the ratio of the observed survival and expected survival and a model based on an excess mortality.

6.1.2.1 Relative survival

Relative survival $S_c(t)$ (or cancer-related survival also called "corrected survival"), may be expressed as the ratio:

$$S_c(t) = \frac{S(t)}{S_p(t)}, \tag{6.1}$$

with $S(t)$ the observed survival and $S_p(t)$ the expected survival (Estève et al., 1990; Hakulinen and Tenkanen, 1987). The expected survival or survival in the population is the survival for a group of the general population with similar characteristics (age, sex, ...) as the study cohort. The expected survival data are obtained from life tables in the population. An example of a mortality table is given in Section 6.1.4. The estimation of the expected survival will define the estimation method of the relative survival. This approach does not need to know the exact cause of death, it is only needed to know whether the subject has been diagnosed with disease and if he or she was alive or dead at a specific time. It allows to separate the impact of prognostic factors on the specific mortality from their effects on other causes of death.

6.1.2.2 Excess death rate

Another formulation using an additive model for the death rate was proposed:

$$\alpha(t, a, x, z) = \alpha_p(a + t, z) + \alpha_c(t, x), \tag{6.2}$$

where $\alpha_c(t, x)$ is the excess death rate (due to the cancer) and $\alpha_p(a+t, z)$ is the death rate from other causes, that is the mortality in the general population for a given time since diagnosis of cancer t, a set of covariates z, for a given age at diagnosis a, from causes other than the cancer under study; x is a vector of explanatory variables. This mortality rate is assumed fixed and known. The survival function derived from the excess death rate $\alpha_c(t, x)$ is called "net survival." This decomposition (6.2) can be done if the illness-related death times and the death times linked to other causes are independent conditional on a set of explanatory variables.

In most cases the relative survival and the net survival coincide and the relative survival may be used to estimate the net survival. However, this equivalence holds only when the excess death rate (risk associated with the net survival) does not depend on demographic covariates. This is no longer verified when the excess mortality rate is related to the age at diagnosis.

The literature on the relative survival refers most often to the additive model (6.2) and applications on cancer. However, multiplicative models have also been proposed (Andersen et al., 1985) :

$$\alpha(t, a, x, z) = \alpha_p(a, t, z) \times \alpha_c(t, x).$$

Multiplicative models do not assume that the observed risk $\alpha(t, a, x, z)$ is greater than the expected risk $\alpha_p(a+t, z)$ unlike the additive model presented in (6.2). However, interpretation of multiplicative models is quite difficult.

6.1.3   Inference

The estimation of the relative survival can be done by calculating the observed survival in the sample and the expected survival from the mortality tables. A standard method to calculate the observed survival is the one that uses the Kaplan-Meier estimate (see Chapter 3). The two most common methods for estimating the expected risk $\alpha_p(\cdot, \cdot)$ associated with the expected survivals $S_p(t)$ are the Ederer II method (Ederer and Heise, 1959) (different from the method Ederer I (Ederer et al., 1961)) and the method of Hakulinen (1982). The expected survival is calculated using the national life tables for individuals from the general population, matched by age, sex, race and time period of the cancer patients under the study. These three methods differ by the choice of the period at risk for each patient. In the method of Ederer I, matched individuals are considered at risk regardless of observation time (even after the end of study). The time of death or censoring for a patient with cancer has no influence on the expected survival. In the method of Ederer II, matched individuals are considered at risk until their time of censoring or death. Finally, in the method of Hakulinen, if the survival time is censored, then it is the same for the survival time of the matched subject. However, if a patient dies, the matched individual is assumed to be at risk until the end of the study.

Several approaches have been proposed to estimate the specific mortality $\alpha_c(t, x)$ from the model (6.2) (Dickman et al., 2004; Remontet et al., 2006). Initially, Estève et al. (1990) assumed a proportional hazards model for the excess mortality rate $\alpha_c(t, x)$: $\alpha_c^i(t) = \sum_{k=1}^{K} 1_{\{t \in [t_k; t_{k+1})\}} \alpha_k \exp(\beta' X_i)$, with

α_k a stepwise-constant Baseline hazard function with jumps at K predefined times t_k for $k = 1, \ldots, K$. The parameters are estimated by maximizing a total log-likelihood over the N individuals of the study:

$$L = \sum_{i=1}^{N} \left\{ \delta_i \log[\alpha_p(a, t, z) + \alpha_c^i(t, x)] - \int_0^{t_i} \alpha_p(a, s)ds - \int_0^{t_i} \alpha_c^i(s)ds \right\}.$$

The estimators based on relative survival for estimating net survival are often biased because of an informative censoring, particularly related to age. When the excess risk and the risk in the population are not affected by common factors, then the time to cancer deaths and those of other causes are independent and the proposed estimators for the net survival are unbiased. This is, however, rarely the case in practice since the excess mortality almost always depends on socio-demographic variables (e.g., age). Recently, Perme et al. (2012) proposed an unbiased estimator of the net survival without modeling and using weighted estimators based on the Inverse Probability Weigthing (IPW) (Klein and Andersen, 2005). The alternative is to use multivariate models with parametric excess risks (Danieli et al., 2012; Dickman et al., 2004; Estève et al., 1990) or non-parametric (Perme et al., 2009) which is also unbiased assuming a well-specified model.

Relative survival or excess survival can be implemented by any software that offers the possibility to fit generalized linear models. Using the R software several packages propose to model the excess survival (packages `Relsurv` of Pohar and Stare (2006) or the package `RSurv` (Giorgi et al., 2003)), using `SAS` software procedure `proc NLMIXED` may be used.

6.1.4 Illustration

In this section we present an example of survival data (Table 6.1) included in the R package `Relsurv`. This is a study on the survival of patients who had a myocardial infarction (n=1040) between 1982 and 1986 and were followed until 1997 in Ljubljana (Slovenia) (Pohar and Stare, 2006). During this follow-up, 547 deaths were observed and the exact cause of death being unknown, we have to use a method of relative survival to investigate the proportion of deaths attributable to the disease. The follow-up times are represented by `time`, and the censoring or death indicators are represented by `cens`. The other variables are age at study entry in days, sex, year (in days since January 1, 1960). We illustrate here a multivariate modeling of an additive relative survival (Estève et al., 1990), with a proportional hazards model to the excess mortality (6.2) with jumps at 1, 2, 3, 4 and 5 years; we focus on the first 5 years of follow-up. The parameters are estimated by maximum likelihood.

In this application, we use the mortality tables from Slovenia between 1930 and 2009 available from the R package `survexp.fr`. Table 6.2 presents an extract of the output for given sex, age and year.

TABLE 6.1

Example of survival data for patients with myocardial infarction: illustration with relative survival.

time	cens	age	sex	year	agegr
2657	1	68	2	8210	62-70
1097	1	63	2	8278	62-70
3764	1	60	1	8254	54-61
3724	1	66	2	8054	62-70
5076	0	57	2	8224	54-61
139	1	57	2	8233	54-61

TABLE 6.2

Extract of a mortality table in three dimensions (sex, age, year) used in relative survival.

Age	Sex	Years			
	female				
		2006	2007	2008	2009
0		9.929247e-06	8.281024e-06	6.301721e-06	7.133348e-06
1		0.000000e+00	1.889816e-06	3.176169e-07	3.176169e-07
2		3.285699e-07	0.000000e+00	3.176169e-07	3.176169e-07
...					...
102		3.403777e-03	1.505997e-03	1.081815e-02	8.920369e-03
103		3.403777e-03	1.505997e-03	1.081815e-02	8.920369e-03
	male				
		2006	2007	2008	2009
0		9.352256e-06	7.759293e-06	8.462280e-06	6.614580e-06
1		9.036621e-07	1.204949e-06	5.996698e-07	8.981845e-07
2		6.024083e-07	3.011876e-07	8.927069e-07	0.000000e+00
...					...
102		1.897780e-03	1.286832e-03	1.897780e-03	3.795561e-03
103		1.897780e-03	1.286832e-03	1.897780e-03	3.795561e-03

The results are detailed in Table 6.3. We can see that gender significantly influences the excess risk of deaths, with a better survival for men ($\hat{\beta} = 0.90$). Age does not appear to be a major factor of cancer-related death. Thus, in a standard survival analysis, the differences in survival as a function of age are in fact due to a difference in mortality in the population. The coefficients related to variable "fu$[\cdot, \cdot]$" are the coefficients of the hazard function of cancer-related death, piecewise constant, with jumps each year. They are similar on the follow-up period of 5 years, indicating a risk of death from cancer rather stable over these 5 years, except perhaps the first year $(\exp(-4.22) = 0.015$ per year). We detail in the Appendix the program associated with this kind of analysis.

TABLE 6.3
Results of the multivariate additive model (6.2) of mortality in excess for the data "rdata" from the R package `Relsurv`.

Variable	$\hat{\beta}$	S.E.$(\hat{\beta})$	z-value	p-value
gender	0.9020	0.2163	4.169	3.05e-05
agegr54-61	0.1418	0.3165	0.448	0.6542
agegr62-70	0.5379	0.2936	1.832	0.0669
agegr71-95	0.6143	0.3141	1.956	0.0505
fu[0,1)	-4.2188	0.3856	-10.940	< 2e-16
fu[1,2)	-4.9896	0.4276	-11.669	< 2e-16
fu[2,3)	-5.0177	0.4388	-11.436	< 2e-16
fu[3,4)	-5.4453	0.5577	-9.763	< 2e-16
fu[4,5)	-4.9705	0.4433	-11.213	< 2e-16

6.2   Competing risks models

Competing risks models are used when there are several competing events (Putter et al., 2007; Belot et al., 2010), the occurrence of an event type preventing the occurrence of other events. In this section, we first present competing risks examples. Then, we introduce estimators used to describe probabilities of the various events and how to take account of these competing risks for regression models.

6.2.1   Examples

Competing risks relate to the situation where several types of exclusive events are possible. A classic example is the study of the survival of patients exposed to several risks of mortality. If a subject dies of cancer, he does not die from heart disease, thus these events are in competition. One can also envisage a situation of competing risks between the development of disease and death (death being in competition with the disease). For example, if one looks at the onset of dementia in the elderly, death is competing with dementia. The model with competing risks is represented by a state diagram (Figure 6.1) with an initial state ("healthy" or more generally "no event") and different types of terminal events. Note that the types of events in the competing risks differ from recurring events. Indeed, in the situation of competing risks, events correspond to terminal events where the occurrence of an event prevents the occurrence of any other event.

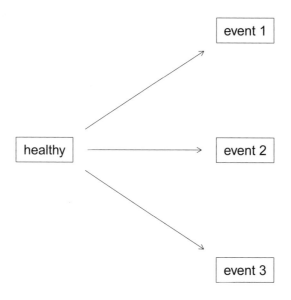

FIGURE 6.1
Diagram of competing risks models with three events.

6.2.2 Specification

In the context of competing risks models (study of K different exclusive events), we denote by T the time to the first event, D the event type, and $X = (X_1, \ldots, X_p)^\top$ possible explanatory variables.

The competing risks model is specified by *cause-specific hazard functions*. For each event k, the hazard rate function is defined by

$$\alpha_k(t) = \lim_{\Delta t \to 0} \frac{\mathrm{P}(t \leq T \leq t + \Delta t,\ D = k \mid T \geq t)}{\Delta t}. \tag{6.3}$$

The function $\alpha_k(t)$ is the instantaneous hazard rate function at time t which is specific to the event k in the presence of the competing events. The term $\alpha_k(t)\Delta t$ represents the probability for a subject to experience the event k between t and $t + \Delta t$ given that this subject is in the risk set at time t. Furthermore, define *the overall hazard rate function:*

$$\alpha(t) = \lim_{\Delta t \to 0} \frac{Pr(t \leq T \leq t + \Delta t, \mid T \geq t)}{\Delta t}. \tag{6.4}$$

This function does not take into account the type of event. It is equal to the sum of the K cause-specific hazard functions: $\alpha(t) = \sum_{k=1}^{K} \alpha_k(t)$. The term $\alpha(t)\Delta t$ represents the probability to experience *any* event between t and $t+\Delta t$ given that no event has occurred before t. From this function, we can define the probability of not having failed from any cause at time t:

$$S(t) = \exp\left(-\sum_{k=1}^{K} A_k(t)\right)$$

where $A_k(t) = \int_0^t \alpha_k(s)ds$ is the cumulative cause-specific hazard. Finally, the *cumulative incidence function of cause k* (also called *crude cumulative incidence function*) is defined by

$$I_k(t) = Pr(T \leq t, D = k) \quad = \quad \int_0^t \alpha_k(u)S(u)du \tag{6.5}$$

$$= \quad \int_0^t \alpha_k(u) \exp\left(-\int_0^u \sum_{k=1}^{K} \alpha_k(s)ds\right) du.$$

This function represents the probability of failing from cause k before time t in the presence of the competing events.

Remark: Note that the naive Kaplan-Meier which treats events from causes other than k as censoring, is estimating

$$1 - S_k(t) = \int_0^t \alpha_k(s)S_k(s)ds.$$

The difference with the cumulative incidence function $I_k(t) = Pr(T \leq t, D = k)$ presented in (6.5) is that the function $S(s)$ is replaced by $S_k(s)$. Since $S(t) \leq S_k(t)$, we have $I_k(t) \leq 1 - S_k(t)$, with equality at t if there is no competition ($\sum_{j=1,j\neq k}^{K} \alpha_j(t) = 0$).

6.2.3 Inference

Let $0 < t_1 < t_2 < \cdots < t_N$ be the ordered distinct time points at which failures of *any cause* occur. Let d_{kj} denote the number of patients failing from cause k at t_j, and let $d_j = \sum_{k=1}^{K} d_{kj}$ denote the total number of failures (from any cause) at t_j. In the absence of ties, only one of the d_{kj} equals 1 for a given j, and $d_j = 1$. The formulas are also valid, however, in the presence of ties. Finally, let n_j be the number of patients at risk (i.e., that are still in follow-up and have not failed from any cause) at time t_j. The overall survival probability $S(t)$ at t can be estimated, without considering the cause of failure, by the Kaplan-Meier estimator

$$\widehat{S(t)} = \prod_{j:t_j \leq t} \left(1 - \frac{d_j}{n_j}\right). \tag{6.6}$$

A discretized version of the cause-specific hazard of Equation (6.3) is also proposed:

$$\alpha_k(t_j) = Pr(T = t_j, D = k \mid T > t_{j-1}).$$

A straightforward estimation is

$$\widehat{\alpha}_k(t_j) = \frac{d_{kj}}{n_j}$$

defined as the proportion of subjects at risk who fail from cause k. Thus, Equation (6.6) can also be written down as

$$\widehat{S(t)} = \prod_{j:t_j \leq t} \left(1 - \sum_{k=1}^{K} \widehat{\alpha}_k(t_j) \right). \tag{6.7}$$

Finally, the cumulative incidence $I_k(t)$ of cause k at t is estimated by

$$\widehat{I}_k(t) = \sum_{j:t_j \leq t} \widehat{p}_k(t_j),$$

where $\widehat{p}_k(t_j) = \widehat{\alpha}_k(t_j)\widehat{S}(t_{j-1})$ estimates $p_k(t_j) = P(T = t_j, D = k)$ which is the product of the hazard and the probability of being event-free at t_j.

6.2.4   Regression models with competing risks

In this section, we are presenting different statistical methods for estimating the effects of covariates. However, just like in standard survival analysis, the effect of one or two binary covariates is most easily investigated by estimating cumulative incidence curves non-parametrically and testing whether the curves differ by covariate value. Gray (1988) developed a log-rank type test for equality of cumulative incidence curves.

6.2.4.1   Regression on cause-specific hazards

If the effect of one or several covariates on a specific event is of interest, a proportional hazards regression on the cause-specific hazards seems the most logical choice

$$\alpha_k(t \mid X) = \alpha_{k,0}(t) \exp(\beta_k^\top X), \tag{6.8}$$

where $\alpha_{k,0}$ is the baseline cause-specific hazard of cause k and $\beta_k = (\beta_{k,1}, \beta_{k,2}, \ldots, \beta_{k,p})^\top$ represents the covariate effects on cause k. The inference is completely standard by considering the other events than the one of interest (event k) as censored observations.

6.2.4.2   Regression for different types of events

Regression for different types of events enables us to test, for example, if the treatment effect is the same for the different types of events. The model is an extended version of the Cox model:

$$\alpha_k(t \mid X) = \alpha_1(t) \exp \left[b_k + \beta_k^\top X + \gamma^\top X \right], \qquad (6.9)$$

with $b_1 = \beta_1 = 0$ and $\gamma = (\gamma_1, \gamma_2, \ldots, \gamma_p)^\top$. In this model, $\alpha_1(t)$ represents the baseline hazard for cause $k = 1$ (covariates $x = 0$) and the baseline hazard for events $k \neq 1$ is defined by $\alpha_k(t) = \alpha_1(t) \exp(b_k)$. Thus, from the term $\beta_k^\top X$ it is possible to test if the effect of a covariate is the same for two different events.

The relative risk for an increment of one unit of a particular covariate (e.g., X_2) from X for the event $k = 1$ is given by

$$\frac{\alpha_1(t \mid X = (x_1, a+1, x_3, \ldots, x_p))}{\alpha_1(t \mid X = (x_1, a, x_3, \ldots, x_p))} = \exp(\gamma_2).$$

For any event $k \neq 1$, the relative risk is $\exp(\gamma_2 + \beta_{k,2})$. Thus, the test on $\beta_{k,2}$ (H_0: $\beta_{k,2} = 0$) enables us to test if the effect of the covariate X_2 is the same for both events 1 and k.

Remark: In these models, we have imposed a proportional hazards assumption between the different events as the baseline hazards have been defined by $\alpha_k(t) = \alpha_1(t) \exp(b_k)$. An alternative approach is to propose a stratified model for each event:

$$\alpha_k(t \mid X) = \alpha_{0k}(t) \exp \left[\beta_k^\top X + \gamma^\top X \right], \qquad (6.10)$$

where the baseline hazard α_{0k} is specific to each event k.

An advantage of the regression for different types of events is the possibility to adjust a model by assuming the same effect of a prognostic factor for different events and then to fit a parsimonious model (Belot et al., 2010).

6.2.4.3   Regression on cumulative incidence functions: Fine and Gray model

Modelling the effect of covariates on the cause-specific hazards implies a complex effects of covariates on the cumulative incidences. Indeed, in order to get the effect of a covariate on the cumulative incidence function for a specific event, we need to combine all the cause-specific hazards (involved in (6.5)).To overcome this issue, Fine and Gray (1999) proposed to model directly the effects of explanatory variables on cumulative incidence functions. In analogy with the relation between hazard and survival, they defined a *subdistribution hazard*:

$$\bar{\alpha}_k(t) = -\frac{\mathrm{d} \log(1 - I_k(t))}{\mathrm{d}t}. \qquad (6.11)$$

This is not the cause-specific hazard. In terms of estimates of this quantity, the difference is in the risk set. For the cause-specific hazard, the risk set decreases at each time point at which there is a failure of another cause. For $\bar{\alpha}_k(t)$, persons who fail from another cause remain in the risk set. If there is no censoring, they remain in the risk set forever and once these individuals are given a censoring time that is larger than all event times, the analysis becomes completely standard. If there is censoring, they remain in the risk set until their potential censoring time, which is not observed if they experienced another event before. Fine and Gray imposed a proportional hazards assumption on the subdistribution hazards:

$$\bar{\alpha}_k(t \mid X = x) = \bar{\alpha}_{k,0}(t) \exp(\beta_k^\top X), \tag{6.12}$$

where $\bar{\alpha}_{k,0}(t)$ is the baseline hazard and $\exp(\beta_k)$ represent the relative risks associated to covariates x on the subdistribution hazard. Estimation follows the partial likelihood approach used in a standard Cox model as the baseline hazard of the subdistribution hazards model is not specified.

6.2.5   Illustration with R

We illustrate these methods using a dataset involving patients affected by prostate cancer. This analysis is performed with the package cmprsk for non-parametric estimation of the cumulative incidence function and the analysis based on the subdistribution hazard function. The package survival is used for the analysis based on cause-specific hazard function. A similar analysis could be performed by using the package mstate (Putter et al., 2007) to estimate the cumulative incidence function and cause-specific hazard function. The various R functions used for this analysis are provided in the appendix of the book. Data come from a randomized clinical trial of patients presenting prostate cancer stages 3 and 4, treated with various doses of diethylstillbestrol. Among the many available informations on 483 patients (Kay, 1986), we only use two prognostic covariates: age (recoded into three categories) and treatment (recoded into two categories: low dose and high dose). Finally, the different causes of death were coded into two categories: death due to cancer and death from other causes.

6.2.5.1   Estimation of cumulative incidence functions

Figure 6.2 presents the estimation of the cumulative incidence function for the two events of interest.

6.2.5.2   Log-rank test for investigating the equality of the cumulative incidence functions

The test proposed by Gray (1988) enables us to investigate the presence of a significant effect for each event of interest. Using cmprsk package, we find

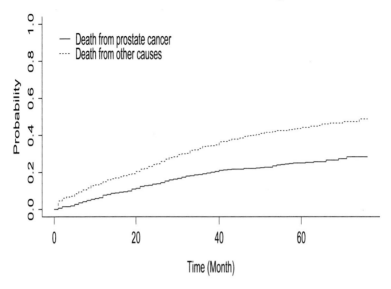

FIGURE 6.2
Cumulative incidence function, Equation (6.5), for the two events using `cmprsk` package.

a significant effect of the treatment on the death by cancer (p=0.003) and a non-significant effect on the death by others causes than prostate cancer (p=0.43).

6.2.5.3 Regression on cause-specific hazards

Regression on cause-specific hazards is defined by:

$$\alpha_k(t \mid \text{Treat,Age}) = \alpha_{k,0}(t) \exp(\beta_{k,1}\text{Treat} + \beta_{k,2}\text{Age}_1 + \beta_{k,3}\text{Age}_2),$$

where Treat is the variable treatment and the variable age has been coded into 3 categories: Age_0 (< 75), Age_1 ([75;80[), Age_2 ($>=80$). Table 6.4 presents the estimations by the cause-specific hazards for death due to prostate cancer($k = 1$). Results for death from other causes than prostate cancer are presented in Table 6.5.

Results from regression on cause-specific hazards confirm the results found by the log-rank tests on the equality of the cumulative incidence function. We find a significant effect (p=0.004) of the treatment on the risk of death from prostate cancer after adjusting on the variable age and a non-significant effect on the death by other causes than prostate cancer (p=0.94).

TABLE 6.4

Results of regression on cause-specific hazards for death by prostate cancer.

	$\hat{\beta}$	$exp(\hat{\beta})$	$S.E.(\hat{\beta})$	z-value	p-value
Treat	-0.53	0.59	0.19	-2.85	0.004
Age_1	0.03	1.03	0.20	0.16	0.88
Age_2	0.11	1.11	0.46	0.23	0.82

TABLE 6.5

Results of regression on cause-specific hazards for death by other types of cancer than prostate cancer.

	$\hat{\beta}$	$exp(\hat{\beta})$	$S.E.(\hat{\beta})$	z-value	p-value
Treat	-0.01	0.99	0.14	-0.08	0.94
Age_1	0.50	1.66	0.15	3.42	$< 10^{-3}$
Age_2	1.16	3.20	0.23	4.96	$< 10^{-6}$

6.2.5.4 Joint model

The proposed model is defined by

$$
\begin{cases}
\alpha_1(t \mid \text{Treat,Age}) = \alpha_1(t) \exp[\gamma_1 \text{Treat} + \gamma_2 \text{Age}_1 + \gamma_3 \text{Age}_2] \\
\alpha_2(t \mid \text{Treat,Age}) = \alpha_1(t) \exp[b_2 + (\beta_{2,1} \text{Treat} + \beta_{2,2} \text{Age}_1 + \beta_{2,3} \text{Age}_2) + \\
\qquad\qquad \gamma_1 \text{Treat} + \gamma_2 \text{Age}_1 + \gamma_3 \text{Age}_2]
\end{cases}
$$

Table 6.6 presents the estimation of this model.

TABLE 6.6

Estimation of the joint model. θ denotes the whole set of the parameters (b, β and γ) defined in the joint model.

	$\hat{\theta}$	$exp(\hat{\theta})$	$S.E.(\hat{\theta})$	z-value	p-value
b_2	0.11	1.11	0.18	0.61	0.54
$\beta_{2,1}(\text{Treat})$	-0.53	0.59	0.19	-2.88	0.004
$\beta_{2,2}(\text{Age}_1)$	0.03	1.03	0.20	0.13	0.89
$\beta_{2,3}(\text{Age}_2)$	0.10	1.10	0.46	0.21	0.83
$\gamma_1(\text{Treat})$	0.53	1.69	0.23	2.28	0.022
$\gamma_2(\text{Age}_1)$	0.48	1.62	0.25	1.93	0.054
$\gamma_3(\text{Age}_2)$	1.07	2.91	0.52	2.07	0.038

The joint model (after adjusting on variable age) shows a significantly different effect of the treatment for the two events of interest (test of $\beta_{2,1}=0$; p=0.004). Relative risk of the treatment effect on the risk of death due to prostate cancer is significantly different from 1 (test on $\gamma_1=0$; p=0.022) while it is non-significantly different from 1 (test on $\gamma_1 + \beta_{2,1}=0$; p=0.96) for the risk of death due to other causes of cancer than prostate cancer.

6.2.5.5   Subdistribution hazards model

Model for subdistribution hazards is defined by:

$$\bar{\alpha}_k(t \mid \text{Treat,Age}) = \bar{\alpha}_{k,0}(t)\exp(\beta_{k,1}\text{Treat} + \beta_{k,2}\text{Age}_1 + \beta_{k,3}\text{Age}_2),$$

where $\bar{\alpha}_{k,0}(t)$ is the baseline hazard. Table 6.7 presents the results of the estimation of the model for the prostate cancer event ($k = 1$). Estimations of models for other events than prostate cancer are presented in Table 6.8.

TABLE 6.7
Results of subdistribution hazard model for death by prostate cancer.

	$\hat{\beta}$	$exp(\hat{\beta})$	$S.E.(\hat{\beta})$	z-value	p-value
Treat	-0.53	0.59	0.18	-2.91	0.004
Age_1	-0.13	0.88	0.20	-0.64	0.52
Age_2	-0.44	0.64	0.46	-0.97	0.33

TABLE 6.8
Results of subdistribution hazard model for death by other types of cancer than prostate cancer.

	$\hat{\beta}$	$exp(\hat{\beta})$	$S.E.(\hat{\beta})$	z-value	p-value
Treat	0.09	1.09	0.14	0.63	0.53
Age_1	0.45	1.56	0.15	3.05	0.002
Age_2	1.07	2.92	0.24	4.40	$< 10^{-5}$

Analyses based on the subdistribution hazards model (after adjusting on age variable) show: (i) a significant treatment effect on the subdistribution hazards associated to death from prostate cancer (p=0.004); (ii) a non-significant treatment effect on the subdistribution hazards associated to death from other cancers (p=0.53).

R codes associated to this illustration using `cmprsk` package are detailed in the appendix.

6.3 Frailty models

6.3.1 Type of data

Correlation of survival times can occur when individuals belong to groups such as families or geographical areas. Alternatively, a correlation may be associated with recurrent events when the subject undergoes the same event several times, such as rehospitalization or heart attacks. In both situations we could adjust directly on the cluster as a fixed effect (e.g., "geographical area" for clustered data, or "subject" for recurrent events). This approach, however, has several disadvantages: the number of parameters to estimate increases with the number of groups, which can lead to numerical problems and jeopardize asymptotic results. The fixed effects approach is suitable only if the sample size is large, with large cluster sizes and small number of clusters.

6.3.1.1 Clustered data

Environmental survival data, by their study design, often lead to particular statistical analysis. Indeed these data are often grouped into geographical areas (e.g., city, state, country) and it is common that the subjects in the same area share unidentified risk factors (genetic and environmental). Unobserved or unmeasured risk factors which are shared in a group induce a dependency of events in each group. In survival analysis, if unobserved heterogeneity is ignored, it can create a significant bias in the estimate of the variance of the regression parameters and the estimate of the hazard function.

6.3.1.2 Recurrent events

In some biomedical studies, individuals may undergo several successive *recurrent* events of interest on a period of observation. These recurrent events can be of the same type, such as repeated hospitalizations or successive asthma attacks. We can also speak of recurrent events of different types, such as local, regional or distant recurrence of breast cancer that patients can develop after localized surgeries. Although recurrent data can be regarded as grouped data where all observations of the same subject are a group, they have a number of characteristics that require specific developments. For example, it is necessary to take into account the timing (the order) of observations for the same subject. In addition, the dependency between these recurrent events should be analyzed, in most cases, together with time-dependent predictors. In some situations (e.g., study of different asthma attacks in children), a patient will have different periods at risk, alternating with periods not at risk. In the analysis of recurrent data, all patients are at risk of developing a new event as long as they are not censored or dead, while in the analysis of conventional survival, patients are no more at risk after a first event. On the other hand, the time scale should be defined (Figure 6.3). It is either the time interval between two events (*"gap-time"*) or the time from study entry until the occurrence of an event (*"calendar-time"*). In the representation in *"gap-time,"* the beginning of the at risk period is 0 and the time for a particular event is the time since the end of the previous event (or the entry into study for the first event) to the new event. And the counters are reset to zero after each event. In the *"calendar-time"* representation, the beginning of the at risk period corresponds to the time of the previous event, the counters are not reset to zero and left truncation must be taken into account. Indeed an individual will be at risk of developing a second event only after developing a first event. In these two time scales, the duration of the at risk periods are the same. These two time scales are related to semi-Markov models, in which the transition probability between two states depends only on the time spent in the state (or *"gap-time"*), while in non-homogeneous Markov models, this transition depends only on the time from the inclusion in the study. The choice of one of these two time scales depends on the application. The formulation in total time (that is, calendar time without taking truncation into account: see Figure 6.3.D) is not a good representation to study recurrent events of the same type, since it assumes that patients are at risk for a second relapse from entry into the study, without already having experienced a first relapse.

The within-subject correlation from recurrent event can come from two sources: the heterogeneity between subjects and the dependence between events (Box-Steffensmeier and De Boef, 2006). The heterogeneity means that different subjects have different risks. Part of this heterogeneity may be explained and taken into account by regression models; part of it may remain unexplained either because some known explanatory factors could not be measured, or because there are unknown factors which modify the risk. Thus, patients with a genetic predisposition for a disease (which may be unmeasured or unknown) will tend to develop more frequently relapses of this disease. On the other hand, the occurrence of an event may cause an increase or decrease in the risk associated with the occurrence of subsequent events. This dependence between events will also be associated with a within-subject correlation.

6.3.2   Principle

Many articles and books have been published to extend the classical survival analysis models to models for correlated survival data using frailty models (Cook and Lawless, 2007; Duchateau and Janssen, 2008; Hanagal, 2011; Wienke, 2010). These approaches are in constant evolution. We will describe the shared frailty models and various extensions: joint frailty models (Rondeau et al., 2007), correlated frailty models, hierarchical models with frailties. We will consider parametric or semi-parametric approaches. Moreover, different distribution functions are possible for the random effects.

Two types of models can be used to model the association between individual survival times in each group: *marginal models* or models with random

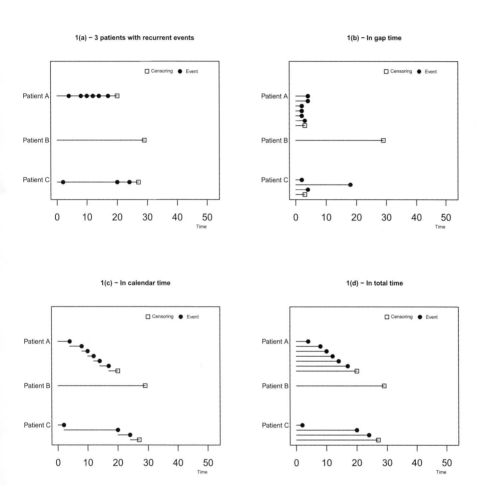

FIGURE 6.3

Illustration of different possible representations for the intervals at risk of a patient: (a) 3 patients with recurrent events; (b) gap-times; (c) time since inclusion; (d) total time.

effects (*"frailty models"*). The marginal approach specifies the marginal hazard function of the multivariate survival times, without modelling explicitly the dependence structure between the survival times. Thus, this method addresses the dependency of the survival times as a nuisance (Wei et al., 1989; Lee et al., 1992). The marginal approach assumes that the risk for each event is described by a classical Cox model. The estimation is performed by the method of generalized estimating equations (GEE) described in Section 4.4 adapted to the Cox model. By this approach the estimators of the regression coefficients are consistent and asymptotically normal. A corrected and robust estimator of the variance-covariance matrix is proposed; it takes into account the correlation between the different members of the same group. We will detail subsequently only frailty models that quantify the intra-group or intra-subject correlation.

We will mainly use the software R to make illustrations on real data, including libraries R packages `frailtypack` and `survival`. Our programs are displayed in the appendix. Stata and `SAS` are also possible softwares to fit frailty models but with fewer options; the proposed approaches are mainly parametric with Weibull Baseline hazard functions. WinBUGS can also be used for Bayesian analysis (Spiegelhalter et al., 2004).

6.3.3   Specification

The frailty model is an extension of the classical Cox model in which we add a frailty variable u_i (or random effect) specific to each group i or each individual i in the context of recurrent events. In the context of clustered data, observations for each subject j ($j = 1, \ldots, n_i$) of the group i ($i = 1, \ldots, G$) are collected; in the context of recurrent data, each subject i has n_i recurrent times, and n_i is random. We observe the time $\tilde{T}_{ij}$, which is the minimum between a censoring time C_{ij} and an event time T_{ij}, and δ_{ij}, a censoring indicator ($\delta_{ij} = I_{\{T_{ij} \leq C_{ij}\}}$). The T_{ij}'s and C_{ij}'s are assumed independent. The hazard function conditional on frailties u_i (identically and independently distributed) for subject j from group i is then expressed by

$$\alpha_{ij}(t \mid X_{ij}, u_i) = u_i \alpha_0(t) \exp(\beta^\top X_{ij}) \tag{6.13}$$

In this model, X_{ij} is the vector of explanatory variables, β is the p-dimensional vector of fixed effects, $\alpha_0(t)$ is the baseline hazard function, the frailty term u_i is a random variable specific to each group. This frailty will represent all the unobserved risk factors common to a group. The model makes an assumption of independence of survival times between groups (i.e., for different values of i). On the other hand, it makes the assumption of independence of survival times in each group conditionally to the frailty u_i. Another formulation of the model (6.13) is as follows:

$$\alpha_{ij}(t \mid X_{ij}, \omega_i) = \alpha_0(t) \exp(\beta^\top X_{ij} + \omega_i). \tag{6.14}$$

The distinction is sometimes made between $u_i = \exp(\omega_i)$ which is described as a frailty variable, while ω_i is described as a random effect.

The model (6.13) is called a "shared frailty model" since all individuals of the same group share the same frailty. A classic choice for the distribution of u_i is the gamma distribution with density $f_{u_i}(u) = \frac{u^{1/\theta-1}\exp(-u/\theta)}{\theta^{1/\theta}\Gamma(1/\theta)}$ ($\Gamma(.)$ being the gamma function), allowing for interesting mathematical simplifications in the writing of the likelihood. Here, $\mathrm{E}(u_i) = 1$ and $\mathrm{var}(u_i) = \theta$. The parameter θ will allow to assess the intra-group association (or equivalently the variability between groups).

In bivariate data, such as the study of couples, another way to quantify the intra-couple dependency is to use the Kendall coefficient of concordance, which is a measure based on ranks (Hougaard, 2000; Kendall, 1938). For two randomly chosen pairs i and i' ($i, i' = 1, \ldots, G; i \neq i'$), event times are (T_{i1}, T_{i2}) and $(T_{i'1}, T_{i'2})$, the theoretical Kendall's tau is:

$$\tau = \mathrm{E}[\mathrm{sign}((T_{i1} - T_{i'1})(T_{i2} - T_{i'2}))] = 2\mathrm{P}((T_{i1} - T_{i'1})(T_{i2} - T_{i'2}) > 0) - 1$$

with, $\mathrm{sign}(x) = \frac{|x|}{x}$ for $x \neq 0$ and $\mathrm{sign}(0) = 0$. Censoring times or equal times do not contribute to this calculation. Another formulation of Kendall's tau is:

$$\tau = 4 \int_0^\infty \int_0^\infty \{f(t_1, t_2)S(t_1, t_2)\} \, \mathrm{d}t_1 \mathrm{d}t_2 - 1.$$

A zero value of τ corresponds to null intra-pair correlation. In the case of shared gamma frailty model (6.13), this measure is estimated by $\hat{\tau} = \hat{\theta}/(\hat{\theta}+2)$. An estimate of the standard deviation of $\hat{\tau}$ can be obtained by applying the delta method (Oehlert, 1992): $\mathrm{Var}(\hat{\tau}) = \mathrm{Var}(\frac{\hat{\theta}}{\hat{\theta}+2}) \approx \frac{4}{\hat{\theta}+2}\mathrm{Var}(\hat{\theta})$.

6.3.4 Inference

In the frailty model, the parameters of interest (the regression coefficients β, the variance of the random effects θ and the baseline hazard function $\alpha_0(t)$ at time t) cannot be estimated by maximizing a Cox partial likelihood. Several estimation approaches have been proposed: the frequentist approach with inference based on the EM algorithm (Klein, 1992), or based on the maximization of a penalized partial likelihood (Therneau and Grambsch, 2000), or the Bayesian representation with inferences using Laplace integrations (Ducrocq and Casella, 1996) or using the MCMC algorithm (Clayton, 1991).

However, even if these methods are relatively simple to implement, they may require relatively long computation times with a large number of iterations. Conceptually, the frailties are unobserved variables, so the EM algorithm (see Section 2.5.3) has been widely used, for instance by Nielsen et al. (1992). The algorithm iterates between two steps. In the first step, an estimate of the expectations of unobserved frailties conditionally on observed data and current parameter values is obtained. Then, the values for these expectations are used in a maximization step to update the parameter values. However, this algorithm can be long and was not proposed in current softwares to estimate frailty models. We present two methods of semi-parametric estimation that are used in R packages. Unlike the parametric approaches, no assumptions about the shape of the baseline hazard function is made.

6.3.4.1 Semi-parametric approach using penalized likelihood

When a gamma distribution for the random effects is chosen, the integration with respect to the frailty u_i of the marginal likelihood takes a simple analytic form and a compact expression of the complete marginal log-likelihood $L(\alpha_0(.), \beta, \theta)$ is obtained. The expression of the marginal log-likelihood in the general context of right-censored survival data is obtained by analytical integration over the random effects and given the independence assumption between clusters (i):

$$L(\alpha_0(.), \beta, \theta) = \log \prod_{i=1}^{G} \int_u V_i(\alpha_0(.), \beta, \theta \mid u) f_{u_i}(u) du \qquad (6.15)$$

$$= \sum_{i=1}^{G} \left\{ \sum_{j=1}^{n_i} \delta_{ij} \{ \beta^\top X_{ij} + \log(\alpha_0(\tilde{T}_{ij})) \} \right.$$

$$- (1/\theta + m_i) \log \left[1 + \theta \sum_{j=1}^{n_i} \alpha_0(\tilde{T}_{ij}) \exp(\beta^\top X_{ij}) \right]$$

$$\left. + I_{\{m_i \neq 0\}} \sum_{k=1}^{m_i} [\log(1 + \theta(m_i - k))] \right\}$$

with $V_i(\alpha_0(.), \beta, \theta \mid u)$ the individual conditional contribution to the likelihood, $f_{u_i}(u)$ the density of the random effects and $m_i = \sum_{j=1}^{n_i} I_{\{\delta_{ij}=1\}}$ the number of observed events in the i-th group.

The parametric models make strong assumptions about the shape of hazard functions. The semi-parametric penalized likelihood methods have been proposed in shared frailty models and a smooth Baseline hazard function was obtained using splines (Rondeau et al., 2003). This penalized likelihood approach (developed in Section 3.4.3) is used to constrain the estimator of the hazard function to be continuous and to have low local variations. The expression of the penalized log-likelihood is as follows:

$$L_{pl}(\alpha_0(.), \beta, \theta) = L(\alpha_0(.), \beta, \theta) - \kappa \int_0^\infty \alpha_0''^2(t) dt \qquad (6.16)$$

where $\kappa \geq 0$, is a smoothing parameter.

Maximizing (6.16) defines the maximum penalized likelihood estimators (MPnLE), $\hat{\alpha}_0(.)$, $\hat{\beta}$ and $\hat{\theta}$. The variance estimator of the parameters can be obtained by $\hat{H}_{pl}^{-1}$, where H_{pl} is minus the Hessian of the penalized log-likelihood.

The estimators $\hat{\alpha}_0(.)$ cannot be calculated explicitly and are approached on the basis of cubic M-spline (a variant of the B-splines) (Ramsay, 1988). I-splines (*Integrated splines*) are used to estimate the cumulative risk functions. The approach allows a good approximation of the estimator of the hazard function by increasing the number of nodes. The smoothing parameter can be selected by using a criterion of approximate cross-validation method as in O'Sullivan (1988) and Joly et al. (1998). Another approach is to set the number of degrees of freedom of the model and deduce the smoothing parameter using the relationship between these two values (Rondeau et al., 2003). For instance, if we want to estimate a straight line, we choose a number of degrees of freedom equal to 2. Marquardt algorithm (Marquardt, 1963) can be used to maximize the penalized log-likelihood (6.16). The first and second derivatives of the penalized log-likelihood $L_{pl}(\alpha_0(.), \beta, \theta)$ or unpenalized log-likelihood $L(\alpha_0(.), \beta, \theta)$, from which the Hessian matrix and therefore the asymptotic variance-covariance are deducted, are computed numerically using finite differences.

It is interesting to test if the variance of the random effects is different from zero or not, i.e., $H_0 : \theta = 0$ *vs.* $H_1 : \theta > 0$. If a Wald test is used, the variance of the random effects are at the limit of the domain of definition: the distribution of the squared Wald test in this case is a mixture of two chi-square distributions with 0 or 1 degrees of freedom (Molenberghs and Verbeke, 2007) where the chi-square distribution with zero degree of freedom is defined by $P(\chi_0^2 = 0) = 1$. Another possible test is the score test of homogeneity based on the marginal partial likelihood (Commenges and Jacqmin-Gadda, 1997); the advantage of the score test is that it does not require fitting the frailty model.

The penalized likelihood approach has been implemented into the R package `frailtypack` (shown in Section 6.3.6).

6.3.4.2 Approach using partial penalized likelihood

Therneau et al. (2003), based on the work of McGilchrist and Aisbett (1991), using the formulation (6.14) of the frailty model, proposed to use a partial penalized likelihood approach with a penalty term based on the distribution of the random effects. It can be shown analytically that estimators obtained using the penalized partial likelihood are the same as those obtained with the EM algorithm for shared gamma frailty models (Duchateau and Janssen, 2008). However, this equivalence is not true for other distributions of the random effects.

By considering the frailty variables as observed parameters, Therneau and Grambsch (2000, Section 9.6.5) proved that the partial penalized likelihood can be written as the product of a partial likelihood (with $u = (u_1, \ldots, u_G)$ as unknown parameters) and the density of the random effects:

$$\mathcal{L}_{ppl}(\beta, \omega, \theta) = \prod_{i=1}^{G} \mathcal{L}_{part}(\beta, \omega_i) \mathcal{L}_{pen}(\omega_i, \theta)$$

$$= \prod_{i=1}^{G} \left(\frac{e^{\beta^\top X_{ij} + \omega_i}}{\sum_{j \in R(t_{ij})} e^{\beta^\top X_{ij} + \omega_i}} \right)^{\delta_i} f(\omega_i; \theta), \qquad (6.17)$$

with R(t) the set of individuals (or rather their indices) that are still at risk to develop the event of interest at time t. In this expression (6.17), the penalization term $\mathcal{L}_{pen}(\omega_i; \theta) = f(\omega_i; \theta)$ associated with the generally unimodal distribution of the random effects ω_i, implies a high penalty for extreme values of the frailty variables. Therefore, the partial penalized log-likelihood can be written as a sum of two terms, one of which does not depend on θ and the other does not depend on β:

$$L_{ppl}(\beta, \omega, \theta) = \log \mathcal{L}_{ppl}(\beta, \omega, \theta) = \sum_{i=1}^{G} \log \mathcal{L}_{part}(\beta, \omega_i) + \log \mathcal{L}_{pen}(\omega_i, \theta).$$

This approach has been implemented into the R package `survival` (shown in Section 6.3.6). Note the difference between the approach of Therneau et al. (2003) where a penalty on frailty variables is used and the approach of Rondeau et al. (2003) where a penalty on the hazard function is used.

6.3.5 Estimation of the random effects

In frailty models the parameters of interest are the fixed effects and the variance of the random effects. However, it may be interesting to also estimate the random effects themselves. This is useful for obtaining individual predictions and to graphically identify groups of patients different from others. It is natural to "estimate" the random effects by a Bayesian approach, considering $f_{u_i}(u \mid \theta) = \frac{u^{1/\theta-1} \exp(-u/\theta)}{\Gamma(1/\theta)\theta^{1/\theta}} \sim \Gamma(1/\theta; 1/\theta)$ as the *a priori* distribution. The *a posteriori* distribution of the random effects is then:

$$f_{u_i}(u \mid \tilde{T}_i, \beta, \alpha_0(\cdot), \theta) = \frac{f(\tilde{T}_i \mid u_i, \beta, \alpha_0(\cdot), \theta) f_{u_i}(u \mid \theta)}{f(\tilde{T}_i, \beta, \alpha_0(\cdot), \theta)}.$$

In this expression, $f(\tilde{T}_i \mid u_i, \beta, \alpha_0(\cdot), \theta) = u_i^{m_i} \prod_{j=1}^{n_i} \alpha_{ij}(t)^{\delta_{ij}} \exp[-u_i \alpha_{ij}(t)]$ is the conditional likelihood of group i.

The expression of the marginal likelihood of group i is:

$$f(\tilde{T}_i, \beta, \alpha_0(\cdot), \theta) = \int_0^{+\infty} f(\tilde{T}_i \mid u_i, \beta, \alpha_0(.), \theta) f_{u_i}(u \mid \theta) du_i$$

$$= \int_0^{+\infty} (u_i^{m_i} \prod_{j=1}^{n_i} \alpha_{ij}(\tilde{T}_{ij})^{\delta_{ij}} \exp[-u_i \alpha_{ij}(\tilde{T}_{ij})])$$

$$\times \frac{u_i^{1/\theta-1} \exp(-u_i/\theta)}{\Gamma(1/\theta)\theta^{1/\theta}} du_i$$

$$= \frac{\prod_{j=1}^{n_i} (\alpha_0(\tilde{T}_{ij}) \exp(\beta^\top X_{ij}))^{\delta_{ij}} \Gamma(m_i + 1/\theta)}{\theta^{1/\theta} \Gamma(1/\theta)(1/\theta + \sum_{j=1}^{n_i} \alpha_0(\tilde{T}_{ij}) \exp(\beta^\top X_{ij}))^{1/\theta+m_i}}.$$

We deduce:

$$f_{u_i}(u \mid \tilde{T}_i, \beta, \alpha_0(\cdot), \theta) = \frac{u_i^{m_i+1/\theta-1} \exp[-u_i(1/\theta + \sum_{j=1}^{n_i} A_{ij}(\tilde{T}_{ij}))]}{\Gamma(m_i + 1/\theta)(1/\theta + \sum_{j=1}^{n_i} \alpha_0(\tilde{T}_{ij}) \exp(\beta^\top X_{ij}))^{-1/\theta-m_i}}.$$

Thus, the *a posteriori* distribution of u_i is a gamma distribution with parameters $m_i + 1/\theta$ and $\sum_{j=1}^{n_i} A_{ij}(t) + 1/\theta$ ($\sim \Gamma(m_i + 1/\theta; \sum_{j=1}^{n_i} A_{ij}(t) + 1/\theta)$), from which one can deduce the *a posteriori* expectation and variance (by replacing θ and $A(\cdot)$ by their estimators):

$$\mathrm{E}_{post}(u_i) = \frac{m_i + 1/\theta}{\sum_{j=1}^{n_i} A_{ij}(t) + 1/\theta} \quad \text{and} \quad \mathrm{var}_{post}(u_i) = \frac{m_i + 1/\theta}{(\sum_{j=1}^{n_i} A_{ij}(t) + 1/\theta)^2}$$

The function `frailty.pred()` of the R package `frailtypack` provides the *a posteriori* estimates of the random effects, $\hat{E}_{post}(u_i)$.

6.3.6 Application with the R package frailtypack

We illustrate the use of the R package `frailtypack`, for fitting shared frailty models to the data of the colorectal cancer study described in Section 1.4.3. The data file "readmission" contains data from a prospective cohort of re-hospitalization after surgery in patients diagnosed with a colorectal cancer (González et al., 2005).

The R package `frailtypack` can estimate gamma or log-normal frailty models by maximizing a penalized likelihood (associated to an approximation on a splines basis for the baseline hazard functions) or by maximizing a classical likelihood (associated with a parametric estimation of the baseline hazard functions). An estimate of the baseline hazard function can be obtained. The script for shared frailty models is given in the appendix. We also illustrate in the appendix the possibility to use the R package `survival`.

The application for readmission data is summarized in Table 6.9, for a semi-parametric shared frailty model with gamma frailties, a gap time-scale and a stratification on sex:

$$\alpha_{ihj}(t \mid X_{ihj}, u_i) = u_i \alpha_{0h}(t) \exp(\beta^\top X_{ihj})$$

with $\alpha_{0h}(t)$ the baseline hazard function for stratum h and X_{ihj} denotes the covariates vector for the jth individual of stratum h and group i. The date of origin is the time of surgery. Advanced stages of the tumor (according to Dukes) and a high Charlson comorbidity index, were associated with a shorter time between two readmissions, increasing the risk of recurrence. The variance of the random effects was significantly different from zero ($\hat{\theta} = 0.68$, $p < 10^{-4}$); this indicates a significant within-subject correlation of the recurrent times, even after taking into account various adjustment variables. In a model stratified on sex, as the one presented here, we assume that the effect of the explanatory variables is the same on each category of the stratification (e.g., same effect of the grade for men and women), but the baseline hazard is different for men and women. Figure 6.4 shows an association between a large number of events and higher frailties. This type of graph also allows identifying extreme values.

TABLE 6.9
Results of the shared frailty model for rehospitalizations associated with colorectal cancer, stratified on sex.

Variables	$\hat{\beta}$	$\exp(\hat{\beta})$	S.E.$(\hat{\beta})$	p-value	global p-value
Dukes stage					
A-B (ref)		1			
C	0.38	1.46	0.15	0.01	$< 10^{-4}$
D	1.12	3.06	0.19	$< 10^{-4}$	
Charlson index					
0 (ref)		1			0.004
1-2	0.41	1.50	0.26	0.12	
≥ 3	0.42	1.52	0.14	0.002	
variance of random effects	0.68 (0.14)				

6.3.7 Models with interaction between frailties and observed explanatory variables

In the previous section we discussed the models with only one random effect. In this section, we discuss the models with two frailties for the same cluster. Research was dedicated to the expansion of shared frailty models to more

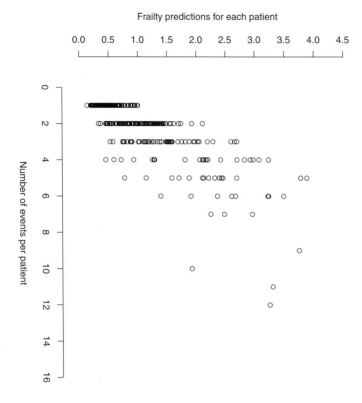

Frailty predictions for each patient

FIGURE 6.4
Individual predictions of the random effects given the number of events per patient.

general approaches which allow for instance an interaction between treatment effect and a center in multicentric clinical trials (Ha et al., 2011; Legrand et al., 2005; Vaida and Xu, 2000; Yamaguchi and Ohashi, 1999), or an interaction between treatment and study in a meta-analysis of survival times (Rondeau et al., 2008). In these situations, two sources of inter-trial heterogeneity of survival times are studied. First, the heterogeneity between trials can be directly attributed to differences in the baseline hazard, due to different study patterns or patient recruitment or different medical practices. Secondly, heterogeneity of the treatment efficacy from one trial to another is possible. It is treated with a random treatment effect specific to each trial. Frailty models are then proposed with several additives random effects: a random intercept for each trial which acts on the baseline hazard and a random trial-specific treatment effect, which allows the treatment effect to vary from one group (or trial) to another.

In additive frailty models, a general formulation of the correlation structure of the random effects can be used including a correlation term between the two random effects. This term reflects a possible dependence between the heterogeneity among trials of the baseline hazard and the heterogeneity of the treatment effect. The hazard function in these models is:

$$\alpha_{ij}(t \mid u_i, v_i, X_{ij}) = \alpha_0(t) \exp(u_i + (v_i + \beta_1)X_{ij1} + \sum_{k=2}^{p} \beta_k X_{ijk})$$

$$u_i \sim \mathcal{N}(0, \sigma^2), \qquad v_i \sim \mathcal{N}(0, \tau^2), \qquad corr(u_i, v_i) = \rho,$$

where, β_k for $(k = 2, \ldots, p)$ are the fixed effects for each explanatory covariate X_{ijk} and β_1 is the effect of the variable of interest (treatment). The random effects u_i and v_i are assumed to have a multivariate Gaussian distribution with mean 0 and covariance matrix $\Sigma = \begin{bmatrix} \sigma^2 & \sigma\tau\rho \\ \sigma\tau\rho & \tau^2 \end{bmatrix}$.

Different estimation methods for this type of models with two independent random effects have been proposed, including a penalized partial likelihood combined with Laplace transform (Ripatti and Palmgren, 2000), a Monte Carlo EM algorithm (Vaida and Xu, 2000), a Bayesian approach combined with a Laplace transform (Legrand et al., 2005). More recently correlated random effects were considered either by a penalized likelihood estimation method (Rondeau et al., 2008) or by hierarchical likelihood ("h-likelihood") approaches (Ha et al., 2011).

In a frailty model with several random effects, integration over the random effects is no longer analytically possible to obtain an expression for the marginal likelihood. The parameters have been estimated using penalized likelihood maximization combined with a Laplace (first order) integration technique to approximate the marginal likelihood. This approach is faster than techniques that use multidimensional numerical integrations such as Gaussian quadrature. A drawback of the approach, related to the asymptotic nature of the Laplace approximation is that, to obtain good estimators, it is necessary to have large group sizes and many groups. Bias on the estimate of the variance of the random effects have been observed by simulations in Rondeau et al. (2008) for 10 groups and 20 subjects per group. This type of model with two correlated shared frailties has been implemented in the package `frailtypack` with the function `additivePenal()`.

6.4   Extension of frailty models

6.4.1   Joint models for recurrent events and a terminal event

In general, monitoring of recurrent events for a subject may be censored by a terminal event such as death. Recurrences of serious events are often associated with a high risk of death. In this context, the presence of the terminal event creates a semi-competing risk problem in the sense that whenever patients are at risk of another recurrent event, they are also at risk of the terminal event. This dependence can be treated by the joint modeling of recurrent events and a terminal event. Again, marginal formulations have been proposed to jointly analyze these survival times (Ghosh and Lin, 2003). A joint shared frailty model and an estimation method based on Monte Carlo EM algorithm was proposed by Liu et al. (2004). An extension of this work was proposed using a penalized likelihood estimation to jointly model recurrent events and death (Rondeau et al., 2007). It has been shown in this article that ignoring the dependence between the recurrence events and the terminal event could lead to bias in the estimation of the regression coefficients.

6.4.1.1 Specification

We note T_{ij} the j-th event time for subject i (i=1,...,G), C_i the corresponding censoring time (different from death), D_i death (or terminal event) time. Each follow-up time corresponds to $\tilde{T}_{ij} = \min(T_{ij}, C_i, D_i)$ and δ_{ij} its binary indicator of censorship, which is zero if the observation is censored or if the patient has died, and 1 if time T_{ij} is observed ($\delta_{ij} = I_{\{\tilde{T}_{ij}=T_{ij}\}}$). Similarly we note $\tilde{T}_i^*$ the last follow-up time for subject i, which is either a censoring time or a death time ($\tilde{T}_i^* = \min(C_i, D_i)$) and $\delta_i^* = I_{(\tilde{T}_i^*=D_i)}$. What we actually observe is $(\tilde{T}_{ij}, \tilde{T}_i^*, \delta_{ij}, \delta_i^*)$. A joint model for recurrent events and a terminal event can be defined by:

$$\begin{cases} \alpha_{ij}^R(t \mid u_i) = u_i \alpha_0^R(t) \exp(\beta_1^\top X_{ij}) = u_i \alpha_{ij}^R(t) \\ \alpha_i^D(t \mid u_i) = u_i^\gamma \alpha_0^D(t) \exp(\beta_2^\top X_i) = u_i^\gamma \alpha_i^D(t) \end{cases} \qquad (6.18)$$

Individual correlation between recurrent events and death is taken into account with a shared frailty term u_i. This frailty term will act differently on recurrent events and death since the effect is modulated by the parameter γ. So when $\gamma = 1$, the effect of the frailty is the same for recurrent events and death. More generally, when $\gamma > 0$, the risks of recurrence and death are positively associated with a different effect of the two frailties on the two hazard functions. In the standard model, the assumption is that $\gamma = 0$ in (6.18), i.e., that $\alpha_i^D(t \mid u_i)$ is independent of u_i and then death (or terminal event) is not informative for recurrence rate $\alpha_{ij}^R(t)$ (i.e., the two rates are not associated). Note that in this model, the interpretation of the value of γ is meaningful only when heterogeneity is present, i.e., when the variance of the random effects is significantly different from zero.

6.4.1.2 Inference

A parametric approach can be used to estimate the parameters of this joint model. Both R package `frailtypack` and procedure `NLMIXED` from `SAS` provide a parametric estimation approach by using maximization algorithms

(Marquardt and Newton Raphson, respectively). The procedure NLMIXED has the advantage of offering two types of distribution for random effects, gamma or log-normal (as shown in Section 6.4.1.3).

An approach by penalized likelihood has been proposed (Rondeau et al., 2007).

$$L_{pl}(\xi) = L(\xi) - \kappa_1 \int_0^\infty \alpha_0^{R''2}(t)\mathrm{d}t - \kappa_2 \int_0^\infty \alpha_0^{D''2}(t)\mathrm{d}t, \qquad (6.19)$$

with $L(\xi)$ the total marginal log-likelihood and ξ the whole set of parameters:

$$
\begin{aligned}
L(\xi) &= \log \prod_{i=1}^G \mathcal{L}_i(\alpha_0^R(.), \alpha_0^D(.), \beta, \gamma, \theta) \\
&= \log \prod_{i=1}^G \int_0^{+\infty} \left\{ \prod_{j=1}^{n_i} \left[\alpha_{ij}^R(\tilde{T}_{ij} \mid u_i)^{\delta_{ij}} \times \exp\left(-u_i \sum_{j=1}^{n_i} \int_{\tilde{T}_{i,j-1}}^{\tilde{T}_{ij}} \alpha_{ij}^R(t)\mathrm{d}t \right) \right] \right. \\
&\quad \left. \times \; \alpha_i^D(\tilde{T}_i^* \mid u_i)^{\delta_i^*} \times \exp\left(-u_i^\gamma \int_0^\infty Y_i(\tilde{T}_i^*)\mathrm{d}A_i(\tilde{T}_i^*) \right) \right\} f(u_i; \theta)\mathrm{d}u_i.
\end{aligned}
$$

In this penalized likelihood (6.19), two penalty terms are used, one for each hazard function. The same basis of splines for the two functions can be used. In this expression, unlike the standard gamma frailty model of Section 6.3.3, there is no analytical solution of the marginal likelihood: the term u_i^γ which appears in the integral prevents analytical simplification of the marginal likelihood. Numerical approximations of the integrals over random effects such as Gaussian quadrature can be used.

In the standard shared frailty model or in the joint frailty model described here, the computations are easier if the random effects have normal distributions. Liu and Yu (2008) proposed to use a transformation of the likelihood in order to use other distributions of the random effects. This transformation allows to use the NLMIXED procedure from SAS (programmed for Gaussian random effects).

6.4.1.3   Application with the R package frailtypack

We illustrate the joint gamma frailty model on rehospitalization data after colorectal cancer (presented in Section 1.4.3). The basic time-scale selected is the time between two readmissions and the parameters are estimated using penalized likelihood (presented in Section 6.4.1.2). Comparing the standard frailty model to the joint frailty model, we see some differences of estimation (see Table 6.4.1.3). The effect of the stage was slightly underestimated in the standard frailty model when association with death was not accounted for. In the joint model, the variance of the random effect is significantly different from zero ($\hat{\theta} = 0.73$); this reflects a dependence between the risk of readmission and the risk of dying. In addition the value of $\hat{\gamma} = 0.74$ ($\hat{\gamma} > 0$) indicates a positive association between these two risks. Thus, in this application it seems that unobserved prognostic factors influence both events (rehospitalization and death) in the same way.

The script for a joint frailty model is given in the appendix for the R package `frailtypack` and for the `NLMIXED` procedure from `SAS`. The `NLMIXED` procedure offers by default a log-normal distribution for the random effects, but a change in the likelihood can be used to utilize also a gamma distribution for the random effects (Liu and Yu, 2008). In the `NLMIXED` procedure, a complete specification of the likelihood is necessary.

6.4.2 Models with nested frailties

Survival data analysis for clustered data by shared frailty models is very useful with multiple application areas (see Section 6.3.3). However, these models are restricted to only one level of data aggregation. More and more, epidemiological studies have a more complex grouping pattern, with several levels of grouping. Nested frailty models are particularly interesting in cohorts where data are naturally grouped in clusters with two hierarchical levels (e.g., families in different cities), or because of the study design, i.e., the data are collected by multiple levels of grouping (e.g., different geographical areas nested in cities). This approach may also be useful in the analysis of recurrent and clustered survival data. We illustrate this model in Section 6.4.2.2 using data from a randomized clinical trial to study the effect of gamma-interferon in chronic granulomatous disease. In shared frailty models, ignoring random components (or data grouping levels) we may get invalid results. *"Nested frailty models"* have been proposed for analysis of hierarchical survival data at multiple levels of grouping.

6.4.2.1 Specification and inference

We define two random effects v_i and w_{ij} and assume that the cluster-level random effects v_i and the sub-cluster random effects w_{ij} are independent and gamma-distributed random effects ($\Gamma(1/\alpha; 1/\alpha)$ and $\Gamma(1/\eta; 1/\eta)$) with $E(v_i) = 1$, $\text{var}(v_i) = \alpha$ and $E(w_{ij}) = 1$, $\text{var}(w_{ij}) = \eta$. For identifiability, they have a mean equal to 1. In the nested frailty models, the hazard function given the two independent random effects v_i and w_{ij} for the k-th subject ($k=1,\ldots,K_{ij}$) from the sub-cluster j ($j=1,\ldots,J_i$) and the cluster i ($i=1,\ldots,G$) is:

$$\alpha_{ijk}(t, X_{ijk} \mid v_i w_{ij}) = v_i w_{ij} \alpha_0(t) \exp(\beta^\top X_{ijk}). \tag{6.20}$$

The two hierarchical levels of data aggregation are considered in models including two nested random effects. The parameters can be estimated using an EM algorithm (Sastry, 1997) or a Bayesian approach (Ducrocq and Casella, 1996). A method of semi-parametric penalized likelihood estimation to estimate the hazard function in nested frailty models from right-censored and

TABLE 6.10
Results of the standard or joint frailty model for the risk of readmission related to colorectal cancer and the risk of death (with the R package `frailtypack`).

Variables	standard model RR (IC 95%)	joint model RR (IC 95%)
Rehospitalisations		
Gender		
Male	1	1
Female	0.60 (0.46-0.79)	0.60 (0.46-0.79)
Dukes stage		
A-B (ref)	1	1
C	1.47 (1.10-1.97)	1.50 (1.11-2.03)
D	3.00 (2.06-4.35)	3.56 (2.41-5.26)
Charlson Index		
0 (ref)	1	1
1-2	1.53 (0.92-2.52)	1.48 (0.90-2.44)
≥ 3	1.52 (1.17-1.99)	1.54 (1.18-2.01)
Variance of the random effects (S.E.)	0.66 (0.14)	
Death		
Gender		
Male		1
Female		0.72 (0.47-1.11)
Dukes stage		
A-B (ref)		1
C		2.50 (1.30-4.82)
D		15.36 (7.35-32.11)
Charlson Index		
0 (ref)		1
1-2		2.06 (0.61-7.00)
≥ 3		3.05 (1.88-4.94)
Variance of the random effects (S.E.)		0.73 (0.11)
γ		0.74 (0.22)

left-truncated data has been proposed (Rondeau et al., 2006). Unlike in shared frailty models, the expression of the marginal likelihood in nested gamma frailty models contains non-analytical integrals over the random effects of the highest level. Gaussian quadrature methods are used to approximate these integrals.

6.4.2.2 Application with the R package `frailtypack`

We illustrate the use of nested gamma frailty models using a penalized likelihood estimation (Rondeau et al., 2006) with data from Fleming and Harrington (1991) (Appendix D.2) available in the R package `survival`. The data come from a randomized trial assessing the effect of gamma interferon (γ-IFN) treatment in chronic granulomatous disease (CGD) *vs.* placebo. Recurrent infection times on 128 patients from 13 hospitals were observed; so these hierarchical data have two levels of grouping. The results presented in Table 6.11 compare standard frailty models, with frailty at patient level or at hospital level, with nested frailty models that take into account two random effects. The results are also presented for two basic time choices (in "gap time" or "calendar time").

Whatever the approach, all analyses concluded that treatment with γ-IFN significantly reduces the risk of serious infections in patients with CGD (e.g., in the nested frailty model with gap times, HR=0.32, $IC_{95\%}$ (0.16-0.63)). In standard shared frailty models, the variance of the random effects specific to each hospital is overestimated (i.e., $\widehat{var}(v_i) = 0.12$ against $\widehat{var}(v_i) = 0.008$ in the nested frailty model) as only one part of the correlation structure of the data is considered. Nested frailty models suggest that the variance between patients is significantly greater than the variance between hospitals.

The models based on times between two visits lead to a similar treatment effect, but to a higher estimate of the sub-cluster heterogeneity compared to the calendar time-based models (i.e., $\hat{\eta} = 1.57$ against $\hat{\eta} = 0.81$, which corresponds to a higher correlation of the times between 2 visits than between the times since entry into the study). AIC criterion (presented in Section 2.4.1) can be used to compare statistically these two models. In both time-scales, a subject is at risk for the same duration and a subject cannot be at risk before the end of the previous event. We have however a difference of interpretation between the two approaches. In the calendar time-scale approach, the hazard does not change after an event occurrence, whereas in the "gap time" approach, the risk depends on the time since the last event and thus, it returns to the initial risk after each event.

Smooth baseline hazard functions estimated by the nested frailty models (results in Table 6.11) are given in Figure 6.5. The data are not shown after 350 days due to a lack of information.

6.5 Cure models

In this section we discuss an extension of survival analysis to "cure models." These models are useful when the population is made up of two unobserved groups, one group at risk and the other has a null risk for the event; so cure

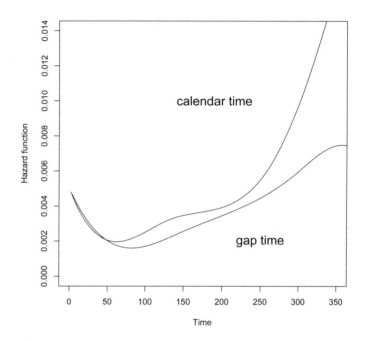

FIGURE 6.5
Baseline hazard functions for CGD data estimated by penalized likelihood in
calendar time-scale or gap time-scale, obtained with the nested frailty model
and the R package `frailtypack`.

TABLE 6.11
Analysis of recurrent events with nested frailty models for CGD data.

	Shared frailty models		Nested frailty models
	Hospital level	*Patient level*	
	$\hat{\beta}$ (S.E.*)	$\hat{\beta}$ (S.E.*)	$\hat{\beta}$ (S.E.*)
Baseline time scale = "gap"			
Treatment (γ-IFN)	-1.12 (0.27)	-1.17 (0.36)	-1.16 (0.35)
$\text{var}(v_i) = \gamma$ (hospital)	0.15 (0.14)	-	0.007 (0.003)
$\text{var}(\omega_{ij}) = \eta$ (patient)	-	1.58 (0.71)	1.57 (0.69)
Penalized Log-likelihood	-530.26	-523.41	-515.04
Baseline time scale = "calendar"			
Treatment (γ-IFN)	-1.10 (0.26)	-1.06 (0.31)	-1.06 (0.31)
$\text{var}(v_i) = \gamma$ (hospital)	0.12 (0.13)	-	0.007 (0.003)
$\text{var}(\omega_{ij}) = \eta$ (patient)	-	0.80 (0.39)	0.78 (0.39)
Penalized log-likelihood	-524.35	-520.32	-513.41

* Standard error of the parameter m estimated with $\sqrt{\hat{H}_{mm}^{-1}}$.

models are mixture models. The terminology to qualify the not at-risk population varies from one application domain to another: "long-term survivors" or "cured" in epidemiology; "non-susceptible" in toxicology and "sterile" in fertility analysis.

In some applications, we can make the assumption that a sub-population of individuals is likely to suffer from a certain type of event while another sub-population is not. Thus, a significant number of patients are called "cured" and are no longer at risk of an event after the first treatment, the population is now a mixture of subjects at risk and not at risk. In this case, conventional survival analysis techniques, such as the Cox proportional hazards model is no longer suitable, since it assumes that all subjects have the same sensitivity to the disease and eventually develop the event of interest if the follow-up period is long enough. Cure models have been extensively developed in recent years (Pocock et al., 1982; Sy and Taylor, 2000); they assume the existence of a cured fraction in the population. A graphical representation of the data is used to identify the presence of these two sub-populations, at risk or not. Then, this will result in a Kaplan-Meier survival curve with a long stable plateau, inducing a significant censoring at the tail of the distribution. Cure models are increasingly used in cancer studies. Cancer treatment has been improved in recent decades, with an increasing proportion of cured patients for many types of cancer. In these studies, the omission of a not at-risk sub-population may lead to underestimate the event hazard and therefore to overestimate the survival function of non-cured patients. Cure models enable us to estimate the probability for a subject to be cured (="incidence") and the distribution of survival times before the event for non-cured subjects (= "latency"). In addition, explanatory variables may have an effect on the probability of being cured and on the hazard of the disease if not cured.

We introduce the following notations: U is an indicator that the subject is at risk for the event of interest ($U = 1$) or not ($U = 0$). We denote $\pi(Z^*) = P(U = 1 \mid Z^*)$ the probability of being at risk to develop the event given the vector of explanatory variables $Z^* = (Z_1^*, \ldots, Z_q^*)^\top$. The cure rate $1 - \pi(\cdot)$ is then defined as the probability that a subject never develops the event of interest. A logistic regression model $\pi(Z^*) = \exp(b^\top Z^*)/(1 + \exp(b^\top Z^*))$ can be used. Let T be the event time defined only when $U = 1$ (i.e., for non-cured patients) with the conditional survival function $S(t \mid U = 1) = P(T > t \mid U = 1)$ with β and Z, the vectors of regression coefficients and explanatory variables associated with latency. Thus, the marginal survival function is:

$$S(t) = 1 - \pi(Z^*) + \pi(Z^*)S(t \mid U = 1).$$

The conditional distribution can have a parametric form (e.g., exponential or Weibull type), or semi-parametric (Peng and Carriere, 2002). In the proportional hazards model the conditional distribution takes the form:

$$S(t \mid U = 1) = S_0(t \mid U = 1)^{\exp(\beta^\top Z)},$$

where $S_0(t \mid U = 1)$ is the survival function. Note $\alpha_0(t \mid U = 1)$ the baseline hazard associated to $S_0(t \mid U = 1)$. If $S_0(t \mid U = 1)$ is left unspecified, the model is defined as a Cox mixture proportional hazards model. Note that the coefficients β and b have different interpretations. A positive β means that the risk of an event (if the subject is susceptible) is higher if Z is increasing, while a positive b means that the probability of being cured is lower if Z increases.

Denoting $f(\cdot) = S(\cdot)\alpha(\cdot)$ the p.d.f. of T, the expression of the total observed likelihood for the mixture model is written:

$$\mathcal{L}(\alpha_0(\cdot), \beta, b) = \prod_{i=1}^{N} (\pi_i(Z_i^*)f(t_i \mid U = 1, Z_i))^{\delta_i} \times (1 - \pi_i(Z_i^*) + \pi_i(Z_i^*)S(t_i \mid U = 1, Z_i))^{1-\delta_i}. \tag{6.21}$$

When all individuals are supposed at risk, $\pi_i(Z_i^*) = 1$ for each Z_i^* and the likelihood (6.21) reduces to the likelihood for a standard survival model.

We defined the random variable U in order to know if an individual i is at risk ($U_i = 1$) or not ($U_i = 0$). It follows that if $\delta_i = 1$, then $U_i = 1$, and if

$\delta_i = 0$ then U_i is not observed. Given the U_i's, the full likelihood (6.21) is:

$$\mathcal{L}(\alpha_0(.), \beta, b, u_i) = \prod_{i=1}^{N} (\pi_i(Z_i^*))^{u_i} (1 - \pi_i(Z_i^*))^{1-u_i} \qquad (6.22)$$

$$\prod_{i=1}^{N} (\alpha_0(t_i \mid U = 1) \exp(\beta^\top Z_i))^{\delta_i u_i} S_0(t_i \mid U = 1)^{u_i \exp(\beta^\top Z_i)}$$

$$= \mathcal{L}_1(b, u) \times \mathcal{L}_2(\alpha_0(.), \beta, u).$$

The EM algorithm has been widely used to maximize this likelihood that decomposes into a part which depends only on b and another part that depends on β and on $\alpha_0(\cdot)$ (Sy and Taylor, 2000).

This modelling can be easily implemented by the `NLMIXED` procedure from `SAS` (Corbière and Joly, 2007) using a parametric approach. Extensions of cure models have been proposed for the analysis of clustered survival data (Chatterjee and Shih, 2001; Locatelli et al., 2007; Peng and Zhang, 2008; Wienke et al., 2003) or recurrent events (Price and Manatunga, 2001; Rondeau et al., 2013). They involve random effects in both the incidence part and in the latency part.

7

Multistate models

7.1 Introduction

Survival analysis addresses a problem where one is interested in an event, typically death. Statistical models for survival can be described by a model for the distribution of the time of occurrence of this event, T. A more theoretical, and more powerful way to describe the occurrence of an event is in terms of a counting process $\{N(t), t \geq 0\}$, where $N(t)$ counts the number of events up to t (see Section 3.7.1). Another perspective is to describe survival as a multistate process. We can consider that the event "death" is defined by the change from the biological state "alive" to the state "dead." Figure 7.1 gives a graphical representation of this perspective. The instantaneous risk of transition from the state "alive" to the state "dead" is quantified by the hazard function conventionally used in survival problems. In the most general case, we speak of *transition intensities*. The state at time t can be represented by a random variable $X(t)$ which can take two values here, 0 if the subject is alive, 1 if he/she is dead, and the trajectory can be described by the process $\{X(t), t \geq 0\}$. In the case of survival, there is not much difference between the two points of view because we have $X(t) = N(t)$. When there are more than two states, one needs a multivariate counting process for representing $X(t)$ as described in Section 7.8.

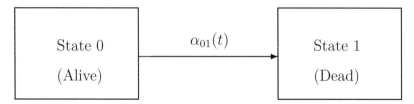

FIGURE 7.1
Graphical representation of a survival process as a two-state process; $\alpha_{01}(t)$ is the transition intensity between state 0 and state 1, corresponding here to the hazard function.

We are often interested in events that are not death but, for example, the occurrence of disease. In the case of chronic illness among the elderly, the risk of dying is also important. It is therefore useful to model the two possible important events: occurrence of disease and death. This can be represented by two counting processes (or a bivariate process). In terms of states, two events define three states: "healthy," "ill," "dead." We can encode these states by values $0, 1, 2$ and represent the evolution of the state by a process $\{X(t), t \geq 0\}$ where $X(t)$ can take the values $0, 1, 2$. Such a process is called a multistate process. This three-state model is the most widely used in epidemiology and is called the illness-death model. We see that there is a duality between event representation and representation by states: an event leads to a different state while a transition from one state to another is an event. In this chapter, we will focus on the multistate point of view which is often more attractive, but the event point of view is more general and will also be discussed.

We can obviously generalize to a larger number of events that define a larger number of states. The number of events or states is however limited in practice because highly complex models raise problems of identification and interpretation, and also numerical problems. Once states are defined, we make a number of assumptions to make inference and interpretation possible. The first assumptions define which transitions are possible. For example in the illness-death model we consider that transitions $2 \to 0$ and $2 \to 1$ are impossible (there is no resurrection!). It is said that transitions $0 \to 2$ and $1 \to 2$ are irreversible. The second class of required assumptions specify how the transition intensities depend on the past. Here the Markov assumption is fundamental. We have also to model the effect of explanatory variables on the transitions intensities. Finally, we can develop parametric, non-parametric or semi-parametric models.

Several books deal with multistate models: Andersen et al. (1993), Hougaard (2000) and Aalen et al. (2008).

7.2 Multistate processes

7.2.1 Definition

Here we describe *multistate processes* which are mathematical objects that will serve us to develop *multistate models*. A multistate process is a process $\{X(t), t \geq 0\}$, where $X(t)$ can take a finite number of values $0, 1, \ldots, K$. One can see a process as a family of random variables indexed by t: for fixed t, $X(t)$ is a random variable. In many applications, the index t represents time.

The first question relates to the discrete or continuous nature of t. If t is discrete, it takes integer values $0, 1, 2, \ldots$; if t is continuous, it takes real values of $\mathbb{R}^+$: $t \geq 0$. Stochastic processes, and in particular multistate processes can be described for discrete or continuous time settings. Some properties can be set in the same manner in both cases, but the theories differ, especially when we introduce transition intensities which take an important role in the continuous-time setting.

The transition probability from state h to state j between time s and $t > s$ is the probability that the process is in state j at time t given that he was in state h at time s and conditionally on the past trajectory until time s:

$$P_{hj}(s, t; \mathcal{F}_{s-}) = P[X(t) = j \mid X(s) = h, \mathcal{F}_{s-}], h, j = 0, \ldots, K, \qquad (7.1)$$

where $\mathcal{F}_{s-}$ represents the past up to s. In mathematical terms, $\mathcal{F}_{s-}$ is the sigma-field of all events that may happen strictly before s. The law of a multistate process may be defined by the transition probabilities for all h, j, s, t.

7.2.2 Markov property and Chapman-Kolmogorov equation

The Markov property for the law of a multistate process is that the events $\{X(t) = j\}$, $j = 0, \ldots, K$, are independent on the past $\mathcal{F}_{s-}$ given $X(s)$: the future path of X after s depends only on the state of X at s and not on the past trajectory.

Definition 4 (Markov property) *X is a Markov process if for all s, t such that $0 \leq s < t$:*

$$P[X(t) = j \mid X(s) = h, \mathcal{F}_{s-}] = P[X(t) = j \mid X(s) = h]; h, j = 0, \ldots, K. \qquad (7.2)$$

$P[X(t) = j \mid X(s) = h]$ is called "transition probability" and is denoted by $P_{hj}(s, t)$. The matrices with entries $P_{hj}(s, t)$ are the transition probability matrices and are noted $\boldsymbol{P}(s, t)$.

A subclass of Markov processes are homogeneous Markov processes.

Definition 5 (homogeneous Markov processes) *A homogeneous Markov process is a Markov process whose transition probabilities satisfy: $\boldsymbol{P}(s, t) = \boldsymbol{P}(0, t - s)$, for all s, t such that $s < t$.*

For Markov processes, the transition probability matrices satisfy the Chapman-Kolmogorov property:

Property 3 (Chapman-Kolmogorov)

$$\boldsymbol{P}(s, t) = \boldsymbol{P}(s, u)\boldsymbol{P}(u, t), s < u < t \qquad (7.3)$$

If $P_{hj}(s, t) = 0$, $0 \leq s < t$, the process can never go from h to j. A state h is absorbing if for all $j \neq h$, $P_{hj}(s, t) = 0, 0 \leq s < t$. If a state is not absorbing, it is transitory.

7.2.3 Discrete-time processes

A discrete-time multistate process is a family of random variables $\{X(0), X(1), \ldots\}$, where each of these variables can take integer values from 0 to K. The law of the process is given by $P(X(t+1) = j \mid X(t) = h, \mathcal{F}_{t-1})$ for all t, h, j. The Markov property can be expressed by:

$$P(X(t+1) = j \mid X(t) = h, \mathcal{F}_{t-1}) = P(X(t+1) = j \mid X(t) = h).$$

A discrete-time multistate Markov process is called a "Markov chain." Note $\alpha^d_{hj}(t) = P(X_{t+1} = j \mid X_t = h)$. The superscript d recalls that this applies to the discrete-time case. The matrix with entries $\alpha^d_{hj}(t)$, $\boldsymbol{\alpha}_d(t)$, called *transition matrix*, characterizes the dynamics of the process in the same way that the matrix of transitions intensities $\boldsymbol{\alpha}$ in the continuous-time case that we will see in Section 7.2.4. However, this is also a transition probability matrix and it can be noted: $\boldsymbol{\alpha}_d(t) = \boldsymbol{P}(t, t+1)$. As such, the sum of the terms of each row of these matrices is equal to 1, since $\sum_{j=0}^{K} P_{hj}(s, t) = 1$ (matrices with this property are called "stochastic matrices"). Knowing the transition matrices, the transition probability matrices can be calculated by using the Chapman-Kolmogorov equation:

$$\boldsymbol{P}(s, t) = \boldsymbol{\alpha}_d(s)\boldsymbol{\alpha}_d(s+1) \ldots \boldsymbol{\alpha}_d(t-1), t > s \geq 0.$$

For homogeneous Markov process, the transition matrices do not depend on time: $\boldsymbol{\alpha}_d(t) = \boldsymbol{\alpha}_d(s) = \boldsymbol{\alpha}_d$. The transition probability matrix is then:

$$\boldsymbol{P}(s, t) = \boldsymbol{\alpha}_d^{t-s}.$$

Discrete-time homogeneous processes have been used in particular in MCMC (Markov Chain Monte Carlo) algorithms; see Brémaud (1999). These algorithms use the existence of stationary distributions of these processes. Let $\nu^0 = (\nu_0^0, \ldots, \nu_K^0)^\top$ be a vector characterizing the probability distribution of $X(0)$, i.e., $\nu_h^0 = P(X(0) = h)$. The distribution in t is given by $\nu^t = \nu^0 \boldsymbol{\alpha}_d^t$ (where $\boldsymbol{\alpha}_d^t$ is $\boldsymbol{\alpha}_d$ at the power t). Under certain conditions, there is a stationary distribution π such that $\pi = \pi\boldsymbol{\alpha}_d$, and ν^t converges to the stationary distribution. See also the algorithms for hidden Markov models that have had many uses, such as speech recognition (Rabiner, 1989) and genetics. We do not develop these themes because we are interested in multistate processes for modeling in epidemiology, while discrete-time homogeneous processes are not very suited for this purpose. Indeed both features—discrete aspect of time and homogeneity over time—are not very realistic for biological processes, although they may be adopted in some applications for the sake of simplicity.

7.2.4 Continuous-time processes

Transitions intensities are defined as a probability limit of transitions between times t and $t + \Delta t$, when Δt tends to zero. We assume that these limits exist.

Where they do not exist, this means that there are probability masses at certain times; the study of such probability laws is particularly interesting to study the properties of non-parametric estimators, which often put masses at observed event times. We do not develop this study in this book, except for the description of non-parametric estimators in Section 7.5.2. We assume here that the limits exist, which is reasonable to model many real-world phenomena. The transition intensity from h to j is:

$$\alpha_{hj}(t) = \lim_{\Delta t \to 0} P_{hj}(t, t + \Delta t)/\Delta t. \qquad (7.4)$$

We define $\alpha_{hh}(t) = -\sum_{j \neq h} \alpha_{hj}(t)$, and $\sum_{j \neq h} \alpha_{hj}(t)$ is the hazard function associated with the distribution of the sojourn time in the h state. Specifically, conditionally on the entry time in the state h, T_h, the process will stay a certain time in the state h; sojourn time noted $T(h)$ is equal to the output time from h minus T_h. The hazard function of the distribution of this time is $\alpha_{T(h)}(u) = \sum_{j \neq h} \alpha_{hj}(u + T_h), u \geq 0$. We also define the cumulative transition intensities: $A_{hj}(t) = \int_0^t \alpha_{hj}(u)du$.

The set of transition intensities forms the matrix of transition intensity: $\boldsymbol{\alpha}(t)$. The sum of the terms of each row of these matrices is equal to zero (this is in contrast with the discrete-time case where $\boldsymbol{\alpha}_d$ has sums of rows equal to 1). Note that if the law of the process is not Markovian, transition intensities depend on the past (hence they are random), while in the Markov case, they are deterministic functions. It is easier to describe the law of the process in terms of transition intensities rather than transition probabilities. One reason is that the transition intensities are functions of time t, while the transition probabilities depend on two times s and t. Another reason is related to the interpretation of the dynamics of the process: we consider that the transition intensities describe the instantaneous dynamics of the process and the transition probabilities are derived from this dynamics. In a survival problem, there is a transition intensity, $\alpha_{01}(t)$ which is the hazard function, simply denoted $\alpha(t)$. In the Markov case, the equations for calculating the transition probabilities from the transition intensities are given by the forward Kolmogorov equation (there is also another form, the backward Kolmogorov equation):

Property 4 (Forward Kolmogorov equation)

$$\frac{\partial}{\partial t} \boldsymbol{P}(s, t) = \boldsymbol{P}(s, t) \boldsymbol{\alpha}(t); \boldsymbol{P}(s, s) = \boldsymbol{I}, 0 \leq s < t, \qquad (7.5)$$

where $\boldsymbol{I}$ is the identity matrix.

This is actually a system of differential equations (in t for all fixed s) formed by all the equations of the type:

$$\frac{\partial}{\partial t} P_{hj}(s, t) = \sum_{k=1}^{K} P_{hk}(s, t) \alpha_{kj}(t); P_{hk}(s, s) = \delta_{hk}, 0 \leq s < t,$$

where $\delta_{hk} = 1$ if $h = k$, and $\delta_{hk} = 0$ if $h \neq k$ (the Kronecker symbol). In a survival problem, this equation gives the relationship between the survival function and the hazard function. Indeed, the survival function is $S(t) = P_{00}(0, t)$. Kolmogorov equation writes: $\frac{dS(t)}{dt} = S(t)\alpha(t)$ with $S(0) = 1$. The solution is: $S(t) = \exp[-\int_0^t \alpha(u) \, du]$.

It is not always easy to solve the forward Kolmogorov equation. A solution is given by the product-integral (see Andersen et al., 1993, Section II.6):

$$\boldsymbol{P}(s, t) = \prod_s^t [\boldsymbol{I} + \boldsymbol{\alpha}(u)du], \tag{7.6}$$

defined by

$$\lim_{\max |s_i - s_{i-1}| \to 0} \prod [\boldsymbol{I} + \boldsymbol{A}(s_i) - \boldsymbol{A}(s_{i-1})],$$

where $s = s_1 < \ldots < s_{i-1} < \ldots = t$ is a partition of the interval $[s, t]$ and where $\boldsymbol{A}(s)$ is the matrix of cumulated transition intensities with entries $A_{hj}(s)$.

However, this expression does not necessarily lead to a simple calculation. For homogeneous Markov processes, transitions intensities do not depend on time: $\alpha_{hj}(t) = \alpha_{hj}(s) = \alpha_{hj}$ for all h, j, t, s. In this case, the solution of the forward Kolmogorov equation gives the matrix of transition probabilities $\boldsymbol{P}(t)$ as a function of the exponential of a matrix:

$$\boldsymbol{P}(t) = e^{t\boldsymbol{\alpha}}. \tag{7.7}$$

The exponential of a matrix is calculated relatively easily, particularly when the matrix can be diagonalized. If $\boldsymbol{\alpha}$ has eigenvalues which are all different, it can be written as $\boldsymbol{\alpha} = VDV^{-1}$, where D is the diagonal matrix of eigenvalues, and V is the matrix of eigenvectors. In this case, $\boldsymbol{P}(t) = Ve^{tD}V^{-1}$; the exponential of a diagonal matrix D is a diagonal matrix whose diagonal terms are the exponential of terms of D.

7.2.5 Graphical representation

The transition intensities are also used to represent some features of the laws of multistate processes graphically. If $\alpha_{hj}(t) = 0$ for all t, a direct transition from h to j is not possible. This does not imply that $P_{hj}(s, t) = 0$ for all s, t (because it can be allowed to go from h to j through other states). If both direct transitions of h to j and j to h are possible, we say that there is reversibility. Reversibility induces cycles; cycles involving more than two states are possible but rarely encountered in epidemiological applications. Graphically, states are generally represented by rectangles, and we put an arrow between h and j if the direct transition is possible, that is to say, $\alpha_{hj}(.) \neq 0$. Figure 7.2 represents a progressive irreversible three-state model for which direct transition $0 \to 2$ is not possible; this process is called "progressive." State 2 is absorbing.

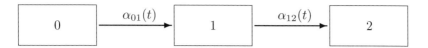

FIGURE 7.2
Graph of a progressive three-state process.

7.2.6 The illness-death model

Figure 7.3 graphically represents an irreversible illness-death model. State 2 is absorbing. For the Markov irreversible illness-death model, probabilities matrix takes the form:

$$\boldsymbol{P}(s,t) = \begin{pmatrix} P_{00}(s,t) & P_{01}(s,t) & P_{02}(s,t) \\ 0 & P_{11}(s,t) & P_{12}(s,t) \\ 0 & 0 & 1 \end{pmatrix},$$

and the transition intensity matrix takes the form:

$$\boldsymbol{\alpha}(t) = \begin{pmatrix} -(\alpha_{01}(t) + \alpha_{02}(t)) & \alpha_{01}(t) & \alpha_{02}(t) \\ 0 & -\alpha_{12}(t) & \alpha_{12}(t) \\ 0 & 0 & 0 \end{pmatrix}.$$

The forward Kolmogorov equation gives, for each s, a system of differential equations in t. There is a solution using the product-integral that we do not give here. One can actually solve the system directly. In particular, one obtains the three differential equations (in t for given s) below:

$$\frac{dP_{00}(s,t)}{dt} = -P_{00}(s,t)(\alpha_{01}(t) + \alpha_{02}(t))$$

$$\frac{dP_{11}(s,t)}{dt} = -P_{11}(s,t)\alpha_{12}(t)$$

$$\frac{dP_{12}(s,t)}{dt} = P_{00}(s,t)\alpha_{01}(t) - P_{11}(s,t)\alpha_{12}(t)$$

It is easy to solve the first two equations. The third is a bit more difficult, but one can check that the following solutions are obtained, giving the transition probabilities as a function of the transition intensities:

$$P_{00}(s,t) = e^{-A_{01}(s,t) - A_{02}(s,t)}$$

$$P_{11}(s,t) = e^{-A_{12}(s,t)}$$

$$P_{01}(s,t) = \int_s^t P_{00}(s,u)\alpha_{01}(u)P_{11}(u,t)du$$

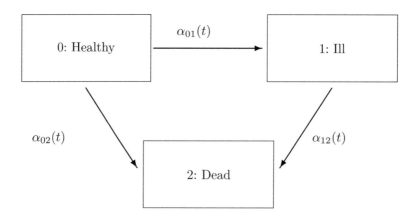

FIGURE 7.3
Irreversible illness-death model.

The formulas for $P_{00}(s,t)$ and $P_{11}(s,t)$ are similar to the formula relating the survival function for the hazard function in a survival problem, which is $S(t) = e^{-A(t)}$, since $S(t)$ is the probability of remaining in state 0 between times 0 and t. These formulas say that the probability of not leaving a state during the period (s,t) is equal to the exponential of minus the cumulative risk over the period. The formula for $P_{01}(s,t)$ involves an integral over the transition time $0 \to 1$. This formula obtained rigorously by solving the Kolmogorov equation can be intuitively understood: for going from 0 to 1 between times s and t, one must make a transition at a time u such that $s < u < t$; one remains in 0 between s and u with probability $P_{00}(s,u)$, one goes to 1 with a risk $\alpha_{01}(u)$ and remain in 1 until t with probability $P_{11}(u,t)$; this must be integrated over u between s and t. To complete the description of the probabilities of possible events, we note that $P_{02}(s,t) = 1 - P_{00}(s,t) - P_{01}(s,t)$, $P_{12}(s,t) = 1 - P_{11}(s,t)$ and $P_{22}(s,t) = 1$ (absorbing state).

7.2.7   Semi-Markov processes

A relaxation of the Markov property is allowed by considering semi-Markov processes. The class of semi-Markov processes is defined by the fact that only the chain of states is Markov: intuitively this means that the probability that the next transition is to state j depends only on the state in which the process is; note that the sojourn times may depend on other characteristics of the trajectory and therefore a semi-Markov process is not necessarily a Markov process. The most widely used sub-class of semi-Markov processes is defined by the constraint that the events $\{X(t) = j\}$ are independent on the past conditionally on $\{X(s) = h\}$ (for all h and j) and the last time of transition in h, T_h, or equivalently conditionally on the time spent in the state h, $t - T_h$. We formally define this sub-class. For all $h, j = 0, \ldots, K$ and $0 \leq s < t$, we have:

$$P[X(t) = j \mid X(s) = h, \mathcal{F}_{s-}] = P[X(t) = j \mid X(s) = h, T_h] \qquad (7.8)$$

We will not present other semi-Markov processes than this sub-class. The transition intensities of such processes can be written $\alpha_{hj}(t; T_h)$. This double dependence of the transition intensities on the current time and the last time of transition is quite complex to manage in applications; this can be simplified by a time homogeneity assumption, saying that the transition intensities depend only on the time spent in the current state. These transition intensities are written $\alpha_{hj}(t - T_h)$. For such processes, the sojourn times in the different states are independent. These processes are sometimes called "clock reset" because everything happens as if, at each transition to a new state, one puts the time to zero.

7.3 Multistate models: generalities

7.3.1 General assumptions

We use the theory of multistate processes to build statistical models. We consider that interesting characteristics of the history of individuals in a population can be described by multistate processes. So for each subject i, we define a process X_i. We generally assume that the X_i's are independent, but this can be relaxed by introducing shared frailties in groups.

The first thing, of course, is to define what are the interesting states that these processes X_i's represent.

Then, as in survival problems, it is important to define what is the "time" t that indexes these processes. First, there is a choice between a discrete or continuous time. Discrete time processes have been used to build models in two different cases: (a) the relevant time is really discrete, and (b) observations are regularly spaced. An example of a really discrete-time problem is the occurrence of a pregnancy after *in vitro* fertilization attempts. For a naturally infertile couple, pregnancy can only start at times of attempts. An example of regularly spaced observations can be given by some studies of nosocomial infections, where the events of interest are collected every day. Although infection can occur in continuous time (i.e., at any time of the day), a discrete-time approximation is reasonable in this case. However, it is often more realistic to consider that the phenomena evolve in continuous time. In the following, we describe processes based on continuous time models. Another very important aspect in the definition of time is the choice of origin: calendar time is the basic time-scale if we choose a common origin of time for all subjects; the time from the start of treatment and the time from birth (age) may be relevant, and in this case, the event which defines the origin of time is specific to the subject.

The next step is to define which are the possible transitions. Finally, we must make restrictive assumptions on the dependence on the past. In practice, it is a choice between Markov or semi-Markov assumptions. There is also the possibility of making an assumption of homogeneity in time. For modeling in epidemiology, this assumption is often too rigid, but it may be acceptable to assume that the transition intensities are piecewise constant. The law of each process X_i can be characterized by the matrix of transition intensities $\boldsymbol{\alpha}^i(t)$.

7.3.2 Models for transition intensities

The final aspect of the modeling is to specify the transition intensities. The population is homogeneous if $\alpha_{hj}^i(t) = \alpha_{hj}^{i'}(t) = \alpha_{hj}(t)$ for all i, i'. The model is completed by assumptions on $\alpha_{hj}(t)$. If one makes no assumption, this is a non-parametric approach. For parametric models we can use the same family of distributions as for the survival problems. The main families of distributions used are the exponential, Weibull, and Gamma distributions. The difference with survival problems is that one considers some parametric form for the transition intensity, while the distribution function which has this hazard function is generally not that of an observable time. For example, in a competing risks model, the transition intensity α_{0j} is the hazard function associated with the distribution of the transition time in the state j if there were no other risks. We can say that it is a latent time. For example, the age at which each subject develops Alzheimer's disease may be considered as a latent time: many subjects die without developing Alzheimer's disease. In fact it is not necessary to assume that each individual has a latent time of onset of the disease: one can simply characterize the model by the transition intensities.

The choice of constant transition intensities (the hazard function of an exponential law) is a special case because it defines a homogeneous Markov model. One can also choose models with piecewise constant intensities. The relatively simple relationship between intensities and transition probabilities makes these models interesting, especially in the case of interval-censored observations. Alioum et al. (2005) have used such an approach in a complex model (10 states) with interval-censored observations.

Among the parametric models of continuous transition intensities, the intensities of Weibull type are the most used. The Weibull transition intensity for $h \to j$ is:

$$\alpha_{hj}(t, \gamma_{hj}, \rho_{hj}) = \rho_{hj}\gamma_{hj}^{\rho_{hj}}t^{\rho_{hj}-1},$$

where γ_{hj} and ρ_{hj} are parameters. One can choose Weibull transition intensities for all possible transitions. Therefore, this introduces two parameters for each possible transition (as opposed to one parameter in the case of constant intensity transition). Of course, nothing prevents choosing different families for different transitions, for instance Weibull intensities for some transitions and gamma intensities for other transitions, although this is rarely done.

7.3.3 Models for variability: fixed effects and frailties

The inter-individual variability can be explained by explanatory variables in a manner similar to what is done in survival models. The generalization of the proportional hazards model is the proportional intensities model:

$$\alpha_{hj}^i(t) = \alpha_{hj}^0(t) \exp(\beta_{hj}^\top Z_{hj}^i), \qquad (7.9)$$

where the $\alpha_{hj}^0(t)$s are the baseline transition intensities and the Z_{hj}^is are the explanatory variables. The explanatory variables and their effects depend on the transition $h \to j$ considered. We can, as in survival, consider time-dependent variables. The model is completed by assumptions on $\alpha_{hj}^0(t)$.

The Aalen additive model, presented for the survival Section 3.8, was also extended to the multistate case (Aalen et al., 2001).

It is also possible to introduce random effects to account for non-independence of subjects. Joly et al. (2012) developed a fairly complex multistate model for the history of teeth that can undergo several events. The trajectories of the teeth of the same subject cannot be considered independent, and this is modeled by shared random effects (or frailties) for some transitions.

7.3.4 The illness-death model

The most used multistate model in epidemiology is the illness-death model shown in Figure 7.3. It is particularly suited to the study of chronic diseases. Indeed, chronic diseases occur mostly among the elderly and therefore, the risk of death unrelated to the disease under study is not negligible. In this model, the states "healthy," "ill," "dead" are coded respectively 0, 1, 2. So there are three possible transitions: $0 \to 1$, $0 \to 2$, $1 \to 2$. If illness and death are studied in a young population, we can neglect the risk of death from the state "healthy." In this case there are only two transitions: $0 \to 1$, $1 \to 2$, which brings us back to the progressive model shown in Figure 7.2. The state 2 representing death is obviously absorbing.

We can also discuss the irreversible nature of the model. One could consider a reversibility of the disease, corresponding to a recovery, and therefore a transition $1 \to 0$. This may be relevant for a relatively mild illness (e.g., diarrhea) but not for severe illnesses. For example, it is believed that dementia is irreversible. Regarding cancer, remissions can often be obtained by treatments but it is more appropriate to construct a model with an additional state "remission" rather than to consider that the subjects in remission come back to the "healthy" state.

7.4 Observation schemes

7.4.1 Truncation

Observations are often incomplete. The first issue is the selection of the observed sample. In the case of survival, right- and left-truncation conditions are known (see Section 3.3). There is left-truncation if the condition for the individual to be selected is $T_i > V_0^i$, where T_i is the survival time and V_0^i is the truncation variable for subject i. In terms of multistate process, the survival process has two states: $X_i(t) = 0$ if the subject is alive in t, $X_i(t) = 1$ if he is dead. Then, the left-truncation condition is expressed by $X_i(V_0^i) = 0$. This condition can be applied in a more general multistate model, but there are more possibilities. For example, applied to the illness-death model with the three states denoted 0, 1 and 2, the condition $X_i(V_0^i) = 0$ means that healthy subjects are selected. If we want to select subjects who are alive in V_0^i, this is expressed by $X_i(V_0^i) = 0$ *or* 1, or equivalently $X_i(V_0^i) \neq 2$.

Right-truncation defined in Chapter 3 for survival models can also be generalized to multistate models. One can also imagine more general conditions of selection. However, such conditions are rarely encountered in applications.

7.4.2 Right-censoring

We generally have incomplete observations of the trajectories of selected subjects. The most common pattern is comparable to the right-censoring that we know in survival: the trajectory of X_i is observed up to time C_i. So we observe $X_i(t), 0 \leq t \leq C_i$. If there is left-truncation in V_0^i, part of the X_i trajectory, $X_i(t)$ for $0 \leq t \leq V_0^i$, is not informative because we condition on this event.

In the case with right-censoring and left-truncation, non-parametric methods yield estimators easy to calculate and have been well studied theoretically (Andersen et al., 1993). It is also fairly easy to adjust parametric models.

7.4.3 Discrete-time observations: interval-censoring

If the date of death is generally observed in continuous time (i.e., exactly observed or right-censored), the date of onset of illness is often observed in discrete time. This is particularly the case in cohort studies where subjects are examined at dates fixed in advance in the study protocol. When the process is observed in discrete time, the observation is $X(V_0^i), X(V_1^i), \ldots, X(V_M^i)$, where $M \geq 0$ may or may not be a random variable. This type of observations is called "panel data." From a statistical point of view, this scheme creates interval-censored observations of transition times.

Often, the observation pattern is mixed; some transitions are observed in continuous time, others in discrete time. For example, in an illness-death model, the transition to the disease is in general observed in discrete time, while death is most often observed in continuous time. In the case where there is one and only one absorbing state K, $\tilde{T} = \inf(T_K, C)$ is observed, where C is a right-censoring variable and T_K is the entry time into the absorbing state. We observe the process at $M+1$ moments $V_0, \ldots, V_M$ in a state other than K (an observation in K contains no additional information since the transition to K is observed in continuous time). Here $M \geq 0$ is a random variable because we must have $V_M \leq \tilde{T}$.

An example that will be discussed in Section 7.6.6 is that of a study on dementia where subjects are seen at planned visit times and a diagnosis of dementia is made during these visits. If diagnosis of dementia is made for the first time at some visit, this means that the subject developed the disease between this visit and the previous visit. On the other hand, if the subject dies, one can know his/her exact date of death.

As with survival issues, cases of interval-censoring are more complex than the case of right-censoring, and new problems for inference in multistate models arise; this will be discussed in Section 7.6.

7.4.4 Ignorability

As in the context of survival, we have to make some assumptions about the laws of the censoring and truncation variables. The simplest assumption is to consider that censoring and truncation times are fixed. If they are random variables, one must in principle have a model for their distributions. In the case of so-called "independent" censoring and truncation, a factorization of the likelihood avoids this modeling. Mechanisms generating incomplete data are then called "ignorable." The simplest case occurs when these variables are independent of the trajectories of the process of interest. The likelihood is then written as if the times were fixed. In a study where times of visit were planned, this assumption holds. However, this is not always the case. For example, if the observations are collected when subjects spontaneously consult a physician, it is likely that the consulting time is not independent of changes in the health status of the subject. Nevertheless, the mechanism leading to incomplete data can be ignorable in cases where it is not independent from the process of interest. See the definition of independent censoring in Andersen et al. (1993), the definition of coarsening at random (CAR) in Heitjan and Rubin (1991) which extends the missing at random (MAR) concept of Rubin (1976), and the general coarsening model for processes (GCMP) proposed in Commenges and Gégout-Petit (2007). A simple example is when a censoring variable depends on a fixed covariate which is taken into account in the model, so that conditionally on this covariate censoring and process of interest are independent.

7.5 Statistical inference for multistate models observed in continuous time

7.5.1 Likelihood

To rigorously prove the formula of the likelihood, it is necessary to use the theory of counting processes (Andersen et al., 1993). However, this formula can be understood intuitively as explained below. Assume that the process X (here we omit the index i) is observed continuously between V_0 and C, and we observe $R \geq 0$ transitions at times $T_1, T_2, \ldots, T_R$. With the convention $T_0 = V_0$, the likelihood (conditional on $X(V_0)$) can be written as a function of transition probabilities and transition intensities:

$$\mathcal{L} = \Big[\prod_{r=0}^{R-1} P_{X(T_r),X(T_r)}(T_r,T_{r+1}-)\alpha_{X(T_r),X(T_{r+1})}(T_{r+1}) \Big] P_{X(T_R),X(T_R)}(T_R,C), \quad (7.10)$$

for $R \geq 1$. For $R = 0$ the first term disappears and the likelihood is simply $P_{X(T_0),X(T_0)}(T_0,C)$, that is, the probability that X stays in the initial state.

This expression can be intuitively explained. For each value of r one observes that the process stays in the state where it was, $X(T_r)$, between T_r and T_{r+1}: this event has the probability $p_{X(T_r),X(T_r)}(T_r,T_{r+1}-)$ and we observe that the process makes a transition from $X(T_r)$ to $X(T_{r+1})$ at time T_{r+1}; this is done with the risk $\alpha_{X(T_r),X(T_{r+1})}(T_{r+1})$. The last term of the equation is the probability that the process remains in the same state since the last transition until the date of censoring.

Example 14 (R=1) *If one observes a single transition from h to j at time T_1 the likelihood is $P_{hj}(T_0,T_1)\alpha_{hj}(T_1)P_{hh}(T_1,C)$.*

Example 15 (Survival) *In a survival problem, the only possible transition is between 0 and 1; moreover, state 1 being an absorbing state $P_{11}(s,t) = 1$ for all s,t. Thus if one observes the transition (uncensored observation) the likelihood writes $P_{00}(0,T)\alpha_{01}(T)$: this is the likelihoood of an uncensored observation in survival since $P_{00}(0,T)$ is the value of the survival function in T, $S(T)$, and $\alpha_{01}(T)$ is the value of the hazard function in T. If one does not observe the transition after a follow-up up to time C (censored case), the likelihood is simply $P_{00}(C) = S(C)$. We thus retrieve the likelihood classically used in survival problems.*

We can show that the likelihood (7.10) is the same as that obtained by considering each transition $h \to j$ as a survival problem. Subjects who have sojourned in h are contributing to this likelihood. We consider that the observation is truncated to the left at time T_h when the subject entered into h; if he has transitioned to j, the time of the event is observed; if he has transitioned to a state other than j, the observation is considered as censored at the time of transition. If there is no common parameter for the different transitions, we can split the problem in as many survival problems as there are possible transitions, thus creating pseudo-datasets that can be analyzed with softwares adapted to survival data. This procedure is well explained in Andersen and Keiding (2002).

7.5.2   Non-parametric inference: Aalen-Johansen estimator

The non-parametric approach for estimating the law of a multistate process in a homogeneous population is an extension of the Nelson-Aalen estimator of survival, itself equivalent to the Kaplan-Meier method. The Nelson-Aalen estimator is an estimator of the cumulative risk. Using the remark at the end of the previous Section (Section 7.5.1), one can estimate the transition intensities by applying the Nelson-Aalen estimator for each transition. Assuming that the events (transitions) arrive at different times T_r the estimator of A_{hj} jumps at these times:

$$\Delta \hat{A}_{hj}(T_r) = \frac{1}{Y_h(T_r-)},$$

where $Y_h(T_r-)$ is the size of the sample at risk, that is to say the number of subjects in the state h just before time T_r. The estimator $\hat{A}_{hj}$ is constant on the intervals where no transition was observed. From estimators of cumulative intensities, one can construct an estimator for the transition probabilities. The relationship between transition intensities and transition probabilities is given by the Kolmogorov equation whose solution can be expressed as a product-integral form. For non-parametric estimators the solution is simple because there are non-zero probability masses at times when transitions were observed and zero probability on intervals containing no observed transition. So the matrix of transition probabilities at time T_r where a transition $h \rightarrow j$ has been observed is equal to the identity matrix except for the element hj is equal to $\frac{1}{Y_h(T_r)}$ and the element hh which is equal to $1 - \frac{1}{Y_h(T_r)}$. We denote this estimator by $\hat{P}(T_r-, T_r)$. For an interval (s, t) containing no observed transition time, the transition probability matrix is the identity matrix. Using the Chapman-Kolmogorov equation, we can deduce the estimator for an interval that contains $M \geq 1$ observed transition times. The estimator, called the "Aalen-Johansen estimator," is:

$$\hat{P}(s, t) = \prod_{r=1}^{M} \hat{P}(T_r-, T_r).$$

The properties of convergence and asymptotic normality can be established in a similar way as for the Kaplan-Meier estimator (see Andersen et al., 1993).

7.5.3   Inference for semi-parametric regression models

If the interest is in the regression coefficients of a proportional intensities model, inference can be achieved by estimating the decoupled survival problems, as explained in Andersen and Keiding (2002): the principle is that each transition hj can be treated as a survival problem with left-truncated observations since subjects are at risk for the hj-transition only from the time where they entered in state h. An extension of the Aalen additive model has also been proposed by Aalen et al. (2001). Asymptotic properties are comparable to what was obtained in the estimators for semi-parametric survival models.

7.5.4   Parametric inference

Parametric families can be used for transition intensities. If there are explanatory variables, we have to choose a regression model and make assumptions about the baseline transition intensities. In this book, we will restrict ourselves to proportional intensities models. The main method used is maximum likelihood, and MLE has the properties of consistency, efficiency and asymptotic normality. The task is therefore to maximize the likelihood given by (7.10). Calculating the likelihood poses no particular problem except in complex models, especially in reversible models, for which the computation of transition probabilities may not be simple. Maximization can be done conventionally by a Newton-type algorithm.

7.5.5   Inference by penalized likelihood

The penalized likelihood approach provides smooth estimators of transition intensities, without a parametric assumption. Estimators of transition intensities and regression parameters are defined as maximizing the penalized log-likelihood:

$$pL(\boldsymbol{\alpha}(.), \beta) = L(\boldsymbol{\alpha}(.), \beta) - \sum_{h,j>h} \kappa_{hj} \int_0^{\infty} [\alpha''_{hj0}(u)]^2 du, \qquad (7.11)$$

where $L(\boldsymbol{\alpha}(.), \beta)$ is the logarithm of the likelihood (7.10) and the κ_{hj}'s are smoothing parameters. There are as many smoothing parameters as possible direct transitions. The solution to this maximization problem can be approximated on a basis of splines, one for each transition intensity. The choice of the smoothing parameters can be done by optimizing a cross-validation criterion, but this may be difficult numerically.

   As for survival problems, the asymptotic properties are complex and not very well known. In practice, the method gives good results, as shown in some simulation studies (Joly and Commenges, 1999). It is particularly useful in the case of interval-censoring where conventional non-parametric methods become very complex.

7.5.6   Ilness-death model applied to bone-marrow graft

We will illustrate the use of multistate models on an example from the book by Klein and Moeschberger (2003). This is a study of bone marrow transplantation in 136 patients with acute leukemia. Several characteristics were collected at the time of transplantation: age and sex of the donor and recipient, the time between diagnosis and transplantation and the type of disease. Patients were classified into three risk groups: 38 patients with acute lymphocytic leukemia (ALL), 54 patients with acute myeloid leukemia in first remission (AML-LR) and 44 patients with acute myeloid leukemia in second remission (AML-HR). After transplantation, several events may occur: immune reconstitution by a return to normal platelet level (platelet recovery), graft-*vs.*-host disease (GVHD) which can be acute or chronic, relapse or death. Prophylaxis can be administered to prevent and control GVHD. It can be expected that the platelet recovery improves the prognosis and that GVHD deteriorates it, but GVHD can also have a positive impact. Relapse and death can also be considered as competing events. Several multistate models have been considered in the literature to study the problem of bone marrow transplantation (Keiding et al., 2001; Klein and Shu, 2002; Putter et al., 2007). In this section, we will consider an illness-death model: state 0 is the state after transplantation with no platelet recovery, state 1 is obtained after platelet recovery, and state 2 is relapse or death; see Figure 7.4.

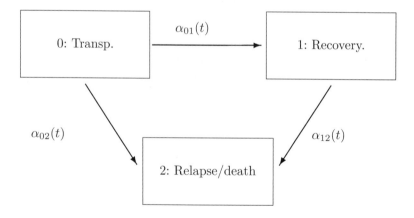

FIGURE 7.4
Irreversible illness-death model.

The objective is to estimate the transition intensities and to study the role of explanatory variables on these intensities. Three explanatory variables are considered: type of disease (ALL, AML-LR or AML-HR), patient's age and presence of prophylaxis against GVHD. In this example, the transitions are assumed to be observed in continuous time and we are interested in the non-parametric and semi-parametric estimation under the proportional intensities model. It is interesting to note that for continuous observation time, estimates can be computed by considering separately each of the three transitions and using conventional analysis techniques for survival data, taking into account right-censoring and left-truncation. We wish here to treat the problem in its entirety using the estimation methods for multistate models. We make a Markov assumption but we assume that all transition intensities may depend on the time since transplantation; this defines a non-homogeneous Markov model. We used the `mstate` package (De Wreede et al., 2010). Patients had an average of 28 years of age at the time of transplantation and 29% of them received prophylaxis against GVHD. For 119 of the 136 patients (87%), platelets returned to normal levels after transplantation; 53 of these 119 patients (44%) subsequently relapsed or died, the other 66 patients (56%) were alive and have not relapsed at the end of the study. Sixteen patients (12%) relapsed or died without having had a platelet recovery and one patient had no event during follow-up. At first, if we do not take into account the explanatory variables, we can estimate the cumulative transition intensities using the Nelson-Aalen estimators:

$$\hat{A}_{hj}(t) = \sum_{t_r \leq t} dN_{hj}(t_r)/Y_h(t_r) \qquad (h \neq j)$$

where the t_r are times of events, $dN_{hj}(t_r)$ is the number of transitions from h to j at time t_r, and $Y_h(t_r)$ the number of at-risk subjects for transition from h to j at time t_r. As mentioned in Section 7.5.2, the Nelson-Aalen estimator has jumps $\Delta\hat{A}_{hj}(t_r) = dN_{hj}(t_r)/Y_h(t_r)$ at event times t_r. Estimates of the three cumulative transition intensities are shown in Figure 7.5. In the first months after transplantation, patients are more likely to restore their immune system by getting their platelets to a normal level than to relapse or die.

From estimators of cumulative intensities $\hat{A}_{hj}(t)$, one can obtain the estimators of transition probabilities $\hat{P}_{hj}(s,t)$ for $s < t$ using Aalen-Johansen formulas as described in Section 7.5.2. Figure 7.6 represents estimated transition probabilities $\hat{P}_{01}(0,t)$, $\hat{P}_{02}(0,t)$ and $\hat{P}_{00}(0,t)$. The transition probabilities do confirm that during the first year after transplantation, patients are more likely to replenish their platelets than to relapse or die.

We can also look at what happens after a short post-transplantation period. For example, we may want to compare the prognosis of patients according to whether they have recovered their platelets to a normal level 100 days after transplantation. To do this, we can compare the probabilities $\hat{P}_{02}(t_{100},t)$ and $\hat{P}_{12}(t_{100},t)$, where $t_{100} = 100/365.25$ represents the 100-day period in years (since we took the time scale in years). Figure 7.7 displays the estimated transition probabilities $\hat{P}_{01}(t_{100},t)$, $\hat{P}_{02}(t_{100},t)$ and $\hat{P}_{00}(t_{100},t)$, on the left, and on the right, the probabilities $\hat{P}_{11}(t_{100},t)$ and $\hat{P}_{12}(t_{100},t)$, for $t > t_{100}$. As was expected $\hat{P}_{01}(t_{100},t)$ is zero, because all patients who have recovered their platelets did it within 100 days post-transplantation. We also note that

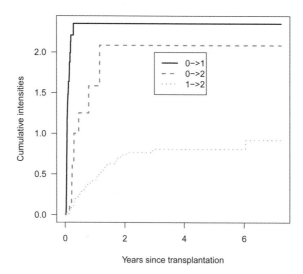

FIGURE 7.5
Estimated cumulative transition intensities for the transplantation study.

the prognosis of patients who have recovered their platelets at 100 days post-transplantation is better than that of patients who have not.

To investigate the role of explanatory variables on the transition intensities, we consider a proportional intensities model $\alpha_{hj}(t) = \alpha_{hj}^0(t) \exp(\beta_{hj}^\top Z_{hj})$, where the $\alpha_{hj}^0(t)$ are the baseline transition intensities and Z_{hj}'s the vectors of explanatory variables. The explanatory variables and their effects depend on the transition $h \to j$ considered. Table 7.1 presents the results obtained with the model with three explanatory variables: type of disease, patient age and prophylaxis against GVHD.

TABLE 7.1
Estimated relative risks of factors associated with platelet recovery and relapse/death in transplanted patients; the relative risks which are significantly different from 1 at the 5% level are indicated by an asterisk.

| | Type of disease (reference : ALL) | | | |
Transition	AML-LR	AML-HR	Age	Prophylaxis
$0 \,--> 1$	0.95	0.63	1.01	0.38*
$0 \,--> 2$	8.95*	7.43*	0.99	4.89*
$1 \,--> 2$	0.43*	1.21*	1.01	1.19*

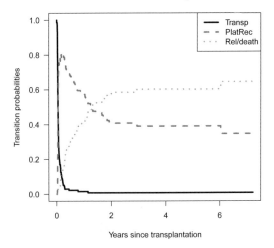

FIGURE 7.6
Estimated probabilities to be in states 0 (Transp), 1 (PlatRec) and 2 (Rel/death).

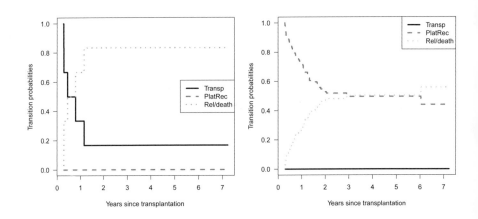

FIGURE 7.7
Estimated transition probabilities starting from state 0 (left) and from state 1 (right) 100 days after transplantation.

The results indicate that the risk of relapse/death without platelet recovery was higher in patients with myeloid leukemia (AML-LR and AML-HR) compared to those with a lymphoid leukemia (ALL): $\widehat{\text{HR}} = 8.95$ for AML-LR patients and $\widehat{\text{HR}} = 7.43$ for patients AML-HR. Patients who received prophylaxis were surprisingly less likely to retrieve their platelets to normal levels and had an increased risk of direct relapse/death.

7.6 Inference for multistate models from interval-censored data

7.6.1 Likelihood

When the multistate process is observed in discrete time, the likelihood is easy to write in terms of transition probabilities. Obtaining the likelihood poses no theoretical problem because in this case the observed events have non-zero probability. If one observes X at $V_0, V_1, \ldots, V_M$, assuming that the mechanism generating these times is ignorable, the general formula for the probability conditional on $X(V_0)$ is:

$$\mathcal{L} = \prod_{m=0}^{M-1} P_{X(V_m), X(V_{m+1})}(V_m, V_{m+1}). \tag{7.12}$$

Even if the likelihood is easy to write, it is not necessarily easy to calculate because the relationship between transition probabilities and transition intensities may not be simple. Note that in this case we cannot factorize the likelihood such that each factor contains only one transition intensity; thus it is not possible to decouple the problem in several survival problems as in the continuous observation case (Section 7.5.1).

The most common observation scheme is actually a mixed observation scheme where some transitions are observed in continuous time and others in discrete time. If death is represented by an absorbing state K, the transition to this state is most commonly observed in continuous time. Transitions to other states related to a disease can often be observed only in discrete time. Suppose we observe $(\tilde{T}, \delta)$ where $\tilde{T} = \inf(T_K, C)$ and $\delta = 1_{\{T_K \leq C\}}$, and where T_K is the time of death and C a right-censoring variable; moreover X is observed in M occasions $V_0, V_1, \ldots, V_M < \tilde{T}$. For such an observation scheme, it is necessary to use the theory of counting processes to rigorously establish the likelihood and this demonstration is more difficult than in the case of continuous observation time (Commenges and Gégout-Petit, 2007).

Still assuming an ignorable mechanism for generating such observation times, the probability conditional on $X(V_0)$ is, for $M \geq 1$:

$$\mathcal{L} = \prod_{m=0}^{M-1} P_{X(V_m),X(V_{m+1})}(V_m, V_{m+1}) \sum_{j \neq K} P_{X(V_M),j}(V_M, \tilde{T}-)\alpha_{j,K}(\tilde{T})^\delta. \qquad (7.13)$$

The first term is similar to the likelihood for discrete-time observation. The last term expresses the fact that the process could pass through any state other than K between V_M and $\tilde{T}$; according to the value of δ one observes whether it transited to state K or not before $\tilde{T}$. As in the previous case, the computational difficulty lies in the difficulty of computing the transition probabilities.

7.6.2 Non-parametric inference

Here, non-parametric inference is much more difficult than for continuous-time observation. We can try to extend the approach of Peto-Turnbull to the multistate case. The difficulty is that there is no simple estimator of cumulative transition intensities here. Moreover, for non-progressive multistate models, it is not only the transition times which are not known exactly, but the states visited between two observation times may also be unknown. Frydman (1995) and Frydman and Szarek (2009) proposed non-parametric estimators for the illness-death model, but the great complexity, both theoretical and numerical, of this approach makes it difficult to use.

7.6.3 Parametric inference

In the case of parametric models, there is no particular theoretical difficulty. The only difficulty may be due to computing the transition probabilities involved in the likelihood. The formulas can be more or less complex depending on the complexity of the model and often involve numerical integrals.

A special case is that of homogeneous Markov models for which one can obtain the transition probabilities easily by Formula (7.7). This property has been exploited to perform inference in models with piecewise constant intensities that are less rigid than homogeneous models (Alioum and Commenges, 2001). This approach was used to model the evolution of HIV-infected subjects by Alioum et al. (2005).

An approximate approach has been proposed by Jackson (2011) and implemented in R in the msm package. The approximation assumes that the intensities are constant between two observations of the process. This assumption greatly simplifies the calculations because we know which state the process is in when the intensities change. However, this is not really correct because in principle the model should not depend on the observations. If times of change of intensity values depend on the observations, it means that they should be considered as parameters; anyway, there is no reason why these changes occur at observation times. However, the msm package now allows defining periods when intensities are constant regardless of the observations, at the price of heavier computations.

7.6.4 Inference by penalized likelihood

As in the case of continuous-time observation, penalized likelihood is given by the Formula (7.11). The difference is that the likelihood itself is calculated using Formulas (7.12) or (7.13) as appropriate. The advantage of the penalized likelihood is that it can be applied without difficulty to the additional problems raised by interval censoring. The only additional difficulty is, as in the parametric case, the more difficult computation of transition probabilities.

It has been applied especially in a progressive three-state model, shown in Figure 7.2, that represents the trajectory of hemophiliacs who could be infected with HIV and develop AIDS (Joly and Commenges, 1999). It has also been applied in the context of an illness-death model and even in an extension of this model to a five-state model by Joly et al. (2009).

7.6.5 Inference for the illness-death model in case of interval censoring

7.6.5.1 The illness-death models with a mixed observation scheme

The illness-death model is particularly suitable for modeling chronic diseases where death is represented by the absorbing state 2. It is very common that the occurrence of the disease is observed in discrete time and death is observed in continuous time. It is a mixed observation pattern. When the number of observations M is greater than 1, the likelihood takes the form:

$$\mathcal{L} = \prod_{m=0}^{M-1} P_{X(V_m),X(V_{m+1})}(V_m, V_{m+1}) \sum_{j \neq 2} P_{X(V_M),j}(V_M, \tilde{T}-)\alpha_{j,2}(\tilde{T})^\delta. \quad (7.14)$$

Here, $X(V_M)$ may be equal to 0 (no observation in the disease state) or equal to 1 (at least one observation in the disease state). This formula takes specific forms depending on the observations and we can distinguish two cases.

- $X(V_M) = 0$: the subject stays in state 0 until V_M. The likelihood is thus:

$$\mathcal{L} = P_{00}(0, V_M)[P_{00}(V_M, \tilde{T}-)\alpha_{02}(\tilde{T})^\delta + P_{01}(V_M, \tilde{T}-)\alpha_{12}(\tilde{T})^\delta]. \quad (7.15)$$

- $X(V_M) = 1$: the subject stays in state 0 until V_l and is observed in state 1 in V_{l+1}, until V_M. The likelihood is thus:

$$\mathcal{L} = P_{00}(0, V_l)P_{01}(V_l, V_{l+1})P_{11}(V_{l+1}, \tilde{T}-)\alpha_{12}(\tilde{T})^\delta. \quad (7.16)$$

Note that in the first case (unobserved disease) it is not known if the disease has occurred or not between the last observation time and the follow-up time

$\tilde{T}$, and one sees in the likelihood the sum of two terms corresponding to the two possible paths. This is a novelty compared to survival problems. It is not only that the transition time is not observed exactly, we do not know if the transition took place or not.

7.6.6 Application of the illness-death model to dementia

The illness-death model was used by Joly et al. (2002) to model the onset of dementia in the elderly. In this work, the transition intensities were estimated by penalized likelihood because the goal was mainly descriptive: to estimate the incidence of dementia according to age. Leffondré et al. (2013) compared the estimators of relative risks of three explanatory variables (education, hypertension, smoking) on the transition to dementia obtained with a survival model and an illness-death model.

We will illustrate the use of the illness-death model through a random sub-sample of the Paquid cohort presented in the introduction Section 1.4.1. The sample consists of 1000 subjects. The event of interest in this example is the occurrence of dementia that is competing with death, and the 20 years follow-up of the cohort was chosen as the date of analysis. The basic time-scale used for all transitions is age. So there is left-truncation because the subjects were selected as alive and without dementia at entry into the cohort. The age of onset of dementia is interval-censored, while the date of death is exactly known, or right-censored. Interval-censoring has two consequences in this example, as it was presented in the previous paragraph. The first is that for subjects diagnosed with dementia, the age of onset of dementia is not known but is between the subject's age at the last visit without dementia and age at the diagnostic visit. The second is that for all deceased individuals who were non-demented at their last visit, we have to take into account the possibility that they could develop dementia between their last visit and death. In this sample 186 subjects were diagnosed with dementia during the follow-up and 724 died, and among them 597 died without a diagnosis of dementia. Because of interval-censoring, it is likely that more than 186 of the 1000 subjects became demented during follow-up. There are two explanatory variables in the sample: sex and educational level. There were 578 women and 422 men; 762 subjects had a primary education level and 238 did not. We used the R Package SmoothHazard to fit the model (this sample is provided with the package). We tried two approaches: parametric, with Weibull intensities, and penalized likelihood. For each subject there is an indicator of dementia, an indicator of death, age at study entry (for left-truncation), age at the last visit without dementia (possibly equal to age at entry), age at diagnosis of dementia (not used if the indicator of dementia is zero), age at death or right-censoring, and finally the value of the two binary explanatory variables. The variable sex is coded 1 for men and 0 for women and educational level is coded 0 if the subject had a primary educational level, 1 otherwise.

We used proportional intensities models. There are three transition intensities and both explanatory variables are included for all transitions. In Table 7.2 we present the results in terms of hazard ratios for all transitions and for both approaches.

TABLE 7.2
Analysis of risk factors for onset of dementia and death in 1000 subjects of the Paquid cohort: relative risk (HR) estimates, confidence intervals 95%(CI), HR for illness-death models with a parametric approach (Weibull) or penalized likelihood.

		Weibull		Penalized likelihood	
Transition	Variables	$\widehat{HR}$	CI 95%	$\widehat{HR}$	CI 95%
$0 \longrightarrow 1$	Sex	0.89	[0.65 ; 1.21]	0.95	[0.68 ; 1.32]
	Primary level	0.59	[0.40 ; 0.88]	0.61	[0.40 ; 0.91]
$0 \longrightarrow 2$	Sex	1.71	[1.35 ; 2.16]	1.64	[1.29 ; 2.08]
	Primary level	1.13	[0.89 ; 1.45]	1.13	[0.88 ; 1.46]
$1 \longrightarrow 2$	Sex	1.78	[1.24 ; 2.57]	1.92	[1.31 ; 2.82]
	Primary level	0.81	[0.52 ; 1.28]	0.81	[0.51 ; 1.30]

As can be seen in Table 7.2, the estimated values of the relative risks of the two approaches are close. In terms of interpretation, men are more likely to die (transitions to state 2) at any age than women, whether demented or not, and those with primary educational level have less risk, at any age, to develop dementia than those who do not have it.

Figures 7.8 and 7.9 show the three estimated transition intensities for the two approaches. These transition intensities were estimated with models without explanatory variables. Here, the difference between the parametric model and the penalized likelihood approach is more visible. The mortality rate of demented estimated by the penalized likelihood is not compatible with a parametric Weibull assumption.

In addition to the transition intensities and regression parameters, many other quantities can be estimated from an illness-death model. For example, cumulative incidences as presented in Chapter 6 or life expectancies presented in the following Section 7.8. This topic is developed in Andersen and Keiding (2012) and Touraine et al. (2013). In this application we will first present the cumulative incidences.

Figures 7.10 and 7.11 present the "cumulative incidences", defined in the context of competing risks by Equation (6.5), and which can be applied to the

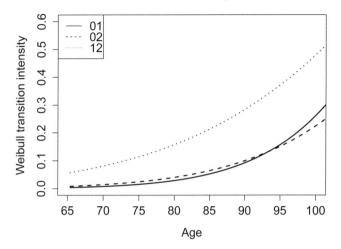

FIGURE 7.8
Estimated transition intensities with Weibull intensities obtained from a sample of 1000 subjects from the Paquid cohort.

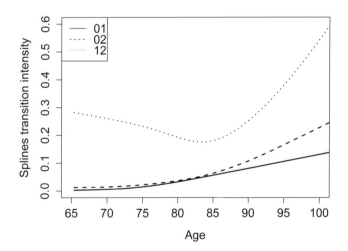

FIGURE 7.9
Penalized likelihood estimates of transition intensities obtained from a sample of 1000 subjects from the Paquid cohort.

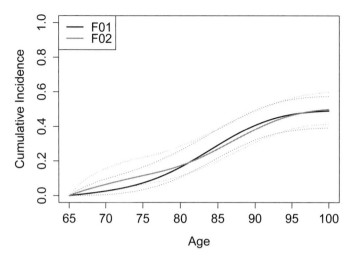

FIGURE 7.10
Estimated cumulative incidences and their 95% confidence intervals, with a penalized likelihood approach for an alive and not demented 65-year-old woman.

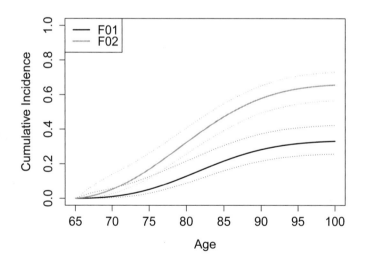

FIGURE 7.11
Estimated cumulative incidences and their 95% confidence intervals, with a penalized likelihood approach for an alive and not demented 65-year-old man.

present model with the following definition:

$$F_{01}(65, t) = \int_{65}^{t} e^{-A_{01}(65,u)-A_{02}(65,u)} \alpha_{01}(u)du$$

$$F_{02}(65, t) = \int_{65}^{t} e^{-A_{01}(65,u)-A_{02}(65,u)} \alpha_{02}(u)du$$

with $A_{01}(s, t) = \int_{s}^{t} \alpha_{01}(u)du$ et $A_{02}(s, t) = \int_{s}^{t} \alpha_{02}(u)du$.

These functions are interpreted as follows: for a subject living and not demented at age 65, $F_{01}(65, t)$ is the probability that he/she became demented between 65 years and t, and $F_{02}(65, t)$ the probability that he/she dies without having been demented between 65 years and t. For this, we estimated the intensities of transitions for an illness-death model separately for men and women, and then we computed the desired functions. All these calculations were made with the SmoothHazard R package, and using a penalized likelihood approach. In theory $F_{01}(+\infty) + F_{02}(+\infty) = 1$. In this example, the calculations were made up to 100 years because there was little information after this age, and so we did not have exactly $F_{01}(65, 100) + F_{02}(65, 100) = 1$. It may be noted in Figures 7.10 and 7.11 that the probability for a man to become demented before death is less than 0.4 (actually 0.34 at 100 years) and is lower than for a woman. For women, on the contrary we see that the probability of becoming demented before dying is close to 0.5.

Another way to represent the "cumulative incidences" is to interpret them as "absolute risks." For this, we plot the following function for men and women:

$$F_{01}(t, 100) = \int_{t}^{100} e^{-A_{01}(t,u)-A_{02}(t,u)} \alpha_{01}(u)du \quad \text{with } t > 65.$$

This function is interpreted as the probability that a subject becomes demented between t and 100 years knowing that the subject is alive and not demented at age t. In fact to calculate the "true" "absolute risks," one must compute it until $+\infty$.

It may be noted in Figure 7.12 that the "risk" for a man alive and not demented to develop dementia before dying grows slowly until about 92 years, before declining sharply. For women it is higher than for men up to 90 years; it began to decline at 75 years.

As presented in Section 7.2.6, it is possible, from the transition intensities to compute the probability of being in a certain state at any time. To illustrate this with the example used in this paragraph, the probabilities $P_{00}(65, t)$, $P_{01}(65, t)$, $P_{02}^{1}(65, t)$ and $P_{02}^{0}(65, t)$ were calculated. They represent the probability for a subject alive and not demented at 65 years, to be respectively alive and non-demented, alive and demented, dead after having been demented, and

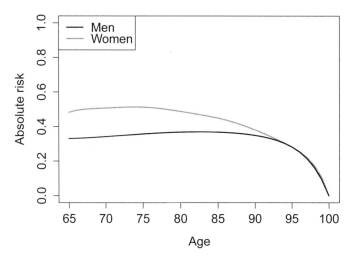

FIGURE 7.12
Penalized likelihood estimates of absolute risks (up to 100 years) for men and women according to age where they are alive and non-demented.

dead without having been demented, at age t. Their expressions are:

$$P_{00}(s,t) = e^{-A_{01}(s,t)-A_{02}(s,t)},$$

$$P_{01}(s,t) = \int_s^t e^{-A_{01}(s,u)-A_{02}(s,u)}\alpha_{01}(u)e^{-A_{12}(u,t)}du,$$

$$P_{02}^1(s,t) = \int_s^t e^{-A_{01}(s,u)-A_{02}(s,u)}\alpha_{01}(u)\int_u^t e^{-A_{12}(u,v)}\alpha_{12}(v)dudv,$$

$$P_{02}^0(s,t) = \int_s^t e^{-A_{01}(s,u)-A_{02}(s,u)}\alpha_{02}(u)du,$$

with $A_{12}(s,t) = \int_s^t \alpha_{12}(u)du$.

In Figure 7.13 are represented (in aggregate form) the estimates of probabilities $P_{00}(65,t)$, $P_{01}(65,t)$, $P_{02}^1(65,t)$ and $P_{02}^0(65,t)$ for women aged 66 to 100 years. In this figure, for each age for an alive and not-demented 65-year-old woman, the probability of being alive and not demented is represented in lighter gray. The little less clear gray part is the probability of being demented, then one has the probability of being dead after being demented; and finally, in dark gray, the probability of being dead without having been demented. With the illness-death model, these four probabilities sum to 1, and we notice that at 100 years the probability of being dead (represented by the 2 darker

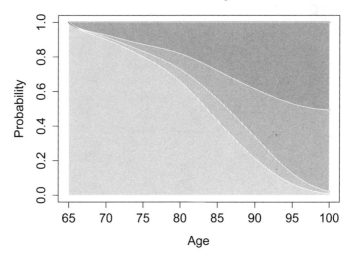

FIGURE 7.13
Estimated transition probabilities $P_{00}(65,t)$, $P_{01}(65,t)$, $P_{02}^1(65,t)$ and $P_{02}^0(65,t)$ for women, with a penalized likelihood approach.

parts) is close to 1. The corresponding probabilities for men are presented in Figure 7.14.

Finally, it is also possible to calculate the overall life expectancy, the disease-free life expectancy and the life expectancy of a demented subject; these computations are detailed in Section 7.7. For example in Figure 7.15 are plotted overall life expectancies of alive and non-demented men and women. This corresponds to the following function:

$$\mathrm{E}[T \mid X(s) = 0] \quad = \quad \int_s^\infty [P_{00}(s,u) + P_{01}(s,u)]du,$$

Note in Figure 7.15 that the life expectancy for women is greater than the life expectancy of men aged 65 to 88 years. Then life expectancies differ little from each other, even if that for men is slightly higher. These estimators were calculated separately for men and women with two illness-death models using a penalized likelihood approach.

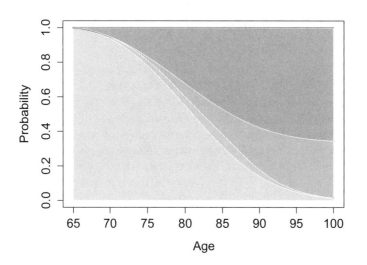

FIGURE 7.14
Estimated transition probabilities $P_{00}(65, t)$, $P_{01}(65, t)$, $P_{02}^1(65, t)$ and $P_{02}^0(65, t)$ for men, with a penalized likelihood.

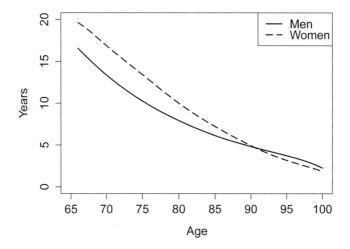

FIGURE 7.15
Estimates of overall life expectancies (in years) for non-demented men and women as a function of age (penalized likelihood approach)

7.7 Complex functions of parameters: individualized hazards, sojourn times

Uses of multistate models are discussed in Andersen and Perme (2008) and Putter et al. (2007); Touraine et al. (2013) focused on this issue for the illness-death model. The approaches presented in the previous sections provide estimators of transition intensities and transition probabilities for models with proportional intensities and these estimators have a direct interest. From these estimators, however, we can estimate other interesting quantities. An interesting property of the maximum likelihood is that if $\gamma = g(\theta)$, and $\hat{\theta}$ is the MLE of θ, $g(\hat{\theta})$ is the MLE of γ. A first application is to estimate the transition intensities for an individual with explanatory variables Z_i:

$$\hat{\alpha}_{hj}^i(t) = \hat{\alpha}_{hj}^0(t) \exp(\hat{\beta}_{hj}^\top Z_{hj}^i), \qquad (7.17)$$

Transition intensities (together with the initial state) characterize the law of the multistate process. So all the interesting quantities can be estimated by substituting in the relations $\hat{\alpha}_{hj}^i(t)$ for $\alpha_{hj}^i(t)$. In particular one can estimate the transition probabilities. Among the transition probabilities, $P_{hj}(0,t)$ gives the probability that the process is in state j at time t, given it was in the state h at start. If one assigns a probability to the initial state $\pi_h(0)$ the probability of being in state j at time t, or state occupation probability, is $\pi_j(t) = \sum_{h=0}^K \pi_h(0) P_{hj}(0,t)$. However, in many medical applications it is assumed that subjects start from state 0, i.e., $\pi_0(0) = 1$, so the probability of being in state j in t is simply $P_{0j}(0,t)$.

We can obviously individualize these calculations, since if there are explanatory variables different subjects do not have the same transition intensities. Some of these explanatory variables may depend on time. In general, it is possible to make personalized prediction at any time u and for any event A^i (relative to subject i), i.e., estimate the probability:

$$P_i(A^i \mid \mathcal{H}_u^i),$$

where $\mathcal{H}_u^i$ represents the available information at u for subject i; for a Markov process, this information reduces to $X_i(u)$, the state of the subject at time u and this probability depends on the values of the explanatory variables. If there are time-dependent explanatory variables, we can still do this calculation if the future values of these variables are known. Otherwise, it leads to more complex models (joint models, see Chapter 8) because one must also model the evolution of these variables.

Another interesting application is to calculate the distribution of the sojourn time in a given state. The sojourn time in state j can be written $T(j) = \int_0^\infty 1_{X(t)=j} dt$. If $A_v = \{T(j) < v\}$, we can estimate its probability. Knowing the probabilities A_v for all v is to know the distribution of sojourn time in j. However, this calculation is difficult in the general case. Fortunately, expected sojourn time is often sufficient in applications. Its calculation is quite simple because we have:

$$\mathrm{E}[T(j)] = \int_0^\infty \mathrm{E}[1_{X(t)=j}]\mathrm{d}t = \int_0^\infty \mathrm{P}[X(t) = j]\mathrm{d}t.$$

It is therefore necessary to integrate the probability of being in state j, which, if the initial state is 0, is equal to $P_{0j}(0,t)$. A special case of this equation is the life expectancy in a survival model, which is equal to $\int_0^\infty S(t)\mathrm{d}t$.

We can also estimate expected sojourn times conditionally on $X(u)$. Joly et al. (2009) have calculated the life expectancy for healthy, demented or institutionalized subjects for different ages.

Example 16 (Life expectancy of a subject diseased at time s.) *In a Markov illness-death model, the expected (future) sojourn time in the diseased state knowing that the subject is in the diseased state at time s is*

$$\int_s^\infty \mathrm{P}(X(t) = 1)\mathrm{d}t = \int_s^\infty P_{11}(s,t)\mathrm{d}t = \int_s^\infty e^{-A_{12}(s,t)}\mathrm{d}t,$$

where $A_{12}(s,t) = \int_s^t \alpha_{12}(u)\mathrm{d}u$ is the cumulative death intensity for diseased subjects between s and t. For a homogeneous model where α_{12} is constant, this integral is easy to calculate and we obtain $1/\alpha_{12}$. In other cases, the integral can be difficult to calculate analytically and is computed numerically.

Example 17 (Life expectancy without disease at time s.) *In a Markov illness-death model the expected (future) sojourn time in the healthy state knowing that the subject is healthy at time s is $\int_s^\infty \mathrm{P}(X(t) = 0)\mathrm{d}t = \int_s^\infty P_{00}(s,t)\mathrm{d}t = \int_s^\infty e^{-A_{02}(s,t)-A_{01}(s,t)}\mathrm{d}t$. The disease-free life expectancy at time 0, for a subject healthy at time 0, is given by this expression taking $s = 0$.*

Example 18 (Expectation of sojourn time in the diseased state.) *The calculation of the expected sojourn time in the diseased state is more complex because the entry time in the diseased state is random and the subject may die before becoming ill. However, we can apply the general formula:*

$$\mathrm{E}[T(1)] = \int_0^\infty \mathrm{P}(X(t) = 1)\mathrm{d}t = \int_0^\infty P_{01}(0,t)\mathrm{d}t.$$

The computation appears more complex because $P_{01}(0,t)$ already involves an integral, which leads to a double integral. This computation is feasible numerically. This expectation can also be expressed as: $\mathrm{E}[T(1)] = \mathrm{E}[T(0) + T(1)] - \mathrm{E}[T(0)]$. $\mathrm{E}[T(0)+T(1)]$ is the overall life expectancy. This yields a simple approach to compute $\mathrm{E}[T(1)]$ because there are simple formulas for $\mathrm{E}[T(0)]$ and $\mathrm{E}[T(0) + T(1)]$.

The variance of the estimates of the expected sojourn times may be computed either by the delta method in simple cases or by simulation (see Section 2.3.2.2). In the simulation procedure, the parameter values (i.e., transition intensities) are generated from the asymptotic distribution of the MLE, and the expected sojourn times are then calculated for these values. This generates a sample of the distribution of the estimates of the expected sojourn time and one can thus evaluate the standard error associated with this estimate.

7.8 Approach by counting processes

As we mentioned in the introduction, a multistate process can be represented by a counting process, in general a multivariate counting process. There are two ways. The first is to associate with every possible hj transition a counting process N_{hj} which counts the hj transitions performed by the process. If the multistate process does not involve recurrent states, the N_{hj} is a $0-1$ counting process. The second way is more parsimonious in the number of processes; we consider that the states are the intersection of several counting processes. For example, in the illness-death model, we are interested in two events: occurrence of disease and death. We can represent each of these events by a $0-1$ counting process. Therefore, we consider a bivariate counting process $N = (N_1, N_2)$, where N_1 counts the occurrence of the disease and N_2 counts the death. The law of the Markov illness-death process with transition intensities $\alpha_{01}(t), \alpha_{02}(t), \alpha_{12}(t)$ can be described by a bivariate counting process $N = (N_1, N_2)$ with intensities:

$$\lambda_1(t) = 1_{\{N_{1t-}=0\}} 1_{\{N_{2t-}=0\}} \alpha_{01}(t) \tag{7.18}$$

$$\lambda_2(t) = 1_{\{N_{2t-}=0\}} [1_{\{N_{1t-}=0\}} \alpha_{02}(t) + 1_{\{N_{1t-}=1\}} \alpha_{12}(t)]. \tag{7.19}$$

In this case a three-state process is represented by a bivariate counting process. The intersection of two $0-1$ processes should create four states, but in the multistate process we do not distinguish between states "death with disease" and "death without disease." Joly et al. (2009) used a five-state process, with eight possible transitions to jointly model dementia, institutionalization and death. This process can also be represented by a three-variate counting process. When more than two events are involved, there is an advantage to model as a counting process because the associated multistate processes have many states and many possible transitions. This approach has not been much used in modeling; see examples in Andersen et al. (1993) and Arjas (Arjas).

Another advantage is the direct link with Jacod formula which enables to rigorously establish the likelihood of observation of these processes (Commenges and Gégout-Petit, 2007).

7.9   Other approaches

Because of the complex relationship between the transition intensities and transition probabilities, the effects of explanatory variables on certain quantities of interest (such as the probability of occupation of a given state) are themselves complex and can be difficult to interpret. One can make curves of probabilities to be in particular states for different profiles of explanatory variables. For ease of interpretation, summaries of these effects should be developed, a development which has not yet been done. In order to obtain estimates of the effects of explanatory variables which are easy to interpret, several authors have proposed models for direct regression of quantities of interest. Fine and Gray (1999) proposed such an approach for competing risks problems. We briefly present two approaches that have been proposed for multistate models: the landmark approach and the pseudo-values approach.

7.9.1   Prediction by "landmarking"

van Houwelingen and Putter (2008) proposed a "landmarking" approach for predictions, as an alternative to the use of multistate models. The authors illustrate the approach in a study of bone marrow transplantation. A full description of the problem lends itself to representation by a multistate model, as we have seen in Section 7.5.6. A seven-state model can be built, where the states are generated by the events graft against host disease (GVHD), platelet recovery (two categories) and failure (death or relapse). However, the objective here is to make a dynamic prediction of the probability of failure-free survival of transplantation at a horizon of 5 years, and the aim of the landmarking approach is to avoid the development of a complex multistate model. The method is to build Cox models for predictions at a number of times, called "landmarks." In this example, the authors propose to take 25 landmark times spread over the first year: $t_{LM} = 0, 1/24, 2/24, \ldots, 1$. For all these time points, the sample consists of individuals at risk, and the explanatory variables take the values they have at these times. The regression coefficients depend on the prediction time. In this example, a linear model is proposed to describe the evolution of the coefficients with time: $\beta(s) = \beta_0 + \beta_1 s$. All data are pooled, and to estimate the variances of the estimators, the sandwich estimator of Lin and Wei (1989) is used. The authors show that the predicted survival probabilities at different times are close to those obtained by using a multistate model.

7.9.2   Pseudo-values approach

Andersen and Klein (2007) proposed a pseudo-value approach to study the effect of (not time-dependent) explanatory variables on certain quantities of interest. The pseudo-value approach is a general method to perform rather simple regression analyses in complex cases with incomplete data. If X is the observable random quantity, we are interested in the quantity $f(X)$ and we want to make a regression of this quantity, i.e., estimating a model for $E[f(X_i) \mid Z_i]$, where Z_i is a vector of explanatory variables. To do this, one can consider a generalized linear model of the form:

$$g\{E[f(X_i) \mid Z_i]\} = \beta^\top Z_i.$$

If one observes X_i, this regression can be directly performed by using maximum likelihood or estimating equations (GEE). In cases where we do not observe X_i (censored data) the pseudo-value approach (Andersen and Perme, 2010) replaces $E[f(X_i) \mid Z_i]$ by an estimate $\hat{\theta}_i$. If the expectation of this pseudo-value $\hat{\theta}_i$ equals $E[f(X_i) \mid Z_i]$, it satisfies the same regression model as $f(X_i)$ since we have: $E(\hat{\theta}_i) = E[f(X_i) \mid Z_i] = g^{-1}(\beta^\top Z_i)$. We therefore have a model for the expectation of $\hat{\theta}_i$; if one does not know the other moments of the distribution, one cannot estimate the regression model by maximum likelihood, but it can be done by GEE. The estimating equation is:

$$\sum_i [\frac{\partial g^{-1}(\beta^\top Z_i)}{\partial \beta}]^\top V_i^{-1} \frac{\partial g^{-1}(\beta^\top Z_i)}{\partial \beta} = 0,$$

where the V_i's are working covariance matrices. To calculate the pseudo-values, we must have an unbiased estimator $\hat{\theta}$ of $\theta = E[f(X)]$ (the marginal expectation of X: $E(\hat{\theta}) = \theta = E[f(X)]$). The pseudo-value $\hat{\theta}_i$ is defined by:

$$\hat{\theta}_i = n\hat{\theta} - (n-1)\hat{\theta}^{-i},$$

where $\hat{\theta}^{-i}$ is the estimator $\hat{\theta}$ applied to the initial sample deprived of observation i.

Andersen and Klein (2007) have shown that this approach can be applied to a regression of the variable indicating state occupation by a multistate process. For example, in the illness-death model the variable $f(X)$ can be $f(X) = 1_{\{X(75)=1\}}$. In this case, the expectation of this variable is the probability of being in the diseased state at time $t = 75$. The marginal unbiased estimator of this probability is the Aalen-Johansen estimator of $P_{01}(0, 75)$, assuming that individuals start from state 0 in $t = 0$. They applied this approach in a study of patients who received a bone marrow transplant to treat leukemia. They considered a model with six states, including two remission states, and were interested in the effects of variables on the probability of remission states. This approach makes it easier to demonstrate the effect of these variables than modeling transition intensities and is relatively easy to implement.

8

Joint models for longitudinal and time-to-event data

8.1 Introduction

The previous chapters of this book focused on models for the two major types of data collected in longitudinal studies. Chapters 4 and 5 describe models for longitudinal data defined as repeated measurements of quantitative or categorical variables, while Chapters 3 and 6 cover models for censored time-to-events. In cohort studies, these two types of data are frequently collected during the follow-up and their joint modelling is useful for various purposes.

Joint models for longitudinal data and censored time-to-events have been developed since the late 1990s; however, they were little used until the late 2000s because of their complexity and the lack of software. The situation changed with the release of several R packages dedicated to these models (JM, JMbayes, joineR and lcmm), and also of some functions in general statistical software (such as stjm in Stata or JMFit in SAS) and the publication of a monograph on some of these models (Rizopoulos, 2012b).

Much remains to be done to promote the dissemination of joint models. The aim of this chapter is to contribute to give a full description and comparison of the value and limitations of each of the two major types of joint models (shared random effects models and latent class models) as well as illustrations using the R packages JM and lcmm.

Joint modelling of repeated measurements of a marker and the risk of an event is useful in three situations:

(1) to study the trajectory of a marker when subject follow-up is censored by the event;

(2) to predict the risk of the event based on repeated measures of the marker;

(3) to explore the association between the marker change over time and the risk of the event.

Objective (1) addresses the problem of non-random missing longitudinal data briefly discussed in Section 4.5.3. The objective is to estimate without bias the mean marker change over time and the effect of factors on this change by jointly modelling either directly the dropout risk or the risk of an event that may cause the stop of the observation of repeated measurements of the marker (when the event is death, for example) or a major change in the dynamics of the marker (when the event is a change of treatment or some clinical events for instance).

For example, repeated measures of the prostate specific antigen (PSA) are used to monitor patients treated for prostate cancer. When cancer relapse occurs, the regular collection of PSA measurements can be continued, but because of the relapse and the set-up of new treatments, the dynamics of the PSA is completely changed. Similarly, the trajectory of the two major biomarkers (CD4 counts and HIV viral load) for monitoring HIV patients changes dramatically after switching to the AIDS stage or after the initiation of antiretroviral treatments.

In both examples, the most common strategy of data analysis is to eliminate the marker measures posterior to the occurrence of the event (relapse, AIDS, or change of treatment) in order to study the marker trajectory before the event (the post-event changes possibly being studied separately). Thereby, the measures collected after the event are thought of as missing. As the event changes the dynamics of the marker, the distribution of the missing data is different from that of the observed data knowing the past measures. These missing data are thus *informative* or *Missing Not At Random* (MNAR, see Section 4.5.3). Remember that the maximum likelihood estimator of a mixed model provides unbiased estimates only under the MAR assumption, that is assuming that the trajectory of the marker is not changed by the occurrence of the event that terminates the observation of the marker. Joint modelling is one of the approaches proposed for estimating without bias the evolution of the marker using incomplete informative data. It also allows estimating the marker change over time for subjects free of the event or conditionally on the time of the event.

Objective (2) (prediction of the risk of the event according to repeated measures of the marker) could be reached by using a time-to-event model (for instance, a Cox model) with time-dependent explanatory variables. However, this approach suffers from several limitations. First, the marker is usually measured with error and only at discrete times, while estimating a Cox model by the partial likelihood requires the knowledge of the exact values of explanatory variables at each time of event for all the individuals at risk. Imputation of the marker value for each subject and each time of event is therefore necessary. Typically the last observed value is imputed. It is not advised to interpolate between the previous value and the first value measured after the event-time because this would introduce a dependence of the current risk on future values of the marker. However, when the intervals between measurements are large, the assumption of constancy between two measurements is not plausible and the estimated parameter associated with the marker in the survival model are biased. This bias also increases when the measurement error is large (Prentice, 1982). On the other hand, as discussed in Section 3.5.7, Cox model with time-dependent covariate is suitable only for *exogeneous* or *external* variables. Exogenous variables must remain measurable and their distributions must be unchanged after the occurrence of the event. If $Y(t)$ is the time-dependent variable at time t, $\mathcal{H}(s)$ the set of measures of Y until time s and T the time-to-event, $Y(t)$ is exogeneous if:

$$f_{Y(t)}(y \mid T \geq s, \mathcal{H}(s)) = f_{Y(t)}(y \mid T = s, \mathcal{H}(s)) \text{ for } t \geq s$$

or

$$
\begin{aligned}
\alpha(s \mid \mathcal{H}(s)) &= \mathrm{P}(s \leq T < s + ds \mid T \geq s, \mathcal{H}(s)) \\
&= \mathrm{P}(s \leq T < s + ds \mid T \geq s, \mathcal{H}(t), t \geq s).
\end{aligned}
\tag{8.1}
$$

In most cases, biomarkers and measurements collected on the subject are not exogenous variables because their distribution is affected by the occurrence of the event. These variables are called *endogenous* or *internal*. When a treatment depends on time following an established protocol independent of the patient's progression, it is an exogenous variable. It becomes endogenous when treatments are adaptive and initiated according to the patient's response. In this case, it raises difficulties in the causal interpretation that dynamic models can help solve. This issue will be discussed in Section 9.6. Air pollution levels, outside temperature and seasons are examples of exogenous variables.

The joint models are used to study the risk of an event according to longitudinal endogenous variables. In the recent years, they have proved to be particularly useful for developing dynamic prediction tools for clinical events (relapse of cancer, AIDS, Alzheimer's disease, death, etc.) from repeated measurements of quantitative markers (biomarkers such as PSA, viral load or CD4 count, cognitive tests, etc.) (Proust-Lima and Taylor, 2009; Blanche et al., 2015).

Finally, in Objective (3), the objective of joint modelling may be a more general exploration of the dependence between the event and the time-trend of the marker. It may therefore be interesting to investigate if there are different profiles of change in the marker associated with different profiles of risk for the event or if the risk of the event depends mainly on the current marker value or on the slope of the marker trajectory over time.

To reach these objectives, two types of joint models have been proposed: the shared random effects models which will be described in the next section and the latent class models detailed in Section 8.3. In both cases, the joint model combines a mixed model for the evolution of the marker and a survival model for the time-to-event. The difference lies in the latent structure that defines the association between the marker and the event. In shared random effects models, random effects or functions of random effects are introduced as explanatory variables in the survival model. In latent class models, the population is assumed to be heterogeneous and therefore composed of sub-populations with different patterns of change for the marker and different risk profiles for the event. In practice, the parameters of the two sub-models are class-specific. The advantages and limitations of each approach will be detailed in the next two sections. Then, Section 8.5 focuses on dynamic prediction tools built from joint models and Section 8.6 is devoted to recent extensions of joint models including simultaneous modelling of several longitudinal markers and/or several events.

8.2   Models with shared random effects

8.2.1   Specification

Joint models have first been developed for one longitudinal Gaussian variable and one right-censored time-to-event. Models for non-Gaussian longitudinal variables will be discussed in Section 8.6. We assume that the evolution in time of a quantity of interest (for instance, cholesterol concentration and cognitive ability) can be represented by a continuous-time Gaussian stochastic process $\{Y(t), t > 0\}$ and we will denote by Y_{ij} an observation of this process at time t_{ij} for subject i, $i = 1, ..., N$, and occasion j, $j = 1, ..., n_i$. Let us denote T_i the time of occurrence of the event and C_i the right-censoring time. The observations are $\tilde{T}_i = \min(T_i, C_i)$ and δ_i is the indicator of events; $\delta_i = 1$ if $T_i \leq C_i$ or $\delta_i = 0$ if not. A shared random-effects joint model combines a linear mixed model and a time-to-event model, most often a proportional hazard model. It may be defined as:

$$Y_{ij} = X_{Yij}^\top \beta + Z_{ij}^\top b_i + \epsilon_{ij} = \tilde{Y}_{ij} + \epsilon_{ij} \tag{8.2}$$

with $\epsilon_{ij} \sim \mathcal{N}(0, \sigma^2)$, $b_i \sim \mathcal{N}(0, B)$ and

$$\alpha_i(t) = \alpha_0(t) \exp(X_{Ti}^\top \gamma + g_i(b_i, t)^\top \eta). \tag{8.3}$$

where $\alpha_i(t)$ is the hazard function, X_{Yij} and X_{Ti} are vectors of explanatory variables and Z_{ij} a sub-vector of X_{Yij}; Z_{ij} and X_{Yij} include especially functions of time for modelling the change of $\mathrm{E}(Y)$ over time and inter-individual variations with time. The conditional expectation, $\tilde{Y}_{ij} = \mathrm{E}[Y_{ij} \mid b_i] = X_{Yij}^\top \beta + Z_{ij}^\top b_i$, is the value of Y for subject i at t_{ij} free of measurement error. It is usually referred to as the *true marker value*. In the following, we denote $X_{Yi}(t)$, $Z_i(t)$ and $\tilde{Y}_i(t) = \mathrm{E}[Y_i(t) \mid b_i]$ the values of X_{Yi}, Z_i and $\tilde{Y}_i$ at any time t.

The baseline risk function $\alpha_0(t)$ may be a parametric function chosen among the hazard functions of standard distributions such as Weibull or Gamma distribution but piecewise constant functions or spline functions allow greater flexibility while avoiding numerical difficulties of semi-parametric approaches. The two sub-models are linked by the function $g_i(b_i, t)$ which may be uni- or multidimensional and by the parameter vector η.

Shared random-effects joint models are identical to random-effects dependent selection models in the terminology used for incomplete longitudinal data and are sometimes misnamed shared parameter models. The latter name is inappropriate since the two sub-models share random variables (the random effects) and not parameters.

The function $g_i(b_i, t)$ defines the dependence structure between the time-to-event and the time-course of the marker. Any function of the random effects can be considered. It is selected depending on the context and the purpose of the study. The main types of formulation for $g_i(b_i, t)$ are the following:

(a) $g_i(b_i, t) = \tilde{Y}_i(t) = X_{\tilde{Y}i}^\top(t)\beta + Z_i^\top(t)b_i$

This is the most common model which assumes that the instantaneous risk of event at t depends on the marker value at t free of measurement error. A transformation of the current value is sometimes used instead of the crude value, such as a logistic transformation that reduces the impact of extreme values of the marker (Sene et al., 2014).

(b) $g_i(b_i, t)^\top = (\tilde{Y}_i(t), \tilde{Y}_i'(t))$

where $\tilde{Y}_i'(t)$ is the derivative of the function $\tilde{Y}_i(t)$ with respect to t at time t. This model is more flexible than the previous one because it assumes that the instantaneous risk of event t depends both on the true current value of the marker and on the slope at t. For instance, the risk of prostate cancer relapse depends both on the current PSA level and the recent change in PSA level (see Section 8.2.4). The same type of dependence may be considered by introducing a delay: $(\tilde{Y}_i(t - \tau), \tilde{Y}_i'(t - \tau))$. In this case, the risk at t depends on the marker value and slope at $t - \tau$.

(c) $g_i(b_i, t) = \tilde{Y}_i(t) = Z_i^\top(t)b_i$

This variant of model (a) assumes that the event risk at t is a function of the individual deviation of the marker at t (that does not include fixed effects of the mixed model) rather than of the marker expectation at t as in model (a). This model is useful to separate the impact of explanatory variables X_i on the event risk from the impact of individual variations of the longitudinal marker. The time-to-event model takes the following form:

$$\alpha_i(t) = \alpha_0(t) \exp(X_i^\top \gamma + Z_i^\top(t)b_i\eta). \tag{8.4}$$

and makes it possible to test the contribution of the individual longitudinal trend of the marker for predicting the risk after adjustment for the explanatory variables X_i.

(d) $g_i(b_i, t) = b_i$

In this model, the risk of event depends only on the individual random effects (intercept and random slope, for example). Let us note that the function g_i does not depend on time here; the excess of risk (or the decrease of risk) associated with the marker is thus constant over time regardless of the marker trajectory.

(e) $g_i(b_i, t)^\top = (b_{0i} Z_{i1}(t), ..., b_{qi} Z_{iq}(t))$

In this case, the risk depends on each random effect multiplied by the associated element of the vector $Z_i(t)$. The interpretation of this type of formulation is detailed in the example below.

Example 19: *Let us assume that the time-course of the longitudinal marker can be described by a linear model with random intercept and slope and a single explanatory variable X associated with the initial level and the slope of the marker:*

$$Y_{ij} = \beta_0 + \beta_1 t_{ij} + \beta_2 X_i + \beta_3 X_i t_{ij} + b_{0i} + b_{1i} t_{ij} + \epsilon_{ij} = \tilde{Y}_{ij} + \epsilon_{ij} \qquad (8.5)$$

with $\epsilon_{ij} \sim \mathcal{N}(0, \sigma^2)$ and $b_i = (b_{0i}, b_{1i})^\top \sim \mathcal{N}(0, B)$.

Several joint models corresponding to the above types (a) to (e) may be defined:

(a) $\alpha_i(t) = \alpha_0(t) \exp(X_i \gamma + \eta \tilde{Y}_i(t))$

When X is the indicator variable for a treatment, this model can be used to evaluate the quality of the marker Y as a surrogate marker for the clinical event in clinical trials for treatment X. A surrogate marker is an intermediate variable between the treatment and the event, which, ideally, captures the full effect of the treatment on the event. It can therefore be used as the criterion to evaluate the treatment effect instead of the event, especially when the time of event occurrence may be very long. If the surrogate marker was good, the parameter γ would be zero indicating that the treatment effect on the event is entirely mediated by its effect on the marker. Most of the time, γ is not null and the change in γ estimates when adjusting on $\tilde{Y}_i(t)$ or not quantifies the performance of the surrogate marker. Note that thorough validation of a surrogate marker requires a meta-analysis and the evaluation of how the treatment effect on the marker predicts the treatment effect on the event.

(b) $\alpha_i(t) = \alpha_0(t) \exp(X_i \gamma + \eta_1 \tilde{Y}_i(t) + \eta_2 \tilde{Y}_i'(t))$

The test $\eta_2 = 0$ shows whether, after adjustment for the current value of the marker, the risk also depends on the dynamics of the marker. Note that according to the definition of model (8.5), the derivative of $\tilde{Y}_i(t)$ is $\tilde{Y}_i'(t) = \beta_1 + \beta_3 X_i + b_{1i}$ for all t. This model is thus equivalent to the following:

$\alpha_i(t) = \alpha_0^*(t) \exp(X_i \gamma^* + \eta_1 \tilde{Y}_i(t) + \eta_2 b_{1i})$ *with* $\alpha_0^*(t) = \alpha_0(t) \exp(\eta_2 \beta_1)$ *and* $\gamma^* = \gamma + \eta_2 \beta_3$.

(c) $\alpha_i(t) = \alpha_0(t) \exp(X_i\gamma + \eta(b_{0i} + b_{1i}t))$

This model allows assessing whether, after taking into account the effect of the treatment, the individual deviation of the marker relative to its estimated value at t given the treatment group is a predictor of the event. The main difference between models (c) and (a) regards the interpretation of the parameter γ: in (c), γ measures the global association between the risk and the treatment, whereas, in (a), γ measures the direct effect of the treatment on the risk of the event which is not explained by the effect of the treatment on the evolution of the marker.

(d) $\alpha_i(t) = \alpha_0(t) \exp(X_i\gamma + \eta_0 b_{0i} + \eta_1 b_{1i})$

Here, η_0 and η_1 measure the association between the event risk and the individual deviations on the initial level of the marker and on the slope of the marker after adjustment for treatment.

(e) $\alpha_i(t) = \alpha_0(t) \exp(X_i\gamma + \eta_0 b_{0i} + \eta_1 b_{1i}t)$

In this last model, η_0 and η_1 measure the association between the event risk and the individual deviations on the initial level of the marker and the change in the marker between time 0 and time t.

The R package JM (Rizopoulos, 2012b) estimates joint models of type (a) and (b) while the R package joineR estimates joint models of type (c) and (e). The function stjm of stata (Crowther et al., 2013) estimates models (a), (b) and (d). Finally, the package JMbayes is designed to estimate models depending on any function of the random effects.

Henderson et al. (2000) proposed a more general form for the joint model by introducing two correlated Gaussian processes with zero expectation, $W_{1i}(t)$ and $W_{2i}(t)$:

$$Y_{ij} = X_{Yij}^{\top}\beta + W_{1i}(t_{ij}) + \epsilon_{ij} \text{ with } \epsilon_{ij} \sim \mathcal{N}(0, \sigma^2) \text{ and } b_i \sim \mathcal{N}(0, B), \quad (8.6)$$

and

$$\alpha_i(t) = \alpha_0(t) \exp(X_{Ti}^{\top}\gamma + W_{2i}(t)). \quad (8.7)$$

The process $W_{1i}(t)$ may for instance be defined by:

$$W_{1i}(t) = Z_i^{\top}(t)b_i + w_i(t)$$

where $w_i(t)$ is an autoregressive process or a Brownian motion. These models account more flexibly for the intra-individual variations of the marker change over time but the estimation is much more cumbersome. When

$$W_{1i}(t) = Z_i^{\top}(t)b_i \quad (8.8)$$

and

$$W_{2i}(t) = \eta W_{1i}(t), \quad (8.9)$$

this model is identical to model (c).

8.2.2 Estimation

8.2.2.1 Estimation in two stages

Initially, some authors have suggested estimating joint models in two stages, that is, first, fitting the mixed model to derive estimates of $g_i(b_i, t)$ for each subject, and then fitting the time-to-event model (8.3) adjusted for $\hat{g}_i(b_i, t)$. The mixed model may be estimated on all available data, regardless of the time of event. The most serious drawback of this approach is that the estimation of the mixed model is performed under the assumption of missing at random data while, if the risk depends on the trajectory of the marker through $g_i(b_i, t)$, it follows that the missing data after the event are informative. By denoting $t_{(k)}$ for $k = 1, ..., K$, the ordered observed event times, this problem can be circumvented by estimating a mixed model for each $t_{(k)}$ using only data collected before $t_{(k)}$ on subjects at risk at time $t_{(k)}$; $g_i(b_i, t_{(k)})$ is then estimated from $\hat{E}(b_i \mid \mathcal{H}(t_{(k)}), T_i \geq t_{(k)})$ (Tsiatis et al., 1995). This approach, much more numerically cumbersome than the previous one, led to a less biased estimate of $g_i(b_i, t)$ but generally more variable due to changes in the estimation sample size and in the number of available measures at each time $t_{(k)}$. Moreover, it does not completely remove the bias of naive approaches described in the introduction to this chapter (which consist of imputing the last observed value of the marker in the time-to-event model) (Dafni and Tsiatis, 1998). Indeed, the sequential two-stage approach relies on the Gaussian distribution assumption for the random effects and the residual error that cannot hold for all times $t_{(k)}$ since the analyzed samples are increasingly selected over time (subjects at risk at $t_{(k)}$). It is therefore advised to estimate joint models by maximizing the joint likelihood of Y_i, T_i, δ_i for $i = 1, ..., N$ as described in the next section. This procedure is now easier since software is available. Two-step approaches remain useful for semi-parametric joint models because their estimation by maximizing the joint likelihood is particularly time consuming (Ye et al., 2008). In addition, improvements of the two-step estimation procedure have been proposed to reduce the bias (Albert and Shih, 2010).

8.2.2.2 Estimation by joint likelihood

When the baseline risk function $\alpha_0(t)$ is parametric, the shared random effects joint models are usually estimated by maximizing the joint likelihood. Let us denote θ, the vector including the parameters from the two sub-models (8.2) and (8.3), that is the regression parameters β, γ and η, the variance parameters from the mixed model (σ and those involved in matrix B), and the parameters for the baseline risk function $\alpha_0(t)$. As demontrated by Tsiatis and Davidian (2004), taking advantage of the conditional independence between the marker

Y and the event time T, the log-likelihood is written:

$$
\begin{aligned}
L(\theta) &= \sum_{i=1}^{N} \log \mathcal{L}(Y_i, T_i, \delta_i) \\
&= \sum_{i=1}^{N} \log \int \mathcal{L}(Y_i, T_i, \delta_i \mid b) f_{b_i}(b) db \\
&= \sum_{i=1}^{N} \log \int f_{Y_i \mid b_i}(Y_i \mid b) S_i(T_i \mid b) \alpha_i(T_i \mid b)^{\delta_i} f_{b_i}(b) db, \quad (8.10)
\end{aligned}
$$

with

$$
f_{Y_i \mid b_i}(Y_i \mid b) = \prod_{j=1}^{n_i} f_{Y_{ij} \mid b_i}(Y_{ij} \mid b)
$$

and

$$
S_i(T_i \mid b) = \exp\left(-\int_0^{T_i} \alpha_i(s \mid b) ds\right).
$$

This likelihood relies on the assumption that the observation process is not informative. Tsiatis and Davidian (2004) discuss thoroughly the meaning of these assumptions. Briefly, this means that the measurement times for the marker before the event and the censoring time for the event must depend neither on the time of occurrence of the event nor on the unobserved values of the marker. If there are any missing marker measures other than those induced by the occurrence of the event, they must be missing at random (MAR), that is, not dependent on the current or future value of the marker.

Computation of the integral on the random effects in Equation (8.10) is the main difficulty since it has no closed form. It may be computed by Gaussian quadrature (see Section 4.2.5), by MCMC or by Laplace approximation when the model includes many random effects (Rizopoulos et al., 2009). With the exception of some special cases (model of type (d) or exponential baseline risk function for instance), the univariate integral over time in the survival function has no analytical solution. It can also be computed by quadrature. The structure of the likelihood being similar to that of non-linear mixed models, the same estimation algorithms can be used. Thus, the likelihood can be maximized by Newton-like algorithms (Newton-Raphson or Quasi-Newton) or by the EM algorithm by considering the random effects as missing data.

The R package JM uses a hybrid algorithm combining the EM algorithm for a fixed number of iterations and then a Quasi-Newton algorithm when convergence is not reached to remedy the slowness of the EM algorithm. The integrals over the random effects in (8.10) or its derivatives are computed by standard or *pseudo-adaptive* Gauss-Hermite quadrature. In an *adaptive quadrature*, the quadrature points are centered at each iteration around the current estimate of the random effects b_i obtained by maximizing $\log \mathcal{L}(Y_i, T_i, \delta_i \mid b) f_{b_i}(b)$ and they are rescaled according to its Hessian. This reduces the number of iterations but requires the estimation of b_i at each iteration. Assuming that $\hat{b}_i$ is close to the empirical Bayesian estimate $\hat{b}_i^y$ of the random effects of the mixed model defined in Section 4.1.6 (because repeated measures of Y bring more information than the censored time-to-event), Rizopoulos (2012a) proposed a *pseudo-adaptive* algorithm where the quadrature points are centered and rescaled according to $\hat{b}_i^y$ and the Hessian matrix of $\log \mathcal{L}(Y_i \mid b) f_{b_i}(b)$ computed previously. This avoids estimating b_i at each iteration. The second derivatives are computed by finite differences and the variance estimator is estimated by the inverse of the Hessian of (8.10).

The R package `joineR` uses Gauss-Hermite quadrature and the EM algorithm suggested by Wulfsohn and Tsiatis (1997) for estimating model (c) when $\alpha_0(t)$ is non-parametric. The variances are estimated by parametric bootstrap. Replacing the quadrature by a Monte Carlo integration and estimating variance parameters by the simplex algorithm, this EM algorithm has been extended to estimate the semi-parametric model defined by (8.6) and (8.7) which includes Gaussian processes in the dependence structure between the two response variables. The `stjm` module in stata combines the Newton-Raphson algorithm and adaptive quadrature (Crowther et al., 2013) while `JMFit` macro in SAS uses the optimization and integration techniques of `proc NLMIXED`.

Others have opted for a Bayesian approach (Brown and Ibrahim, 2003). Guo and Carlin (2004) proposed an implementation with Winbugs while the R software package `JMbayes` uses several implementations of the Gibbs sampler.

Overall, these estimation procedures may require large computation time. To estimate only the parameters of the sub-model for the time-to-event, Tsiatis and Davidian (2001) developed the conditional score approach that is less computationally demanding but requires a large number of measurements per subject.

8.2.3   Assessment of the fit

In joint models, assumptions and adjustment of the two sub-models, and, if possible, the latent structure linking the two response variables, must be evaluated. As in all statistical models, comparing observed values with estimated values and a visual exam of conditional residuals are the two main tools.

For the mixed model, it is possible to represent the mean of the observed values Y at every time (and the associated confidence interval) and the trajectory of the average marginal predictions $\hat{E}(Y_i(t) \mid X_{Yi}(t))$ or the trajectory of the average conditional predictions $\hat{E}(Y_i(t) \mid X_{Yi}(t), b_i)$ calculated on all individuals observed at the considered times. If necessary, observations and predictions are gathered by time intervals. By definition of shared random effects models, the dropout following the event occurrence depends on the random effects from the mixed model. Thus, $\hat{E}(Y_i(t) \mid X_{Yi}(t))$ represents the expectation of Y at time t for a subject with a covariate vector equals to

$X_{Yi}(t)$ and $b_i = 0$, whereas the expectation of b_i in the selected sub-sample still in the study at t is not 0. It is therefore better to evaluate the fit with the conditional predictions given the random effects because differences between observations and marginal predictions may be only the consequence of the association between dropout and marker change over time. Similarly, analyses of conditional residuals described in Section 4.1.9 remain useful in the context of joint models.

The random effects are estimated by empirical Bayes estimator, that is, by the expectation of their posterior distribution (knowing the data and the estimated parameters), namely:

$$\mathrm{E}(b_i \mid Y_i, T_i, \delta_i; \hat{\theta}) = \int b \frac{\mathcal{L}(Y_i, T_i, \delta_i \mid b; \hat{\theta})}{\mathcal{L}(Y_i, T_i, \delta_i; \hat{\theta})} f_{b_i}(b; \hat{\theta}) db$$

that may be approximated by the mode of $\mathcal{L}(Y_i, T_i, \delta_i \mid b; \hat{\theta}) f_{b_i}(b; \hat{\theta})$, as for generalized linear mixed models. Note that $\hat{b}_i$ can also be estimated by $\mathrm{E}(b_i \mid Y_i; \hat{\theta})$, conditioning only on the observations of the marker. These predictions are useful to propose a prediction tool for the risk of event based on the estimates from the joint model as this will be detailed in Section 8.5.

To assess the fit of the time-to-event sub-model, the predicted survival curve may be compared to the Kaplan-Meier estimate of the survival curve. The predicted survival curve is estimated by

$$\frac{1}{N} \sum_{i=1}^{N} S_i\left(t \mid \hat{b}_i, X_{Ti}; \hat{\theta}\right).$$

Furthermore, analyses of residuals described in Section 3.5.8 are used to evaluate departures from some model assumptions. Graphical comparison of the distribution of Cox-Snell residuals,

$$A_i\left(\tilde{T}_i \mid \hat{b}_i, X_{Ti}; \hat{\theta}\right) = \int_0^{\tilde{T}_i} \alpha_i\left(t \mid \hat{b}_i, X_{Ti}; \hat{\theta}\right) dt,$$

and of the exponential distribution of parameter 1 provides a global assessment of the survival model.

Martingale residuals, $\delta_i - A_i\left(\tilde{T}_i \mid \hat{b}_i, X_{Ti}; \hat{\theta}\right)$, are used to evaluate the dependence structure between Y and T by means of a graphical representation of these residuals *vs.* the predicted values of the function $g_i(b_i, t)$ (or *vs.* its elements if $g_i(b_i, t)$ is a vector). This enables the assessment of the log-linearity assumption in $g_i(b_i, t)$. In addition, it is recommended to compare joint models with different assumptions about the dependence structure between the two response variables, that is with different functions $g_i(b_i, t)$. However, only model formulations that are useful for the purpose of analysis should be considered because, as described above, the interpretation of the parameters of the survival model vary according to the choice of $g_i(b_i, t)$.

8.2.4 Application

Joint shared random effects models are illustrated on a data set of men treated with radiation therapy (RT) for a localized prostate cancer and followed until the occurrence of a clinical relapse. During the follow-up, repeated measurements of Prostate Specific Antigen (PSA) are collected. PSA is the major marker for progression of prostate cancer. Its change after treatment is characterized by a rapid drop followed by stabilization in the long term or by a gradual increase, the latter being often followed by a clinical relapse, up to several years later. The objective of this joint model analysis is to take into account the effect of the dynamics of the PSA for studying the clinical predictors of relapse, particularly in view of developing more accurate prognostic tools for prostate cancer relapse.

The sample, called MICHIGAN, includes 459 men diagnosed with localized prostate cancer at the Hospital of the University of Michigan from 1988 to 2004. Among them, 74 (16.1%) had a clinical relapse, local, distant or metastatic, possibly leading to death. Three standard prognostic factors were considered in addition to the repeated PSA measures: the stage of the tumor that characterizes the tumor size (stage 1 or 2 *vs.* 3 or 4, denoted `stageT`), Gleason score that characterizes aggressiveness of the cancer (score 7 or >7, denoted `gleason7` and `gleason_sup7` *vs.* <7) and pre-RT PSA level (`iPSA`). Among the 459 men, 41 (8.9%) had an initial stage 3 or 4, respectively, 173 (37.7%) and 34 (7.4%) had a Gleason score equal to 7 or above 7, and the mean pre-RT PSA level in logarithmic scale was 2.18 (SD=0.90). A more complete description of the data can be found in several articles (Proust-Lima et al., 2014; Sene et al., 2014).

The post-RT PSA level (`PSA`) is described as a function of time in years since the end of radiation therapy (`time`) by a linear mixed model taking into account the two phases of evolution, the initial drop by the function $f_1(t) = (1 + t)^{-1.5} - 1$ and a long term linear growth thereafter. In the following, `PSA` level is transformed by $\log(\text{PSA} + 0.1)$ to better meet the normality assumption for the dependent variable. For the subject i at measurement j, the model is:

$$
\begin{aligned}
\log(\text{PSA}_{ij} + 0.1) &= \tilde{Y}_i(\text{time}_{ij}) + \epsilon_{ij} \\
&= \left(\mu_0 + X_i^\top \beta_0 + b_{0i}\right) + \left(\mu_1 + X_i^\top \beta_1 + b_{1i}\right) f_1(\text{time}_{ij}) \\
&\quad + \left(\mu_2 + X_i^\top \beta_2 + b_{2i}\right) \text{time}_{ij} + \epsilon_{ij}
\end{aligned}
\tag{8.11}
$$

where $X = (\text{iPSA}, \text{stageT}, \text{gleason7}, \text{gleason\_sup7})$, $\epsilon_{ij} \sim \mathcal{N}(0, \sigma^2)$ and $b_i = (b_{0i}, b_{1i}, b_{2i})^\top \sim \mathcal{N}(0, B)$.

The risk of clinical relapse of prostate cancer is described by a proportional hazards model with a baseline risk defined using a B-spline basis with three internal nodes located at the quartiles of the event times and adjusting on the same explanatory variables:

$$\alpha_i(t) = \alpha_0(t) \exp(X_i^\top \gamma + g_i(b_i, t)^\top \eta). \tag{8.12}$$

Several functions of the random effects were studied to link the risk of cinical relapse and the PSA change over time:

(a) the current level of PSA: $g_{ia}(b_i, t) = \tilde{Y}_i(t)$

(b) the current slope of PSA: $g_{ib}(b_i, t) = \tilde{Y}_i'(t)$

(c) the current level and slope of PSA: $g_{ic}(b_i, t) = \left(\tilde{Y}_i(t), \tilde{Y}_i'(t)\right)^\top$

(d) the random effects: $g_{id}(b_i, t) = (b_{0i}, b_{1i}, b_{2i})^\top$

(e) the current level of PSA transformed by a pre-determined function:
$g_{ie}(b_i, t) = h\left(\tilde{Y}_i(t)\right)$
It was previously found that the transformation
$h\left(\tilde{Y}_i(t)\right) = \text{logit}^{-1}\left(\left(\tilde{Y}_i(t) - 0.71\right)/0.44\right)$, obtained by likelihood profile, better satisfied the log-linearity assumption (Sene et al., 2014)

(f) the current level of transformed PSA and the current slope:
$g_{if}(b_i, t) = \left(h\left(\tilde{Y}_i(t)\right), \tilde{Y}_i'(t)\right)^\top$

Models were estimated by the function `JointModel` of package JM except for Models (e) and (f) which required additional programming. The standard call to the function is described in the appendix.

Table 8.1 summarizes the estimates of the six joint models. According to the AIC, the best model is Model (f) that assumes that the risk of relapse depends on both the transformed current level of PSA and the current slope. Model (a) that assumes that the risk of relapse depends only on current PSA, the most frequent assumption in the literature, appears as the worst model among the six models tested. In particular, Model (b) where the risk depends on the current slope rather than the current value gives a better fit. Table 8.2 summarizes estimates of the survival sub-model for Model (f). Among the classical prognostic factors, only the initial PSA level remains significantly associated with the risk of clinical relapse after adjusting for the dynamics of PSA (p=0.0005). The current transformed PSA level and the current slope are independent predictors of the relapse risk: an increase in current level of PSA and an increase in the slope of PSA are significantly associated with increased risk of clinical relapse after adjustment for the other prognostic factors.

As described in Section 8.2.3, we assessed the goodness of fit of the selected models with different methods. To evaluate the fit of the mixed model, we displayed in Figure 8.1 the average observed values of Y in time intervals defined according to the percentiles of the measurement times, and the mean of the marginal and conditional predictions computed on all subjects observed in these time intervals. The gap between marginal predictions and observations

TABLE 8.1
Summary of the estimated joint shared random effects models: log-likelihood
(L), number of parameters (p), and AIC.

Dependence structure		L	p	AIC
	none	-2708.2	33	5482.3
(a)	$\tilde{Y}_i(t)$	-2644.2	34	5356.3
(b)	$\tilde{Y}_i'(t)$	-2636.0	34	5339.9
(c)	$\tilde{Y}_i(t)$ and $\tilde{Y}_i(t)'$	-2628.6	35	5327.1
(d)	b_i	-2630.7	36	5333.4
(e)	$h(\tilde{Y}_i(t))$	-2611.1	34	5290.1
(f)	$h(\tilde{Y}_i(t))$ and $\tilde{Y}_i'(t)$	**-2605.6**	**35**	**5281.1**

TABLE 8.2
Estimated parameters for the survival sub-model of joint shared random effects Model (f).

Variable	Estimate	Standard error	Wald Statistic	p-value
iPSA	-0.774	0.222	-3.49	0.0005
stageT	0.480	0.451	1.06	0.288
gleason7	0.473	0.364	1.30	0.194
gleason_sup7	0.793	0.553	1.43	0.152
$h(\tilde{Y}_i(t))$	5.450	0.840	6.49	<0.0001
$\tilde{Y}_i'(t)$	1.080	0.319	3.39	0.0007

highlights the subjects' selection over time: subjects who dropped out following cancer relapse are those with the highest PSA levels. By contrast, conditional predictions (that account for the individual random effects) fit very well the observed PSA measures.

To evaluate the fit of the time-to-event model, we compared the mean of the conditional predictions of the survival curve from Model (f) with the Kaplan-Meier estimates of the survival curve. Then, Cox-Snell residuals were displayed. These two graphs are in Figure 8.2. They show a good overall fit of the model to the data.

Finally, we assessed the log-linear hypothesis for the variables that capture the dependence between the longitudinal process and the survival process by comparing martingale residuals between Model (c) and Model (f). Model (c) assumes that the risk of relapse depends on the current level and slope of PSA while Model (f) assumes a dependence through a transformation of the

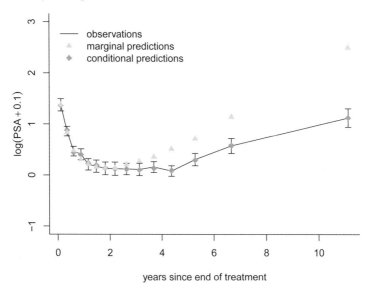

FIGURE 8.1
Mean of the observations (with 95% confidence interval) and of the marginal (triangles) and conditional (diamonds) predictions from Model (f) by time intervals defined according to the percentiles of measurement times.

current level and the current slope. As displayed on Figure 8.3, for Model (c), martingale residuals exhibit a decreasing trend according to the current predicted level of PSA among the high PSA values, which indicates a departure from the log-linearity assumption. This difference disappears when the transformation of the PSA is used in Model (f).

8.3 Latent class joint model

Latent class models are the main alternative to shared random effects models to analyze a longitudinal process and an associated survival process (Lin et al., 2000, 2002; Proust-Lima et al., 2014). While shared random effects models capture the correlation between the two processes through continuous characteristics of the trajectory of the longitudinal marker, the joint latent class models assume that the population is divided in homogeneous groups of subjects with regards to both the marker trajectory and the event risk.

Thus, the latent variable linking the two processes is the discrete random

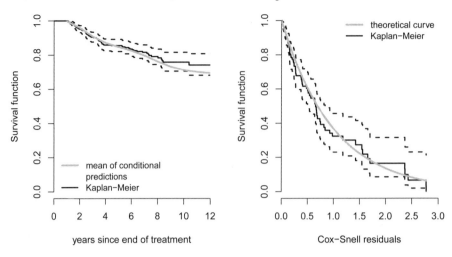

FIGURE 8.2
Mean of the conditional predictions of the survival curve from Model (f) and
the Kaplan-Meier estimates of the survival curve with 95% confidence interval (left). Survival curve for Cox-Snell residuals estimated by Kaplan-Meier
with 95% confidence interval and theoretical survival curve for these residuals
(right).

variable defining the groups or latent classes. This approach can be seen as an
extension of the latent class mixed models described in Section 5.3 for joint
modelling a time-to-event.

8.3.1 Specification

Like for joint shared random effects models, developments of joint latent class
models initially focused on one quantitative longitudinal variable and one
right-censored time-to-event. Extensions to other types of variables will be
discussed in Section 8.6. Let us denote Y_{ij}, the marker Y measured at time
t_{ij} for subject i, $i = 1, ..., N$, and T_i the event time; C_i is the right censoring
time, and we observe $\tilde{T}_i = \min(T_i, C_i)$ and the failure indicator: $\delta_i = 1$ if
$T_i \leq C_i$ and $\delta_i = 0$ if not. Finally, we define the discrete latent variable c_i
which equals g if subject i belongs to the latent class g, $g = 1, ..., G$ where G
is the number of latent classes.

The joint latent class model combines three sub-models, a multinomial
logistic model for the class-membership probability, a linear mixed model for
the trajectory of the marker and a survival model, usually a proportional
hazards model, for the event. The last two sub-models are class-specific. A

Model (c) : current PSA level and current slope of PSA

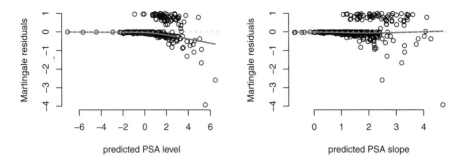

Model (f) : current transformed PSA level and current slope of PSA

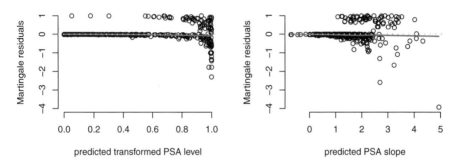

FIGURE 8.3
Martingale residuals *vs.* predicted PSA level (left) or predicted slope of PSA (right) at the time of event or censoring, in Model (c) assuming dependence through the current level and slope (top panel) and in Model (f) assuming dependence through the current tranformed level and the slope (bottom panel).

joint latent class model is thus defined by:

$$\pi_{ig} = \mathrm{P}(c_i = g \mid X_{pi}) = \frac{\exp(\xi_{0g} + X_{pi}^\top \xi_{1g})}{\sum_{l=1}^{G} \exp(\xi_{0l} + X_{pi}^\top \xi_{1l})} \tag{8.13}$$

with $\xi_{0G} = 0$ and $\xi_{1G} = 0$ to ensure identifiability of the model,

$$Y_i(t_{ij}) = Z_{ij}^\top b_i + X_{Yij}^\top \beta_g + \epsilon_{ij} \text{ in latent class } g \tag{8.14}$$

with $\epsilon_i = (\epsilon_{i1}, ..., \epsilon_{in_i})^\top \sim \mathcal{N}(0, \Sigma_i)$, $b_i \sim \mathcal{N}(\mu_g, B_g)$ in latent class g, and

$$\alpha_i(t \mid c_i = g) = \alpha_0(t; \zeta_g) \exp(X_{Ti}(t)^\top \gamma_g) \text{ in latent class } g. \tag{8.15}$$

Vectors X_{pi}, X_{Yij}, Z_{ij} and X_{Ti} are four vectors of explanatory variables. To ensure identifiability of parameters μ_g and β_g, vectors Z_{ij} and X_{Yij} cannot have any variable in common. These vectors usually include functions of time to model the change of $E(Y)$ over time and inter-individual variations with time, while X_{pi} is a vector of explanatory variables that must be time-constant. The random-effects b_i follow a mixture of Normal distributions: given the latent class g, the random effects b_i have a class-specific expectation μ_g and a variance matrix B_g that may be either class-specific, for example by assuming proportionality between the classes, $B_g = \omega_g^2 B$ with B unstructured and $\omega_G = 1$, or common for all latent classes, $B_g = B$. The errors ϵ_i may be independent and homoscedastic with a diagonal variance matrix, $\Sigma_i = \sigma^2 I_{n_i}$, or correlated when they include a Brownian motion or an autoregressive process.

The time-to-event sub-model depends on parameters ζ_g for modelling the baseline risk function and on regression parameters γ_g; both may be class-specific. The survival model may be stratified on the latent classes or proportional class-specific risks may be assumed: $\alpha_0(t; \zeta)e^{\gamma_g}$. All conventional parametric forms can be used for $\alpha_0(t; \zeta_g)$ (Weibull, Gamma, piecewise-constant, splines, etc.).

In both sub-models (8.14) and (8.15), the parameters associated with the explanatory variables β_g and γ_g may also be identical for all classes, to highlight the marginal effect of these explanatory variables adjusted for the latent classes.

8.3.2   Estimation

The estimation procedure of joint latent class models is the same as the one of latent class mixed models described in Section 5.3. Here we focus on an estimation by the maximum likelihood approach but a Bayesian approach could be preferred.

As for latent class mixed models, parameter estimation of joint latent class models by maximum likelihood is performed for a fixed number of latent classes G. Let us denote by θ_G the complete vector of parameters involved in the three sub-models defined in (8.13), (8.14) and (8.15). The log-likelihood of the model can be decomposed thanks to the assumption of conditional independence between the repeated measures of Y and the right-censored event time T given the latent classes defined by c. Thereby,

$$
\begin{aligned}
L(\theta_G) &= \sum_{i=1}^{N} L_i(\theta_G) \\
&= \sum_{i=1}^{N} \log \left(\sum_{g=1}^{G} \pi_{ig} f_{Y_i|c_i}(Y_i \mid c_i = g)\alpha_i(T_i \mid c_i = g)^{\delta_i} S_i(T_i \mid c_i = g) \right)
\end{aligned}
\tag{8.16}
$$

where the probability π_{ig} of belonging to latent class g is defined by (8.13), the instantaneous risk function $\alpha_i(t \mid c_i = g)$ is defined by (8.15) and $S_i(t \mid c_i = g)$

is the survival function specific to class g. The density $f_{Y_i|c_i}(Y_i \mid c_i = g)$ of the repeated marker measures for class g is a multivariate Gaussian density with mean $Z_i\mu_g + X_{li}\beta_g$ and variance matrix $Z_iB_gZ_i^\top + \Sigma_i$; Z_i and X_{li} are matrices with respectively elements $Z_{ij}^\top$ and $X_{lij}^\top$ at line j.

The log-likelihood in (8.16) may be maximized by an iterative algorithm of Newton type. This estimation procedure is implemented in the function Jointlcmm of the R package lcmm (see the appendix for some examples of calls). The optimization algorithm is the Marquardt algorithm as described in Section 2.5.2. Variances of the estimated parameters are obtained by the inverse of the Hessian matrix as for the other families of models.

Parameter estimation raises the same problems as for the latent class mixed models. First, the log-likelihood can be multimodal, so it is highly recommended to estimate a model several times from different initial values to ensure convergence towards the global maximum. Then, each model is estimated for a given number of latent classes but in general, the number of latent classes is unknown and must be determined. Again, the BIC is often preferred to compare models with different numbers of latent classes but other criteria may also be considered including the model goodness-of-fit as detailed in the next section.

8.3.3   Assessment of the fit

The assessment of the fit of a joint latent class model relies both on techniques used in joint shared random effects models to evaluate the fit of the longitudinal sub-model and the survival sub-model, and on techniques used for latent class mixed models including the posterior classification of the subjects and the evaluation of its discriminative power. In addition, the major assumption of conditional independence between the longitudinal process and the survival process given the latent classes must be checked.

Note that in the joint latent class models, measures of fit of the data also provide guidance for choosing the number of latent classes. Indeed, the selection of the optimum number of latent classes may be based on a combination of arguments. In addition to information criteria such as BIC and according to the objectives of the analysis, other criteria may be favored such as the discrimination level between the classes, the accuracy of the predictions, the validation of the conditional independence assumption, and/or the clinical meaning of the latent classes.

8.3.3.1   Posterior classification

We explained in Section 5.3 that a classification could be built and evaluated from latent class mixed models. Such posterior classification can also be derived from joint latent class models but two different posterior probabilities of belonging to the latent classes may be defined:

- either conditionally on the longitudinal data and the time-to-event:

$$\hat{\pi}_{ig}^{Y,T} = P(c_i = g \mid Y_i, T_i, \delta_i; \hat{\theta}_G)$$

$$= \frac{\hat{\pi}_{ig} f_{Y_i \mid c_i}(Y_i \mid c_i = g; \hat{\theta}_G) \alpha_i(T_i \mid c_i = g; \hat{\theta}_G)^{\delta_i} S_i(T_i \mid c_i = g; \hat{\theta}_G)}{\sum_{l=1}^{G} \hat{\pi}_{il} f_{Y_i \mid c_i}(Y_i \mid c_i = l; \hat{\theta}_G) \alpha_i(T_i \mid c_i = l; \hat{\theta}_G)^{\delta_i} S_i(T_i \mid c_i = l; \hat{\theta}_G)} \tag{8.17}$$

where $\hat{\pi}_{ig}$ is the probability of belonging to class g defined by (8.13) and computed with the estimated parameters $\hat{\theta}_G$, and $\alpha_i(T_i \mid c_i = g; \theta_G)$, $S_i(T_i \mid c_i = g; \theta_G)$ and $f_{Y_i \mid c_i}(Y_i \mid c_i = g; \theta_G)$ are defined in Section 8.3.2;

- or conditionally on the longitudinal data only:

$$\hat{\pi}_{ig}^{Y} = P(c_i = g \mid Y_i; \hat{\theta}_G)$$

$$= \frac{\hat{\pi}_{ig} f_{Y_i \mid c_i}(Y_i \mid c_i = g; \hat{\theta}_G)}{\sum_{l=1}^{G} \hat{\pi}_{il} f_{Y_i \mid c_i}(Y_i \mid c_i = l; \hat{\theta}_G)} \tag{8.18}$$

as defined in Section 5.3.3 and computed with the estimated parameters $\hat{\theta}_G$.

From each of these two probabilities, the subject can be *a posteriori* classified in the class to which he/she has the greatest probability of belonging:

$$\tilde{c}_i^{Y,T} = \mathrm{argmax}_g(\hat{\pi}_{ig}^{Y,T}) \text{ and } \tilde{c}_i^{Y} = \mathrm{argmax}_g(\hat{\pi}_{ig}^{Y})$$

Probabilities $\hat{\pi}_{ig}^{Y,T}$ will be preferred to assess the adequacy of the model with the same techniques as those described in Section 5.3.3 for latent class mixed models. The probabilities $\hat{\pi}_{ig}^{Y}$ will be used for the prediction of the event from the repeated measures of the longitudinal marker.

8.3.3.2 Comparison of predictions and observations

Predictions can be calculated from the mixed sub-model defined by (8.14). These predictions are class-specific but may be either marginal or conditional on the random effects. For subject i, measurement j and class g, marginal predictions are

$$\hat{Y}_{ijg}^{(M)} = Z_{ij}^{\top} \hat{\mu}_g + X_{Yij}^{\top} \hat{\beta}_g$$

and conditional predictions are

$$\hat{Y}_{ijg}^{(SS)} = Z_{ij}^{\top}(\hat{\mu}_g + \hat{\tilde{b}}_{ig}^{*}) + X_{Yij}^{\top} \hat{\beta}_g$$

where

$$\hat{\tilde{b}}_{ig}^{*} = \hat{B}_g Z_i^{\top} \hat{V}_{ig}^{-1}(Y_i - X_{Yi} \hat{\beta}_g - Z_i \hat{\mu}_g)$$

is the empirical Bayesian estimator of the centered random effects in class g. Summaries of these predictions are obtained either by averaging over the latent class to get a single prediction for each subject

$$\hat{Y}_{ij}^{(.)} = \sum_{g=1}^{G} \hat{\pi}_{ig} \hat{Y}_{ijg}^{(.)},$$

or by averaging over the subjects to obtain a single prediction for each class at a given measurement time t,

$$\hat{Y}_g(t)^{(.)} = \sum_{i=1}^{N(t)} \hat{\pi}_{ig} \hat{Y}_{ijg}^{(.)},$$

with $N(t)$ the number of subjects with measures at time t (or in a time-interval). Given that predictions are marginal or conditional to the random-effects, the probabilities $\hat{\pi}_{ig}$ are either the marginal probabilities computed by (8.13) with the estimated parameters, or the posterior probabilities given by (8.17).

In practice, the average predictions by class can be compared with the weighted means of the observations $\bar{Y}_g(t) = \sum_{i=1}^{N(t)} \hat{\pi}_{ig} Y_i(t)$. Subject-specific conditional predictions are preferred here because of the withdrawal from the study related to the occurrence of the event. The average predictions by subject may be used to define residuals whose evaluation can be performed as for the joint shared random effects models.

Predictions can also be obtained from the survival sub-model defined by (8.15). These are survival functions conditional to the classes $\hat{S}_{ig}(t)$ which can be averaged by subject or by class as the predictions for Y. The predicted survival curves averaged per class are compared with survival curves estimated by Kaplan-Meier weighted by the probabilities of belonging to the classes. Residuals could also be defined for the survival sub-model as described in Section 8.2.3 for the joint shared random effects models.

8.3.3.3 Conditional independence assumption

The joint latent class model assumes that the latent class structure captures the correlation between the longitudinal marker and the time of event. This central assumption may be evaluated by a score test (Jacqmin-Gadda et al., 2010). This test assesses whether, conditional on the latent class, there is no residual dependence between the longitudinal marker and the time-to-event through shared random effects. Thus, the alternative hypothesis $\mathcal{H}_1$ is defined by a joint latent class model replacing Equation (8.15) by the following that includes shared random effects in addition to the latent classes:

$$\alpha_i(t \mid c_i = g) = \alpha_{0g}(t; \zeta_g) \exp(X_{Ti}^\top(t)\gamma_g + b_{ig}^{*\top}\eta) \qquad (8.19)$$

with η the vector of parameters linking the centered random effects from the mixed model (8.14) ($b_{ig}^* = b_i - \mu_g$) and the time-to-event.

In this model, the null and alternative hypotheses of the test of conditional independence are defined by $\mathcal{H}_0$: $\eta = 0$ (*vs* $\mathcal{H}_1$: $\eta \neq 0$). The score statistic is the derivative with respect to η of the log-likelihood of model (8.19) computed at $\eta = 0$. By denoting θ_G the whole set of parameters of the joint latent class model under $\mathcal{H}_0$, the score statistic has the following form:

$$U(0, \theta_G) = \sum_{i=1}^{N} \sum_{g=1}^{G} \pi_{ig}^{Y,T} \left(\delta_i - A_{ig}(T_i; \theta_G) \right) \mathrm{E}(b_{ig}^* \mid c_i = g, Y_i, \theta_G) \quad (8.20)$$

where the posterior expectation $\mathrm{E}(b_{ig}^* \mid c_i = g, Y_i, \theta_G)$ is estimated by $\hat{b}_{ig}^*$ as explained in the previous paragraph and $A_{ig}(T_i; \theta_G)$ is the cumulative risk function at T_i in class g. The statistic $U(0, \theta)$ is estimated by replacing θ_G by its maximum likelihood estimator under the null hypothesis (thus with the standard joint latent class model). Formula (8.20) shows that the score statistic is an estimate of the covariance between the class-specific residuals of the survival model and the class-specific empirical Bayesian estimators of the random effects weighted by the posterior class-membership probabilities. Under $\mathcal{H}_0$, $U(0, \hat{\theta}_G)^{\top} \mathrm{var}(U)^{-1} U(0, \hat{\theta}_G)$ has asymptotically a χ^2 distribution with m degrees of freedom where m is the size of vector η. The test makes it possible to test either the dependence of the time-to-event on the whole set of random effects from the mixed model or only on some of them (intercept or slope, for example). Two estimators of $\mathrm{var}(U)$ are proposed in Jacqmin-Gadda et al. (2010) and a simulation study showed that this test was more powerful than other procedures of assessment of the conditional independence hypothesis (Lin et al., 2002, 2004; Proust-Lima and Taylor, 2009) even when the alternative hypothesis was misspecified.

8.3.4   Application

The joint latent class models is illustrated on the data set MICHIGAN (on the progression of prostate cancer after radiation therapy). As for the shared random effects models, the change over time of the post-radiotherapy PSA level (PSA) is described according to the time elapsed since the end of radiotherapy (time) using a linear mixed model accounting for the initial drop of PSA level by the function $f_1(t) = (1+t)^{-1.5} - 1$ and the long-term linear growth thereafter. However, in the latent class approach, the change over time is different in each latent class g for $g = 1, ..., G$. The conditional distribution of the transformed PSA given class g for subject i at measurement j is defined by:

$$\log(\mathrm{PSA}_{ij} + 0.1) = \left(\mu_{0g} + X_i^{\top} \beta_0 + b_{0i} \right) + \left(\mu_{1g} + X_i^{\top} \beta_1 + b_{1i} \right) f_1(\mathrm{time}_{ij})$$
$$+ \left(\mu_{2g} + X_i^{\top} \beta_2 + b_{2i} \right) \mathrm{time}_{ij} + \epsilon_{ij}$$

$$(8.21)$$

with $X=(\texttt{iPSA},\texttt{stageT},\texttt{gleason7},\texttt{gleason\_sup7})$, $\epsilon_{ij} \sim \mathcal{N}(0,\sigma^2)$ and $b_i = (b_{0i}, b_{1i}, b_{2i})^\top \sim \mathcal{N}(0, \omega_g^2 B)$ in latent class g, and $\omega_G = 1$.

No predictor is included in the class-membership probability, so that

$$P(c_i = g) = \pi_g = \frac{\exp(\xi_g)}{\sum_{l=1}^{G} \exp(\xi_l)}$$

with $\xi_G = 0$, G being the reference class.

The risk of clinical relapse of prostate cancer in each latent class g is described by a proportional hazards model adjusted for the four explanatory variables $\texttt{iPSA}$, $\texttt{stageT}$, $\texttt{gleason7}$ and $\texttt{gleason\_sup7}$, and assuming a class-specific baseline risk. Thus,

$$\alpha_i(t \mid c_i = g) = \alpha_{0g}(t) \exp(X_i^\top \gamma). \tag{8.22}$$

In this application, the baseline hazard was assumed to be zero in the first year and then was defined according to a Weibull distribution from one year after the end of treatment. We could have also approached the risk of clinical relapse using splines as in the shared random effects model while assuming a proportional risk between latent classes. In this application, however, we found that the class-specific Weibull model fitted the data very well.

Models were estimated with the function $\texttt{Jointlcmm}$ of the package $\texttt{lcmm}$. The standard call of this function is described in the appendix.

TABLE 8.3

Summary of joint latent class models estimated with 1 to 5 classes: log-likelihood (L), number of parameters (p), BIC, Score statistic (ST) and associated p-value for the conditional independence test, and proportion of subjects in each posterior class (%).

G	L	p	BIC	ST (p-value)	Latent class proportion (%)				
1	-2711.6	28	5594.7	134.4 ($<$0.001)	100				
2	-2473.3	35	5161.1	31.4 ($<$0.001)	91.3	8.7			
3	-2419.0	42	5095.4	12.9 (0.005)	85.2	9.1	5.7		
4	-2390.9	49	5082.1	9.3 (0.026)	85.0	8.9	4.4	1.8	
5	-2381.3	56	5105.8	9.6 (0.023)	85.0	9.6	2.2	1.7	1.4

Table 8.3 summarizes the estimates of the joint latent class models with 1 to 5 latent classes. According to BIC criterion, the best model included 4 classes. The mean predicted trajectories of PSA for a subject with $b_i = 0$ and the risk of clinical relapses of cancer in each latent class are displayed in the top of figure 8.4. As the risk of event is very large in classes 2, 3 and 4, the

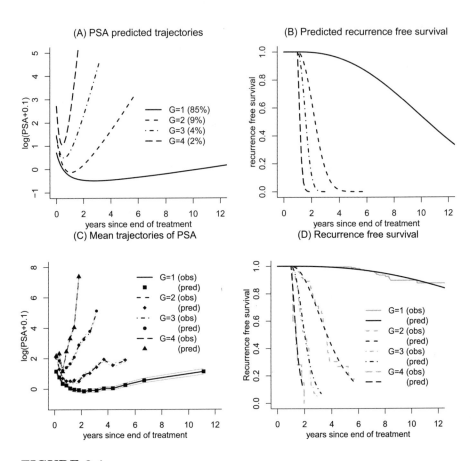

FIGURE 8.4

(A) Mean predicted trajectory of PSA in each latent class and (B) predicted probability of having no clinical relapse in each latent class from the joint model with 4 latent classes for a subject with a T-stage equal to 1, a Gleason score less than 7 and an initial PSA level of 2 ng/mL. (C) Weighted conditional predicted trajectories (pred) and weighted observed trajectories (obs) from the joint model with four latent classes. (D) Weighted average predicted probabilities of having no clinical relapse of prostate cancer (pred) and weighted empirical probability to have no clinical relapse (obs) from the joint model with four latent classes.

predicted trajectories are truncated respectively at 6, 4 and 2 years because very few subjects are still in the sample at these times in these classes.

The sample of 459 men treated for prostate cancer is thus divided into four classes. The main class (Class 1) that gathers 85% of the sample is characterized by a low risk of relapse after initial treatment and a very slow long-term increase of PSA. The other three classes (Classes 2 to 4) are of small sizes. They represent respectively 8.9%, 4.4% and 1.8% of the sample and exhibit long-term PSA increases that could be called respectively "moderate," "strong" and "very strong," associated with moderate to very strong risks of clinical relapses. Note for example in Figure 8.4 (D) that the probability of relapse reaches 1 from 3 years in Class 4, 5 years in Class 3 and 10 years in Class 2.

As described in Section 8.3.3, the fit of the joint latent class model may be assessed by different ways. First, according to the bottom of Figure 8.4, the mean predicted trajectories of PSA in each latent class weighted by the class-membership probabilities show a very good fit of the repeated PSA measures. It is the same for the survival part because the non-relapse predicted probabilities (or progression free survival) averaged and weighted by the posterior class-membership probabilities are very close to the survival curves estimated by the weighted Kaplan-Meier estimator.

Then, the classification issued from the model with four classes is very discriminant. The entropy, as defined in Section 5.3.3, is 0.93 and the classification Table 8.4 shows that the average probability of belonging to the class to which the subject is affected is greater than 90%. In addition, the proportion of men classified with a probability higher than 0.90 reaches almost 3/4 in all classes and about 9/10 in the main class (Class 1).

TABLE 8.4
Number (%) of subjects and mean posterior probabilities (%) of belonging to each class according to the final posterior classification.

Classification	Number of subjects (%)	Mean posterior probabilities of belonging to the class (%):			
		1	2	3	4
1	390 (85.0%)	97.2	2.5	0.3	<0.1
2	41 (8.9%)	7.7	89.4	2.9	<0.1
3	20 (4.4%)	<0.1	5.0	92.9	2.1
4	8 (1.8%)	1.3	0.4	2.3	96.0

The conditional independence hypothesis between the marker and the time of relapse given the latent classes is not valid in the model with four classes (p=0.026, Table 8.3). Nevertheless, the p-value of the test increases substantially when the number of classes rises from 1 to 4. By including additional explanatory variables in the sub-model for the class-membership probability, the conditional independence hypothesis was not rejected (see Proust-Lima et al., 2014).

The fit of the joint latent class model and the joint shared random effects model can be compared, for instance by information criteria, as the two models are not nested. To avoid favoring a model with many parameters, this comparison was done in terms of BIC which promotes more parsimonious models than in terms of AIC. In this application, the best joint random effects model had a BIC of 5425.7, whereas the model with four latent classes had a substantially better BIC of 5161.1. This result is not surprising. First, the joint latent class model better fitted the repeated PSA measures because the latent class mixed model is much more flexible than the standard mixed model used in the joint shared random effects model. Then, the latter includes few parameters to capture the dependence and therefore requires strong assumptions about the dependence structure between the two processes. In contrast, the joint latent class model needs weaker assumptions on the dependence structure and includes many more parameters (49 for the best joint latent class model *vs.* 35 for the best joint shared random effect).

Nevertheless the former should not be systematically favored over the latter: the choice depends on the objective of the analysis. A detailed comparison of the two approaches is given in next section.

8.4   Latent classes *vs.* shared random effects

Comparing the characteristics of the two main types of joint models can be useful to make the choice easier in applications.

First, although both methods take into account the variability of longitudinal profiles thanks to the random effects, joint latent class models (JLCM) are more flexible as they take into account a possible heterogeneity in the population: each latent class corresponds to a sub-population with a specific pattern of change of the marker and a specific risk of the event. In contrast, the shared random effects models (SREM) assume that the population is homogeneous with a single mean trajectory for the marker and a continuous relationship between the marker characteristics and the risk of the event.

Moreover, in standard SREM, the random effects model capture both the correlation between the repeated measurements of the marker and the dependence between the marker and the time of event. Those two dependence structures can be separated in the JLCM since the random effects only account for the correlation between repeated measurements while the latent classes account for the dependence between the marker and the event. To avoid this drawback of SREM, two sets of random effects could be included in SREM, with only one associated with the events but increasing the number of random effects heightens numerical issues of optimization algorithms.

In SREM, the characteristics of the marker trajectory that impact the risk of event are *a priori* chosen by defining the function $g_i(b_i, t)$. Comparing models with different functions $g_i(b_i, t)$ has the advantage to assess different assumptions about the dependence structure between the two processes as has been shown in the application. However, this kind of dependence is usually less flexible than that of latent class models that can highlight sub-populations with risk functions and marker trajectories of various shapes. Such flexibility is nevertheless at the cost of a sharp increase in the number of parameters, and sometimes a difficulty in the interpretation of the latent classes and parameters within each class.

Furthermore, JLCM rely on the assumption of conditional independence given the classes. In each latent class, after adjustment for the explanatory variables, event risk is assumed to be independent of the marker. In SREM, the two processes are assumed to be independent given the shared random effects.

Finally, regarding the estimation process, the calculation of the likelihood of SREM requires a numerical integration on the random effects which may be costly in computation time. This integration is replaced by a sum over the latent classes in JLCM which is less cumbersome. However, the estimation of JLCM is also time consuming because the estimation must be repeated with several starting points to ensure convergence towards the global maximum and with several numbers of classes to choose the optimal number of latent classes.

As a conclusion, SREM are favored to evaluate some hypotheses regarding the dependence between the risk of event and the change over time of the marker and to obtain a quantitative summary of this dependence. The JLCM are more useful to describe this relationship without *a priori* assumptions or when the population is heterogeneous. As they are very flexible, they are also suitable when the main objective is the prediction of the event using the repeated marker measures.

8.5   The joint model as prognostic model

The joint models (with shared random effects or latent classes) can be used to predict clinical events from the dynamics of a marker (Proust-Lima and Taylor, 2009; Rizopoulos, 2011). These predictions define prognostic tools called *dynamic* prognostic tools because they can be updated at each new measurement of the marker. Regardless of the time at which the prediction is made, they give an updated quantification of the risk of event and therefore are potentially more precise compared to conventional prognostic tools using only the information at the beginning of the follow-up. This could be very useful for patients monitoring and for clinical decisions.

The dynamic predictions are usually the predicted probabilities that the event occurs in a window of time $[s, s+t]$ computed using the explanatory variables and the marker measures collected before time s. Time s is often called the "time of prediction" or the "landmark time" while time t is called the "horizon of prediction" $(t \geq 0)$.

For any subject i, let us denote $\bar{Y}_i(s) = \{Y_{ij}, j = 1, ..., n_i, \text{with } t_{ij} \leq s\}$ the vector of marker measures until time s, $\bar{X}_i(s) = \{X_{pi}, X_{Ti}, X_{Yij}, j = 1, ..., n_i, \text{with } t_{ij} \leq s\}$ the vector of covariate measures until time s, T_i the event time to be predicted and θ the vector of parameters of the joint model.

In a joint latent class model, the predicted probability of event in the window $[s, s+t]$ is written (for brevity, we omit dependence on θ in all the functions):

$$P(T_i \leq s+t \mid T_i \geq s, \bar{Y}_i(s), \bar{X}_i(s))$$

$$= \sum_{g=1}^{G} P(T_i \leq s+t \mid T_i \geq s, c_i = g, \bar{X}_i(s)) P(c_i = g \mid T_i \geq s, \bar{Y}_i(s), \bar{X}_i(s))$$

$$= \frac{\sum_{g=1}^{G} \pi_{ig} f_{\bar{Y}_i(s)}(\bar{Y}_i(s) \mid c_i = g, \bar{X}_i(s)) (S_{ig}(s) - S_{ig}(s+t))}{\sum_{g=1}^{G} \pi_{ig} f_{\bar{Y}_i(s)}(\bar{Y}_i(s) \mid c_i = g, \bar{X}_i(s)) S_{ig}(s)}$$

$$(8.23)$$

with $S_{ig}(s) = S_i(s \mid c_i = g, \bar{X}_i(s))$.

In a joint shared random effects model, the event probability has the same form, except that the sum over the latent classes is replaced by an integral over the random effects::

$$P(T_i \leq s+t \mid T_i \geq s, \bar{Y}_i(s), \bar{X}_i(s)) =$$

$$= \int P(T_i \leq s+t \mid T_i \geq s, b_i = u, \bar{X}_i(s)) f_{b_i}(u \mid T_i \geq s, \bar{Y}_i(s), \bar{X}_i(s)) du$$

$$= \frac{\int f_{\bar{Y}_i(s)}(\bar{Y}_i(s) \mid b_i = u, \bar{X}_i(s)) (S_{iu}(s) - S_{iu}(s+t)) f_{b_i}(u) du}{\int f_{\bar{Y}_i(s)}(\bar{Y}_i(s) \mid b_i = u, \bar{X}_i(s)) S_{iu}(s) f_{b_i}(u) du} :$$

$$(8.24)$$

with $S_{iu}(s) = S_i(s \mid b_i = u, \bar{X}_i(s))$.

After the estimation of a joint model, with the estimates $\hat{\theta}$ and their estimated variance $\widehat{V(\hat{\theta})}$, the probability of event may be computed for any subject (including subjects not used for the model estimation). A point estimate is obtained by computing (8.23) or (8.24) with $\hat{\theta}$. Alternatively, the posterior distribution of $P(T_i \leq s+t \mid T_i \geq s, \bar{Y}_i(s), \bar{X}_i(s))$ may be approximated by

Monte Carlo from the asymptotic distribution of the estimates, $\mathcal{N}\left(\hat{\theta}, \widehat{V(\hat{\theta})}\right)$ (Proust-Lima and Taylor, 2009; Rizopoulos, 2011). For this, many vectors of parameters θ_k are generated according to the distribution $\mathcal{N}\left(\hat{\theta}, \widehat{V(\hat{\theta})}\right)$ and the corresponding probabilities $P(T_i \leq s + t \mid T_i \geq s, \bar{Y}_i(s), \bar{X}_i(s); \theta_k)$ are computed. The mean or median of the empirical distribution and its variance can then be calculated.

Figure 8.5 gives an example of dynamic predicted probabilities obtained from a joint latent class model and compared with those obtained by a classical survival model. These are the predicted probabilities of prostate cancer recurrence calculated over a period of 3 years and updated at each new measurement of PSA for a man who had a clinical relapse diagnosed 3.8 years after the end of treatment, a tumor stage equal to 2, a Gleason score of 7 and an initial PSA level of 9,7ng/mL. In the joint latent class model, the probability of event evolves with the increase of PSA over time while the predictions from the classical survival model do not account for this increase in PSA and thus remain very low.

Fixing the time of prediction s and the horizon t, the ability of these estimators for correctly predicting events occurring between s and t may be evaluated using standard criteria such as the ROC curve and the Brier score. Estimators of these criteria accounting for censoring between s and t have been proposed (Proust-Lima and Taylor, 2009; Blanche et al., 2015), as well as summary criteria for a range of prediction times s and tests for comparing several predictors at a given time s or for a set of prediction times s.

8.6 Extension of joint models

Initially the joint models were proposed to simultaneously study the trajectory of a longitudinal marker, assumed to be Gaussian, and the risk of an event. However, cohort studies and clinical trials generally lead to the collection of multiple events and several longitudinal markers, not always Gaussian, and their joint analysis is useful in many health problems. Accounting for these two issues led to the main extensions of joint models briefly described thereafter.

8.6.1 Complex longitudinal data

We described the joint shared random effects models and joint latent class models for a single Gaussian longitudinal marker whose change with time is described by a linear mixed model (see Section 4). But the principle of joint models can also be applied to more complex longitudinal data. According to

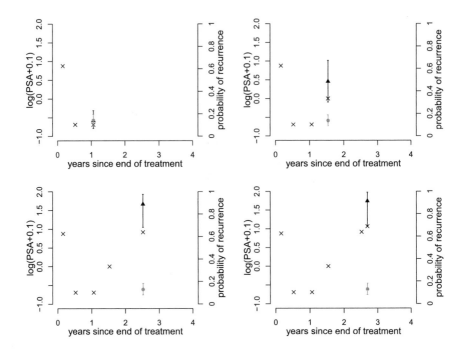

FIGURE 8.5
Individual dynamic predicted probabilities computed for a horizon of 3 years
and updated at each new measurement of PSA (represented by ×) for the
joint model with four latent classes (triangle) and for the model assuming
independence between PSA and risk of relapse (circle) for a man who had
a clinical relapse diagnosed 3.8 years after the end of treatment, a tumor
stage equal to 2, a Gleason score of 7 and an initial PSA level of 9,7ng/mL.
We display the medians and 2.5% and 97.5% percentiles of the predicted
probabilities obtained from 2000 vectors of parameters generated for each
model.

the nature and the number of markers, the linear mixed model is replaced with
a generalized linear mixed model seen in Chapter 4, a curvilinear mixed model
or a multivariate mixed model, with or without underlying latent process, as
described in Chapter 5.

   For example, joint models have been proposed to describe the association
between several longitudinal markers and an event time with a shared random
effects approach (Xu and Zeger, 2001; Song et al., 2002; Lin et al., 2002; Chi
and Ibrahim, 2006; Rizopoulos and Ghosh, 2011; Li et al., 2012; Brown et al.,
2005; Andrinopoulou et al., 2014): the change over time of each marker was
modeled by a mixed model (possibly generalized linear or non-linear) and the
random effects from the mixed sub-models (correlated with each other to take

into account the correlation between the markers) were included as predictors in the survival sub-models to explain the risk of associated clinical events.

These models, estimated in a Bayesian or a frequentist framework, were applied in cancer research to describe the risk of death or of clinical progression from several repeated measures of quality of life (Chi and Ibrahim, 2006), in cardiac surgery to describe the risk of death after replacement of a cardiac valve according to longitudinal indicators of valvar function (Andrinopoulou et al., 2014), or to describe survival after renal transplant (Rizopoulos and Ghosh, 2011). They were also applied in clinical trials (Lin et al., 2002; Xu and Zeger, 2001; Song et al., 2002; Brown et al., 2005), especially for studying surrogate markers.

Using a curvilinear model with latent classes and latent process, Proust-Lima et al. (2009) modeled the change over time of the overall cognitive process underlying three psychometric tests measured repeatedly by linking the latent process to the risk of dementia in the elderly.

8.6.2 Multiple events

As seen in Section 8.6.1, the study of the natural history of a disease or the monitoring of patients often requires the analysis of the evolution of several markers. Similarly, clinical progression may be characterized by the occurrence of multiple events. These events may be either of the same type (successive recurrences of cancer), or may be competing events (deaths from various causes, local or distant metastases) or these may be different events that are correlated but not competing (dementia, loss of autonomy, etc.). Extensions of joint models have been proposed to take into account these different types of multiple events.

For instance, the risk of epileptic seizures has been studied with a joint latent class model for recurrent events by introducing a random effect (frailty) to account for the correlation between events (Han et al., 2007). Recently, joint latent class models for multiple longitudinal markers and competing risks (Proust-Lima et al., 2015) or interval-censored semi-competing risks (Rouanet et al., 2015) have been proposed for studying cognitive decline associated with dementia and death.

However, most joint models for multiple events have been developed in the framework of shared random effects models. Joint models for competing risks have been proposed, where the parameters are estimated either with a Bayesian method (Hu et al., 2009) or by an EM algorithm (Elashoff et al., 2008; Williamson et al., 2008; Li et al., 2012). Chi and Ibrahim (2006) proposed a model for multiple longitudinal markers and multiple events while Liu and Huang (2009) developed a joint model for recurrent events and a terminal event applied to the analysis of the risk of opportunistic infection and death among HIV patients. Joint shared random effects models for competing risks (Yu and Ghosh, 2010) or semi-competing risks (Dantan et al., 2011) including a random change-point for the slope of the marker have also been proposed.

Recently, Ferrer et al. (2015) made available a R function using the JM and mstate packages to estimate joint shared random effects models combining mixed models and multistate models.

9

The dynamic approach to causality

This chapter explores the topic of causality with an emphasis on the dynamical approach; it is more exploratory and research-oriented than the rest of the book. It begins with a general introduction of the topic (Section 9.1), going from philosophical to statistical aspects. Section 9.1.3 gives a gentle introduction of the dynamic approach to causality which may allow readers who are not so much interested in the mathematical and philosophical aspects to skip Sections 9.2 and 9.3. Section 9.2 presents the mathematical definition of influence between stochastic processes. Section 9.3 attempts to ground causality on *physical laws* and using the concept of *system*. Section 9.4 is an application of these concepts to ageing studies. In Section 9.5 the link is made with mechanistic models. Finally, Section 9.6 tackles the problem of dynamic treatment regime.

9.1 Introduction

9.1.1 The causality issue

9.1.1.1 Philosophical aspects

Everybody has an intuitive feeling of the notion of "cause." It is very hard however to define the concept; this is in part due to the fact that it covers several meanings. Aristotle was the first to formalize it. In the *Physics*, he distinguished four types of causes: material, formal, efficient and final (Falcon, 2014). Interestingly he was interested in explaining the movement, or the *change*. The modern use of the word "cause" refers essentially to Aristotle's *efficient cause*: the primary source of change, which precedes the change. Although often neglected, the concept of *final cause* is also interesting in life sciences. A goal which is to be reached in the future explains the succession of events. Interestingly, Aristotle takes a public health example: "I exercise to be in good health." The goal is to be in good health at a time t_2: this goal is the (final) cause of my physical activity at a time $t_1 < t_2$. This does not violate the time-order of efficient causes: exercise is an *efficient cause* of good health, and because I know this fact, I decide to exercise. The final cause applies also to a physician who gives a treatment to a patient, another Aristotle's example.

This example is related to the issue of estimating the effect of a treatment in an observational study, treated in Section 9.6. For the rest of this chapter, we focus on the concept of efficient cause, just keeping in mind that the final cause concept provides another perspective. Many philosophers have worked on the causality issue, and it is not the place here to thoroughly review this topic. In the 18th century, Hume's definition of causality based on regularity and contiguity in time and space was very influential (Hume, 2011). In the 20th century, however, the deterministic view of causality was particularly challenged by the advent of quantum theory. As stated by Bunge (1979), "the principle of causality seemed dead." The same author noted the comeback of causality in the seventies. This is due to a great extent to the allowance of randomness in the appearance of events which are also governed by causal laws: probabilistic causality has been put forward by Reichenbach (1956) and Suppes (1970). Modern approaches have attempted to link causality to the laws of nature (Cartwright, 1979). Another approach defended by Lewis (1973) is to formalize causality in terms of counterfactuals. Other authors such as Woodward (2014) have insisted on the central role of intervention.

9.1.1.2   Causality in the life sciences

Causal issues appear at different levels and hence in different disciplines. Here, we are particularly interested in causal issues in life sciences in general and more specifically in epidemiology. Living beings are complex systems, and this is true at different levels: cells, populations of cells (like the immune system), human beings, etc. Not only are these systems complex, but they have also complex relationships with their environment: cells are part of populations of cells, themselves in relation with other populations of cells, human beings have complex social relationships. The levels of cells or population of cells are the domain of biology and physiology. At these levels, the concept of "mechanism" (Wimsatt, 1994; Machamer, 2004; Craver and Darden, 2013) is used to understand the behaviours of these entities. Attempting to model these mechanisms is the domain of system biology, an example of which will be given in Section 9.5. Health problems of human beings (or animals) are thought to be the result of evolution of biological phenomena: cardiovascular diseases are mainly due to atherosclerosis, which is characterized by atheromatous deposits in arteries: such deposits are favoured by high concentration of LDL (low density lipoproteins) and a context of inflammation and oxidative stress. It is thought that lifestyle factors (such as diet and physical activity) influence this biological context. The same kind of analysis can be done for the most important diseases like cancers or AIDS. It is important to understand the complex causal pathway connecting several factors and the occurrence of the disease. In view of the difficulty of this task, it may also be important to bypass this stage and to directly link a factor (such as physical activity) to the disease. The latter approach has been very fruitful in epidemiology and clinical research.

9.1.1.3 Causality in epidemiology

A large part of the epidemiological endeavor aims at identifying determinants of diseases, and also on a more clinical side, to assess the effect of therapeutic strategies and more specifically the effect of treatments. The goal is to improve public health by trying to modify the distribution of risk factors in the population: lifestyle factors (smoking, diet, physical activity) in particular are thought to be modifiable, although this is not so easy in practice. Prevention is relevant at both population and individual levels. On the clinical side, the goal is to improve therapeutic strategies. So, most of the epidemiological studies have tended to bypass the complex causal pathway leading from risk factors to disease.

Not every person having a particular value of a factor develops a disease: for instance, not all the smokers develop lung cancer. Thus, statistics became the major tool of epidemiology. Correlations or associations between factors and diseases were studied, but it was soon realized that this was not sufficient to deduce causal relation (Wright, 1921). As put by Broadbent (2013), the problem is crudely summarized by the slogan "Correlation is not causation." The main reason for that is that there may be common causes for factor and disease. In epidemiology, these common causes are called "confounding factors."

Statisticians developed two main tools for controlling such factors: randomized trials and regression models. The link between the confounding factors and the factor of interest can be broken by randomization. Randomized controlled trials have become the gold standard for assessing the effect of interventions. They have however a certain number of limitations. First their feasibility: it may not be feasible to control a lifestyle factor. Even when randomized trials are feasible, they often include highly selected subjects and have a short duration; moreover, compliance in taking the attributed treatment may be low and may be different in the different arms of the trial. For all these reasons, observational studies (as opposed to randomized studies) are needed. In observational studies, regression models allow adjusting on potential confounding factors. Linear regression and logistic models were widely used. Since the seventies dynamical regression models for events (Cox model for instance) and quantitative variables (mixed-effect models) were developed. Dynamical models are obviously more apt to grasp causal relationships than static ones. Finally the more elaborate multistate models and joint models are more realistic and thus lend to more reliable causal interpretation. Such models may allow reconstructing part of the causal pathway between factor and disease, thus reducing the gap between epidemiology and system biology. However, the use of such complex dynamical models does not guarantee the validity of a causal interpretation. There is a need to formalize the causality issue in a more general way.

Hill (1965) has proposed criteria for causality in epidemiology, known as the Bradford-Hill criteria. These are nine qualitative criteria: strength of the association, consistency (a concept close to reproducibility), specificity (specific population at risk, specific types of disease), temporality (cause precedes the effect), biological gradient, plausibility, coherence, experiment (availability of experimental or semi-experimental evidence), and analogy (similar effects for other factors). Not all the criteria have the same importance; moreover, some of the criteria (e.g., consistency and experiment) are not at the level of one study but rather pertain to a meta-analysis. These are common sense criteria that may certainly be useful in epidemiology. Statisticians have attempted to develop more formal approaches at the level of one study.

9.1.1.4 Causality in biostatistics

Because of the probabilistic nature of causation, statisticians are naturally involved in the issue of finding causal relationships; however, because of the pitfalls on the way between association and causation, statisticians like epidemiologists have been very cautious on this topic. This is why the term *risk factor* is commonly used and there are very few mentions of causal relationships in the epidemiological literature. In the seventies, however, statisticians began to tackle the causality issue. Jöreskog et al. (2001) developed the linear structural equation models (LISREL) which had been pioneered by Wright (1921). The econometrician Granger (Granger, 1969) formalized the concept of influence of a process on another process, in a time-series framework. Graphical models were developed to represent causal relationships: complete presentations can be found in Spirtes et al. (2000) and Pearl (2000). Rubin (1974) proposed a counterfactual approach for estimating the causal effect of a treatment. The counterfactual approach was further developed by James Robins (Robins, 1986); this approach attracted much attention since then and its principle is briefly described in Section 9.1.2. A general description of statistical approaches to causality can be found in Chapter 9 of Aalen et al. (2008).

9.1.2 The counterfactual approach

9.1.2.1 Principle

One way of representing causal effect is by introducing *potential responses* to the different values of the exposure or treatment of interest. This idea was first proposed by Neyman in 1923 (Splawa-Neyman, 1990) for a field experiment. It was proposed by Rubin (1974) in the context of clinical trials and developed in many other papers. The focus of this chapter is on the dynamical approach to causality. Because of its importance and popularity, we briefly describe the principle of the potential outcome approach for a fixed exposure. The extension to time-varying exposure is also briefly described in Section 9.6 where marginal structural models (MSM) are compared to dynamical models.

Assume that we are interested in the effect of a treatment or an exposure A on an outcome Y. The exposure A can take different values: $A = a$. It is assumed that each subject has a *potential response* Y_a when the exposure takes the value a. Of course, a given subject is exposed to only one particular value a: then the observed outcome is $Y = Y_a$. For instance if the possible values of A are 0 and 1, if a subject has been exposed to the value 1, we observe $Y = Y_{a=1}$, and we do not observe $Y_{a=0}$. This latter value is *counterfactual*, in the sense that $a = 0$ for this subject is counter to the fact that $a = 1$ in reality. If we could know $Y_{a=0}$, we could know the individual causal effect of exposure $Y_{a=1} - Y_{a=0}$. The average or mean causal effect in the population is $E[Y_{a=1} - Y_{a=0}] = E[Y_{a=1}] - E[Y_{a=0}]$. There are three identifiability conditions, called consistency, conditional exchangeability and positivity, under which it is possible to consistently estimate $E[Y_a]$, and thus the average causal effect from observational studies (Robins and Hernán, 2009).

Robins (1986) extended the potential outcome approach to time-varying exposures, further developed in a series of papers. The approach includes different methods (g-estimation of structural nested models, inverse probability of treatment weighting for marginal structural models) and is well summarized in Robins and Hernán (2009). A summary of the history of the developments of these methods can be found in Richardson et al. (2014).

9.1.2.2 Criticism

The potential outcome/counterfactual approach to causality has become very popular. We think, however, that there are several limitations to this approach. One potential problem is that we may have to assume a continuous infinity of potential responses in complex problems where both A and Y are continuous and may vary in continuous time. Another issue is the nature of the randomness of the potential outcomes: they vary in the population, but seem to be fixed for a subject. This has been well analyzed by Dawid (2000) who critiques such a "fatalist philosophy" and notes that "even after treatment has been taken, it seems unrealistic to regard the patient's recovery status as predetermined." One question is how to define causal effect without counterfactuals. The answer is to consider that different regimes can be applied to future patients, corresponding to different probabilities of treatment attribution. This is the approach taken by Arjas and Parner (2004), Geneletti and Dawid (2011) and Commenges and Gégout-Petit (2015). Rather than split the response Y into several potential responses we can consider various regimes, giving rise to different probability laws for Y. This is not counterfactual because for instance an intervention will be made in the future for different individuals. The question is to infer from observational studies what will be the law of Y under this new regime.

9.1.3 The dynamical approach to causality

The dynamical approach to causality uses the formalism of stochastic processes and the concept of system. It has been particularly developed by Aalen (1987), Arjas and Parner (2004) and Didelez (2008); a particular approach called "dynamic path analysis" has been developed by Fosen et al. (2006). The core of the approach presented in this chapter is essentially based on Commenges and Gégout-Petit (2009). There is a mathematical part (Section 9.2) which is to define the *influence* of one component of a stochastic process on another; we resort to the concept of *system* to define "causal influence," which has a physical meaning (Section 9.3). The approach is applied to ageing studies (Section 9.4), mechanistic models (Section 9.5) and dynamic treatment regimes (Section 9.6). The rest of this section 9.1.3 gives an introduction to these topics which may be sufficient to readers not interested in technical developments to directly tackle Section 9.4 and the following sections.

9.1.3.1   Representation by stochastic processes

The starting point of the dynamical approach is to consider that we have a better representation of phenomena and their causal relationship by using stochastic processes than ordinary random variables, and most of the time it is better to consider that these processes live in continuous time. We have already seen examples of this approach in Chapter 7. This leads us to a change of paradigm. In the conventional paradigm, we observe random variables and we search a model that will fit them; in the dynamic paradigm, a system is represented by a stochastic process and we collect observations from this system which will allow estimating the law of the process. Thus, it is useful to distinguish between the model for the system and the model for the observation, a classical distinction in automatics (Kalman and Bucy, 1961; Jazwinski, 1970) but not in biostatistics. To illustrate this different point of view and the further introduced concepts, we will take a toy example. Consider first that we are interested in a physiological quantity, say blood pressure, and how it varies with age. We have observations V_j of blood pressure at age t_j and we may model them by $V_j = \beta_0 + \beta_1 t_j + \varepsilon_j$ with some possible assumptions on the distribution of the ε_j's: this is the conventional approach. In the dynamical approach we have a model for the system which is a model for a stochastic process V in continuous time; this gives justice to the fact that there is some blood pressure at any time. The law of the process can be given by its Doob-Meyer decomposition (see Section 3.7.1) and a possible model is: $V_t = \beta_0 + \beta_1 t + \omega B_t$, where B_t is a Brownian motion or in differential form:

$$\mathrm{d}V_t = \beta_1 \mathrm{d}t + \omega \mathrm{d}B_t,$$

which makes the dynamics of the process more visible. Observations V_j are then noisy observations of the process V at time $t_j : V_j = V(t_j) + \varepsilon_j$. One advantage of this formulation is that it gives a natural correlation structure for the V_j's.

Suppose now that we are interested in the occurrence of a type of event, say dementia. Rather than modeling the distribution of the time of occurrence of the event, we can find the law of a counting process, as was presented in Section 3.7.1. Generally, counting processes are denoted by N_t but since we take here a more general point of view, we denote the process of interest (e.g., dementia) by Y_t. The law of Y_t can be given by its Doob-Meyer decomposition $Y_t = \Lambda_t + M_t$ or its differential form $dY_t = \lambda_t dt + dM_t$. We may have continuous-time observations (with possibly right-censoring) or discrete-time observations (inducing interval-censoring).

Moreover, we shall consider multivariate processes. In the case there are several events, this could be represented by a multistate process; we will prefer a representation by a multivariate counting process as in Section 7.8 because we are interested in the relation between the different components of the multivariate stochastic process. For instance we can be interested in both dementia and death; the interaction of these two events can be represented by an illness-death model. Alternatively, this can be represented by a bivariate counting process.

The multivariate stochastic process X can have components which are counting processes and others which are diffusion processes, allowing us to analyze the relationships between events and continuous phenomena, both typically evolving in continuous time. Suppose we are interested in both blood pressure and dementia, we can consider a joint model for the two processes: $dV_t = \beta_1 dt + \omega dB_t$; $dY_t = \lambda_t dt + dM_t$. The intensity of Y can be modeled as: $\lambda_t = I_{Y_t=0}\alpha_0(t)e^{\gamma V_t}$, where $\alpha_0(\cdot)$ is the baseline hazard function. We may have discrete-time observations of V and continuous- or discrete-time observations of Y, allowing estimating the parameters of this model. The joint models have been presented in Chapter 8. Of course more than two processes can be included and what is interesting is the interaction between the dynamics of these processes.

9.1.3.2 Local influence in stochastic processes

Given a system represented by a multivariate stochastic process X, a criterion of local independence called WCLI (weak local conditional independence) is defined in terms of measurability of processes involved in the Doob-Meyer representation. In our above example of a joint process $X = (Y, V)$ we have:

$$\begin{aligned} dV_t &= \beta_1 dt + \omega dB_t \\ dY_t &= I_{Y_t=0}\alpha_0(t)e^{\gamma V_t}dt + dM_t. \end{aligned}$$

We see that V_t appears in the intensity of Y: if $\gamma \neq 0$, this intensity would not be *measurable* in a filtration not including V. Equivalently we could say that marginally to V, Y does not have the same intensity. On the contrary Y does not appear in the intensity of V: we do not need any information on Y to know the dynamics of V. We shall say that V is WCLI of Y, but that Y is not WCLI of V.

Conversely, if a component of X, X_k, is not WCLI of another component, X_j, we say that X_j has a "direct influence" on X_k, and we note: $X_j \longrightarrow_X X_k$. In our example, we would note $V \longrightarrow_X Y$ and since V is WCLI of Y we can also note $Y \not\longrightarrow_{\boldsymbol{X}} V$. It is important to note that the direct influences depend on both the system $\boldsymbol{X}$ and the probability law.

A graph can then be constructed having the components of the stochastic process as nodes and directed edges where there are direct influences. This is analogous to classical graphical models with the difference that nodes are stochastic processes rather than random variables and the graph may be cyclic; in particular we may have both $X_j \longrightarrow_{\boldsymbol{X}} X_k$ and $X_k \longrightarrow_{\boldsymbol{X}} X_j$. An advantage of these process graphs is that they are more concise than the conventional DAGs and also more concise than the graphs for multistate models. See for instance the graph displayed in Figure 9.3 which features Dementia, Blood pressure, Death and fixed explanatory variables.

In fact, WCLI and influences can be defined on a finite horizon, τ. It could well be that a process has an influence on another process until a certain time only, or that we are not interested in the possible influence after a certain time. This horizon can be fixed or random. A random horizon is particularly interesting when studying the effect of a process which represents a risk factor of a disease, because we are generally not interested in the effect of the disease on the risk factor. Thus in our example, we will study the possible influences on the horizon T_Y, the time of occurrence of dementia. On this horizon, dementia cannot have an influence on blood pressure because by definition this is a period without dementia, while on a fixed-time period, it is not impossible that dementia influence blood pressure; see Section 9.2.3. The case of death is similar, but death is a special event as discussed in Section 9.4. All this is developed in Section 9.2.

9.1.3.3 Systems and causal influences

How can the mathematical property of "direct influence" between components of a process under a particular probability P be used for exploring causality? Answering this question may be possible if we have a definition of "causal influence." We give a definition based on the concept of "system" universally used by physicists, and on the concept of sequence of nested systems. It is postulated that, for a given "level," there exists a sufficiently large system $\boldsymbol{X}^M$ and physical laws allowing to compute the true probability P^* for events of interest. In Section 9.3 we denote the system by $\boldsymbol{S}^M$ to insist on the fact that we are dealing with real systems and not merely with abstract stochastic processes. We give the example of applying the law of gravitation to a system for predicting the movement of earth. A simple system can be formed by Earth and the Sun. Applying the gravitation law to this system will give a prediction of the trajectory of Earth which is not perfect. Including Mars in the system will improve the prediction. Including in addition Venus and Jupiter will yet improve it. So, we tend toward a system in which predictions will be nearly perfect (assuming the gravitation law is correct; for precise computations relativity theory must be used). This principle can be applied to other domains of science and in particular to epidemiology, with the difference that we do not know the physical law but we have rather to estimate it. In our example on dementia we will try to represent all the processes that may influence dementia. Such a system denoted by $\boldsymbol{X}^M$ will be called a *perfect system* for dementia. This allows defining *causal influences*. A direct influence in $\boldsymbol{X}^M$ under P* is called a direct *causal influence*. The causal effects (which are the quantification of causal influences) can be summarized by different contrasts (see Section 9.3.2.1).

Many issues in causality come from the fact that we generally do not work with $\boldsymbol{X}^M$ but with smaller systems. So, we are led to consider a sequence of nested systems and to explore the stability of properties within these sequences. If we do not have a perfect system for Y, by definition there are processes U which influence Y and which are not included in the system. Then the question is whether it is possible to estimate marginal causal effects of a factor V on Y in this system. These processes U are potential unmeasured confounders; they are confounders if they influence V in the larger system $(\boldsymbol{X}, U)$. If they do not influence V, then $\boldsymbol{X}$ is a system with no unmeasured confounders, and marginal causal effects can be estimated.

This is developed in Section 9.3. Also Section 9.6.2 gives assumptions needed for causal interpretation in the context of time-varying exposure. An assumption of *stability*, implicit in Section 9.3, is added, meaning that the different subjects of a population obey the same physical law.

9.1.3.4 Applications

The dynamical approach can be applied at the level of subjects or at the level of populations. In the first case, it is implemented in multistate models and joint models; see Section 9.4. In the second case mechanistic models are developed to represent the dynamic interaction between subpopulations, and this has applications for populations of subjects (like in epidemics models) or for populations of cells within a subject. Mechanistic models are presented in Section 9.5.

The dynamical approach is also useful for estimating the effect of a treatment in observational studies, where the treatment is often attributed in a dynamic way. In this application, this is an alternative to MSM. An example for estimating the effect of HAART on CD4 T-cells population is given. In this case, discrete-time dynamic models as well as mechanistic models can be used. This issue is developed in Section 9.6.

9.2 Local independence, direct and indirect influence

9.2.1 Notations

Consider a filtered space $(\Omega, \mathcal{F}, (\mathcal{F}_t), P)$ and a multivariate stochastic process $\boldsymbol{X} = (\boldsymbol{X}_t)_{t \geq 0}$; $\boldsymbol{X}_t$ takes values in $\mathbb{R}^m$. We have $\boldsymbol{X} = (X_j, j = 1, \ldots, m)$ where $X_j = (X_{jt})_{t \geq 0}$. We denote by $\mathcal{X}_t$ the history of $\boldsymbol{X}$ up to time t, that is $\mathcal{X}_t$ is the σ-field $\sigma(\boldsymbol{X}_u, 0 \leq u \leq t)$, and by $(\mathcal{X}_t) = (\mathcal{X}_t)_{t \geq 0}$ the families of these histories, that is the filtration generated by $\boldsymbol{X}$. Similarly we shall denote by $\mathcal{X}_{jt}$ and $(\mathcal{X}_{jt})$ the histories and filtration associated to X_j. If C is a subset of $(1, \ldots, m)$ we shall call X_C the multivariate process $(X_j, j \in C)$.

9.2.2 Local independence, direct and indirect influence

Let $\mathcal{F}_t = \mathcal{G} \vee \mathcal{X}_t$; $\mathcal{G}$ may contain information known at $t = 0$, in addition to the initial value of $\boldsymbol{X}$ (this will be used to represent fixed variables, like gender, that we call *attributes*). We shall consider the class of special semi-martingales, that is the class of processes which admit a unique Doob-Meyer decomposition in the $(\mathcal{F}_t)$ filtration, under probability P:

$$\boldsymbol{X}_t = \Lambda_t + M_t, t \geq 0, \tag{9.1}$$

where M_t is a martingale and Λ_t is a predictable process with bounded variation. We shall write the Doob-Meyer decomposition of X_j: $X_{jt} = \Lambda_{jt} + M_{jt}$. We shall consider the non-degenerate case in which all the components of M are different from zero; the deterministic case will be studied in Section 9.2.5. We shall assume two conditions bearing on the bracket process (Jacod and Shiryaev, 2003, Chapter I, Theorem 4.2) of the martingale M:

A1 M_j and M_k are orthogonal martingales, for all $j \neq k$;

A2 X_j is either a counting process or is continuous with a deterministic bracket process, for all j.

We call $\mathcal{D}$ the class of all special semi-martingales satisfying **A1** and **A2**. The class of special semi-martingales is stable by change of absolutely continuous probability and this is also true for the class $\mathcal{D}$. This class has been extended by Gégout-Petit and Commenges (2010).

Definition 6 (Weak conditional local independence (WCLI)) X_k *is weakly locally independent of* X_j *in* $\boldsymbol{X}$ *on* $[r, s]$ *if and only if the process* $(\Lambda_{kt} - \Lambda_{kr})_{t \geq r}$ *is* $(\mathcal{F}_{-jt})$-*predictable on* $[r, s]$, *where* $\mathcal{F}_{-jt} = \mathcal{G} \vee \mathcal{X}_{-jt}$ *and* $\mathcal{X}_{-jt} = \vee_{l \neq j} \mathcal{X}_{lt}$.

In the remainder of this chapter we will always take $[r, s] = [0, \tau]$, where τ is a given "horizon;" τ can be a fixed time but can also be a random time (a stopping time); this is developed in Section 9.2.3.

When X_k is WCLI from X_j, it has the same Doob-Meyer decomposition in $(\mathcal{F}_t)$ and in $(\mathcal{F}_{-jt})$, and we will note $X_j \not\longrightarrow_{\boldsymbol{X}} X_k$. The WCLI condition depends on both filtration and probability law. In principle we should refer the WCLI property to the whole filtration rather than only to the filtration generated by $\boldsymbol{X}$. The two filtrations are the same if $\mathcal{G}$ is empty. $\mathcal{G}$ could be used to represent fixed variables, but we can also include them as degenerate processes; thus we may extend the WCLI property to a relationship between a process and fixed variables. Fixed variables are necessarily WCLI from the other components but may influence other components of the process.

Remark 1: Assumption **A2** is necessary for the measurability-based definition of WCLI to be clearly interpreted. If we did not impose **A2** we could find counter-examples in which a WCLI holds while intuitively independence does not hold. Such a counter-example is the process $\boldsymbol{X} = (X_1, X_2)$ which is the solution of the differential equation: $dX_{1t} = a\ dt + b\ dW_{1t}$; $\mathrm{d}X_{2t} = X_{1t}\ \mathrm{d}t + e^{X_{1t}}\ \mathrm{d}W_{2t}$, Where W_1 and W_2 are Brownian motions. We would not like to say that X_2 is WCLI of X_1. However, because X_1 appears in the bracket process of X_2, $\mathcal{X}_{1t}$ is included in $\mathcal{X}_{2t}$ so that Λ_2 is $\mathcal{X}_{2t}$-predictable and thus we would conclude that X_2 is WCLI of X_1.

Remark 2: It is tempting to define WCLI directly in terms of the conditional independence:

$$\mathcal{X}_{kt} \perp_{\mathcal{X}_{Ct-}, \mathcal{X}_{kt-}} \mathcal{X}_{jt-}, 0 \leq t \leq \tau. \tag{9.2}$$

This formula attempts to express non-influence by requiring that X_t is independent of the past of X_j given the past of X_k and X_C. However, this condition is void in general when we consider processes in continuous time. Because conditional independence is defined via conditional probability and in general, events of $\mathcal{X}_{kt}$ have conditional probabilities equal to one or zero given $\mathcal{X}_{kt-}$, the condition always holds.

Remark 3: WCLI is identical with weak instantaneous non-causality of Florens and Fougère (1996).

Definition 7 (Direct influence) *We shall say that if X_k is not WCLI of X_j in $\boldsymbol{X}$, X_j directly influences X_k in $\boldsymbol{X}$ and we will note $X_j \longrightarrow_{\boldsymbol{X}} X_k$.*

Definition 8 (WCLI and Direct influence for set of components) *Let A, B subsets of $(1, \ldots, m)$. We shall say that $X_A \longrightarrow_{\boldsymbol{X}} X_B$ if there is $j \in A$ and $k \in B$ such that $X_j \longrightarrow_{\boldsymbol{X}} X_k$.*

What we call here "direct influence" is the time-continuous analogue of Granger strong causality (Granger, 1969; Florens and Fougère, 1996). We may consider another, stronger, condition of local independence.

Definition 9 (Strong conditional local independence (SCLI)) *X_k is SCLI of X_j in $\boldsymbol{X}$ if and only if $X_j \not\longrightarrow_{\boldsymbol{X}} X_k$ and there is no $X_D \subset \boldsymbol{X}$ such that $X_j \longrightarrow_{\boldsymbol{X}} X_D$ and $X_D \longrightarrow_{\boldsymbol{X}} X_k$. We will note $X_j \not\dashrightarrow_{\boldsymbol{X}} X_k$.*

Definition 10 (Influence) *We shall say that if X_k is not SCLI of X_j, X_j influences (at least indirectly) X_k in $\boldsymbol{X}$ and we will note $X_j \longrightarrow\hspace{-0.5em}\rightarrow_{\boldsymbol{X}} X_k$.*

If X_j influences X_k but X_j does not directly influence X_k, we shall say that X_j indirectly influences X_k.

Definition 11 (Indirect influence) *If $X_j \rightarrow\rightarrow_{\boldsymbol{X}} X_k$ and $X_j \not\mapsto_{\boldsymbol{X}} X_k$ then there is $X_C \subset \boldsymbol{X}$ such that $X_j \longrightarrow_{\boldsymbol{X}} X_C \longrightarrow_{\boldsymbol{X}} X_k$ and we shall say that X_j indirectly influences X_k through X_C in $\boldsymbol{X}$.*

Remark 4: Since the Doob-Meyer decomposition depends on P, so do all the independencies and influences; realizing this fact is crucial for the definition of causal influence in Section 9.3.

9.2.3 Extension to random horizon and the problem of death

The definition of WCLI can be extended without modification to a random horizon τ, where τ is a stopping time. A stopping time τ is such that in the considered filtration $\{\mathcal{F}\}$, the event $\{\tau < t\}$ is included in $\mathcal{F}_t$. As an example, consider a system with two processes V and Y. To fix ideas, V could represent systolic blood pressure and Y dementia; V has a continuous state space, while Y is a $0-1$ counting process. Epidemiologists are interested in knowing whether high blood pressure is a risk factor of dementia. So they are interested in knowing whether Y is WCLI of V, on $(0, T_Y)$, where T_Y is the time of occurrence of dementia. T_Y is a stopping time because in the filtration generated by Y, we know at each time t whether dementia has occurred or not. After Y has jumped, the intensity is null, so that V cannot influence Y after the jump. Note also that in general we are not interested in the effect of dementia on blood pressure, although such an effect is not excluded. If we stop at T_Y, there can be no effect of Y on V because on $(0, T_Y-)$ Y is uniformly zero. Thus, using the random horizon T_Y allows focusing on the effect of V on Y (in our example, of blood pressure on dementia). Another example would be the relation between tobacco consumption and lung cancer. If we are interested in the effect of tobacco on cancer, we define WCLI on $(0, T_C)$, where T_C is the time of occurrence of cancer. There may well be an effect of cancer on tobacco consumption since people with cancer are likely to stop smoking, but this is not of primary interest for epidemiologists.

An example of a random time which is not a stopping time would be the time where the systolic blood pressure reaches its maximum. In the filtration generated by (V, Y), we do not know at time t whether V has reached its maximum; so such a time is not a stopping time and could not be used as a time horizon for defining WCLI.

The case of death is special. This is chiefly relevant for applications where the system represents a subject. In short-term studies or in studies with young subjects, it may not be necessary to model death. In many studies, however, and especially in ageing studies (this will be treated in Section 9.4), this is necessary. Death can be modelled by a $0-1$ counting process. It must be realized that all the other processes are defined for living subjects. Therefore, the maximum horizon for studying WCLI is T_D, the time of death.

9.2.4   Differential equation representation

If Λ_t is differentiable, the Doob-Meyer decomposition can be written in the form of a stochastic differential equation (SDE):

$$\mathrm{d}\boldsymbol{X}_t = \lambda_t \mathrm{d}t + dM_t, \tag{9.3}$$

with $\Lambda_t = \int_0^t \lambda_u \mathrm{d}u$. Differential equations are commonly used in physics, biology and in finance (Øksendal et al., 1992) to describe how physical laws should specify the evolution of $\boldsymbol{X}_t$ as a function of the past plus a random term brought by the martingale. The two main cases, which have been considered in different streams of research, are the case where the trajectories of $\boldsymbol{X}$ are continuous and the case where $\boldsymbol{X}$ is a counting process. In the case of continuous trajectories of $\boldsymbol{X}$ it is common to take for M a Brownian martingale (in which case $\mathrm{d}M_t = f(t)\mathrm{d}W_t$, with $W = (W_t)$ a Brownian motion), and the models considered are Itô processes. In the case where $\boldsymbol{X}$ is a counting process we write:

$$\mathrm{d}\boldsymbol{X}_t = \lambda_t \mathrm{d}t + \mathrm{d}M_t, \tag{9.4}$$

where M is a discontinuous martingale with predictable variation process equal to Λ, and λ is called the intensity of the process. We may consider mixing the two cases, considering that $\boldsymbol{X} = (X_1, X_2)$, where X_1 is an Itô process and X_2 a counting process, each of these processes being possibly multivariate.

9.2.5   The deterministic case

Ordinary differential equation (ODE) models seem to arise as particular cases in which $M = 0$. So one way to apply our definition of WCLI to deterministic models is to consider that these models are in fact stochastic but the martingale has a bracket process which takes small values in regard to Λ. Particular phenomena appear in purely deterministic models, in particular because the concept of *filtration* no longer applies. In that case, the unicity of the differential equation is lost. For instance, consider the process $\boldsymbol{X} = (X_1, X_2)$; consider the case where the process $\boldsymbol{X}$ is deterministic and the trajectories are solutions of the ODE system: $\mathrm{d}X_{1t} = a \, \mathrm{d}t$; $\mathrm{d}X_{2t} = X_{1t}\mathrm{d}t$ with initial conditions $X_{10} = X_{20} = 0$. The trajectories are also solutions of the ODE system: $\mathrm{d}X_{1t} = a \, \mathrm{d}t$; $\mathrm{d}X_{2t} = at \, \mathrm{d}t$ with initial conditions $X_{10} = X_{20} = 0$. One would be tempted to say that X_1 influences X_2 when looking at the first ODE system and but not when looking at the second one. The second ODE system, however, is not time-homogeneous. Unicity can thus be restored if we impose the restriction of time-homogeneity. In view of the unicity of the time-homogeneous differential equation representation, this is the canonical representation, if it exists. The definition of WCLI for stochastic differential equations can then be used to define WCLI for the deterministic case: construct an SDE system by adding to the ODE system orthogonal martingales with deterministic brackets. The influence graph of the time-homogeneous

ODE system is, by definition, the same as that of the derived SDE. In the above example, if we add a standard Wiener martingale to the canonical (time-homogeneous) representation we obtain the SDE: $dX_{1t} = a\, dt + dW_{1t}$; $dX_{2t} = X_{1t}dt + dW_{2t}$, in which it is clear that we have $X_1 \longrightarrow_{\boldsymbol{X}} X_2$.

9.2.6   Graph representation

We may construct a directed graph representing influences between components of $\boldsymbol{X}$. This directed graph has for vertices the components X_j and there is a directed edge (j, k) if and only if $X_j \longrightarrow_{\boldsymbol{X}} X_k$. Note that there can be two directed edges between two vertices, for instance (j, k) and (k, j). A path from X_{j_0} to X_{j_k} is an ordered sequence of directed edges $\{(j_0, j_1), (j_1, j_2), \ldots, (j_{k-1}, j_k)\}$. Influence can be read directly off the graph: $X_j \longrightarrow\longrightarrow_{\boldsymbol{X}} X_k$ if there is a path from j to k.

An example is shown in Figure 9.1 which represents the hypothetical influence graphs for a four-dimensional process $\boldsymbol{X} = (A, V, Y, Z)$. This graph could represent the relationship of processes important in the treatment of HIV infected patients, where Z could represent AIDS (this would be a counting process), Y the CD4+ T-lymphocytes concentration, V the virus concentration and A the treatment process. The graph is not acyclic and in particular we have $A \longrightarrow_{\boldsymbol{X}} V$ and $V \longrightarrow_{\boldsymbol{X}} A$, which reflects the fact that treatment has an effect on virus concentration, and virus concentration in return influences the treatment, an issue which will be tackled in Section 9.6. We see that A indirectly influences Y which we can note: $A \longrightarrow\longrightarrow_{\boldsymbol{X}} Y$. We say that V mediates the effect of A on Y.

9.3   Causal influences

9.3.1   Systems and causal influence

In a scientific problem, there is a set of (real) events of interest, starting from a time origin. As time passes, new events may occur so that it is useful to represent the sets of events of interest for all times by a filtration $(\mathcal{F}_t)$, that we call a *physical filtration*. We mean by this term that in an application (even if here we manipulate an abstract term), each $\mathcal{F}_t$ belonging to the filtration contains real events occurring before or at t, where t is the physical time (and not just a mathematical parameter). It is often useful to distinguish non-dynamical events from dynamical events, which leads to decompose $(\mathcal{F}_t)$ in $\mathcal{G} \vee (\mathcal{X}_t)$.

Example 1: Celestial bodies. At a certain time, we record the masses of the Earth, Sun and Mars; the possible masses form the σ-field $\mathcal{G}$, although

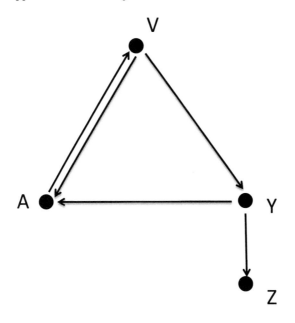

FIGURE 9.1
Example of an influence graph. This is a possible influence graph of important processes for an HIV infected subject: treatment (A), virus concentration (V), CD4 cells concentration (Y), AIDS (Z).

they can also be considered as fixed. The possible locations and speeds of the three celestial bodies up to time t form the σ-field $\mathcal{X}_t$.

Example 2: Population of cells. At a certain time, we consider populations of CD4 T cells and HIV virions in a particular subject; genetic factors may form the sigma-field $\mathcal{G}$. The possible concentrations in the blood up to time t of these two types of particles form the σ-field $\mathcal{X}_t$.

Example 3: Epidemiology. At a certain time, we consider the date of birth and gender of a particular subject; the possible values form the σ-field $\mathcal{G}$. The possible disease and vital status of this subject up to time t form the σ-field $\mathcal{X}_t$.

We generally work with a stochastic process representation of $(\mathcal{F}_t)$, that is a process (G, X). We shall call X the state and G the attribute of the system.

We may distinguish events in which we are directly interested and auxiliary events that we need to incorporate because they are related to the events of interest. For instance, if we are interested in the relative position of the Sun and the Earth, we may have to introduce the position of Mars to make better prediction. It would not be reasonable to include the position of an extra-solar planet nor the concentration of CD4 T cells of a subject: the latter events belong to another level of reality. Since large systems are computationally intractable not only we will not incorporate clearly unrelated events but also events that we think are weakly related; in some cases we will omit related events because we are not aware of them. In order to explore how the influence graph of a system derives from that of a larger system, and also to propose a definition of causal influence it is important to introduce the concept of nested systems. A system $\mathcal{S}^{m'}$ is nested in $\mathcal{S}^m$ if $(\mathcal{F}_t^{m'}) \subset (\mathcal{F}_t^m)$. $\mathcal{S}^{m'}$ can be enlarged by addition of attributes $(\mathcal{G}^{m'} \subset \mathcal{G}^m)$ and/or addition of components $(\mathcal{X}_t^{m'} \subset \mathcal{X}_t^m)$. We can consider a sequence of nested systems $\boldsymbol{S} = \{\mathcal{S}^m\}_{m>0}$ (we note $\mathcal{S}^m \in \boldsymbol{S}$ and $\mathcal{S}^m \subset \mathcal{S}^{m'}$ if $m < m'$). In this case, the family $\{\mathcal{F}_t^m\}_{m>0}$ also forms a filtration (for each t).

Example 4: Immune system-HIV. If we are interested in the population of HIV viruses, we may consider the system $\mathcal{S}^0 = (G_1, X_1, G_2, X_2)$ where X_1 is the concentration of virus and X_2 the concentration of uninfected CD4 T-cells. In this system we cannot express the mechanism of production of viruses by infected cells. A more interesting system is $\mathcal{S}^1$ including virus, uninfected and infected T cells. Still a larger system $\mathcal{S}^1$ is obtained in refining the category "uninfected T cells" by distinguishing quiescent and activated T cells which can be targets for the virus; we have $\mathcal{S}^0 \subset \mathcal{S}^1 \subset \mathcal{S}^2$.

In this sub-section, to emphasize the fact that we are manipulating representations of physical systems, we will speak about direct and indirect influences of X_j on X_k in the system $\mathcal{S}^m$ (and note $X_j \longrightarrow_{\mathcal{S}^m} X_k$ or $X_j \rightarrow\rightarrow_{\mathcal{S}^m} X_k$); these influences correspond to the definitions of influences in $\boldsymbol{X}^m$ in Section 9.2.

We assume that there is a true probability law P^* on $(\Omega, \mathcal{F})$ and we denote its restriction to $\mathcal{F}^m$ by $\mathrm{P}^*_{\mathcal{F}^m}$. The general idea in the following development is that $\mathrm{P}^*_{\mathcal{F}^m}$ can be computed or approximated by applying physical (or natural) laws to a sufficiently rich system. We shall now endeavor to define *physical laws*. Let us first define *mathematical laws*.

Definition 12 (Mathematical laws) *Mathematical laws at a certain level are a set of mathematical procedures that can be applied to any system $\mathcal{S}^m$ of this level to build a probability $\mathrm{P}^{\mathcal{S}^m}$ on $\mathcal{F}^m$.*

Generally the probability $\mathrm{P}^{\mathcal{S}^m}$ will be different from $\mathrm{P}^*_{\mathcal{F}^m}$. Suppose that the events of interest are described in a system $\mathcal{S}^1$, we may have to consider richer systems for making correct predictions. We define *physical (or natural)* *laws* as yielding a probability that may be as close as we wish to $P^*_{\mathcal{F}^1}$, if we can apply them to a correct system.

Definition 13 (Physical laws) *If for any system $\mathcal{S}^1$ of a given level, there exists a sequence of nested systems $\boldsymbol{\mathcal{S}} = \{\mathcal{S}^m\}_{m>0}$ including $\mathcal{S}^1$ and* mathematical laws *such that* $P^{\mathcal{S}^m}_{\mathcal{F}^1}$ *converges weakly toward* $P^*_{\mathcal{F}^1}$, *these mathematical laws will be called* physical laws *at this level, and such a sequence $\boldsymbol{\mathcal{S}}$ will be called an approximating sequence for $\mathcal{S}^1$.*

We may postulate the existence of *physical laws*. This postulate reflects the asymptotic *separability* of the universe; that is, for making good predictions we do not need to take into account the whole universe, but on the other hand, application of the laws (even if we know the correct laws) never leads to perfect prediction, partly because we have isolated a system from the rest of the universe.

The systems may be more or less satisfactory according to the distance to the true probability achieved. For instance we would not call a set constituted of the Earth and Mars a satisfactory system; if we applied Newton's laws to this system, we would see that the observed trajectories would be in large disagreement with the predicted ones; we would thus search for a better set of bodies, for instance the set (Sun, Earth, Mars).

A3. There is a *perfect* system $\mathcal{S}^M$ for $\mathcal{S}^1$ such that $\mathcal{F}^1 \subset \mathcal{F}^M$ and $P^{\mathcal{S}^M}_{\mathcal{F}^1} = P^*_{\mathcal{F}^1}$.

This means that the probability law computed with the physical law applied to system $\mathcal{S}^M$ coincides with the true law P^* on the events of interest $\mathcal{F}^1$.

We assume that **A1** and **A2** hold for all the systems considered; assuming **A3** we can give the following definition.

Definition 14 (Causal influence) *A component j has a causal influence on a component k in $\mathcal{S}^1$ if $X_j \to\to_{\mathcal{S}^M} X_k$ under P^*, if $\mathcal{S}^M$ is a perfect system for $\mathcal{S}^1$.*

Remark 5: The direct influences under the physical law are the same in all the systems and in particular in the perfect system; a direct influence under the physical law is thus always a causal direct influence.

Example 5: Solar system. If we consider a system (Earth, Moon) the law of gravitation tells us that the earth (in our presentation, the position of the Earth) has an influence on the trajectory of the moon; by definition (if we accept that the law of gravitation is a *physical law*), this is a causal influence. Even if this system is not completely satisfactory, the notable fact is that in any richer system, the Earth will have an influence on the Moon; this stability is characteristic of causal influences.

Example 6: Immune system-HIV. The mechanisms which derive from the properties of HIV and CD4 T-lymphocytes are such that HIV can infect CD4 lymphocytes and that infected lymphocytes can produce viruses. The number of viruses produced depends in part on the number of infected lymphocytes. Thus the component of the state "number of viruses" (in a given individual) has a causal influence on the component "number of infected lymphocytes." We can deduce the form of causal influences at the level of concentrations from knowledge of the mechanisms which lead to the replication of the virus and application of diffusion laws. The approach is similar to Boltzman's theory of gases (Strevens, 2005).

9.3.2 Conditional and marginal causal effects

Marginal causal effects have been the target of most counterfactual approaches, and in particular the MSM. On the other hand, the dynamic approach is based on defining conditional effects. The perfect system assumes that all the factors influencing the process of interest have been identified. From this, marginal causal effects can be computed, as we shall see.

9.3.2.1 Conditional causal effects

First let us define conditional causal effects. For the sake of simplicity we will describe these concepts for a simple system $X = (Y, V, C)$, where Y is the process of interest, and we wish to assess the causal effect of V (which is not itself influenced by Y) on Y. We shall assume that X is a perfect system for Y. We assume that C is a process which influences Y. Because of that, the system $X' = (Y, V)$ is not a perfect system for Y. The causal effect is encapsulated in the compensator of Y which can be written: $\Lambda_{Y,t} = \phi_t(\bar{Y}_{t-}, \bar{V}_{t-}, \bar{C}_{t-})$, where $\bar{Y}_{t-}$ is the history (of sigma-field) of Y up to time $t-$ and a similar notation for the other processes. If we fix the trajectory of V to be v, the compensator becomes $\Lambda_{Y,t} = \phi_t(\bar{Y}_{t-}, \bar{v}_{t-}, \bar{C}_{t-})$. This defines a probability law P^v, in which C does not influence V. This is similar to the "do operator" of Pearl (although here in the context of processes): the "do operator" can be interpreted as considering a probability law in which V is not influenced by any other process. The probability law obtained would apply if we could manipulate V. Figure 9.2 represents the influence graphs in the two situations. We can assess the effect of V on Y, conditional on C, by contrasting the compensators of Y for two fixed trajectories of V, v and v'; with the perfect system assumption these conditional causal effects can be estimated from observational studies.

We present two examples: in the first one, Y_t is a quantitative process, in the second, this is a $0 - 1$ counting process, and in both cases the Markov property will hold; to alleviate the notation, we assume that both V and C have continuous trajectories (so we get rid of the $t-$). In a first example Y_t may represent for instance cognitive ability. We assume that the Doob-Meyer decomposition of Y in its differential form is:

$$dY_t = (\beta_0 + \beta_1 V_t + \beta_2 C_t)dt + dM_t. \tag{9.5}$$

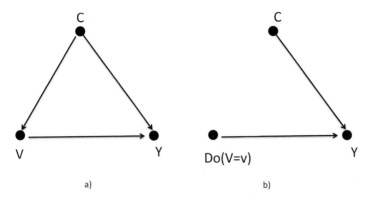

FIGURE 9.2
Influence graph with C a confounding process in the situation (a) which may be that of an observational study; (b) which may be that of an experimental study where V can be manipulated.

The Doob-Meyer decomposition itself (i.e., in a non-differential form) is then:

$$Y_t = Y_0 + \beta_0 + \beta_1 \int_0^t V_u du + \beta_2 \int_0^t C_u du + M_t.$$

A simple contrast between the compensators under $P^{v'}$ and P^v, $\Lambda_{Y,t}^{v'}$ and $\Lambda_{Y,t}^v$ respectively, is the difference of intensities at time t:

$$CE_1(v', v|C) = \frac{\partial \Lambda_{Y,t}^{v'}}{\partial t} - \frac{\partial \Lambda_{Y,t}^v}{\partial t} = \beta_1(v_t' - v_t).$$

If, however, we consider this for different values of t, this is a function. A simpler contrast would be to look at the difference of the compensators themselves at a given time t_f, and because the martingales have zero expectations, this is also equal to the difference of the expectations of Y_{t_f}:

$$CE_2(v', v|C) = \Lambda_{Y,t_f}^{v'} - \Lambda_{Y,t_f}^v = E_{v'}(Y_{t_f}|\bar{C}_{t_f}) - E_v(Y_{t_f}|\bar{C}_{t_f}) = \beta_1 \int_0^{t_f} (v_t' - v_t) dt,$$

where E_v stands for the expectation under the law P^v. These contrasts are in principle conditional on C; in this example the contrast does not in fact depend on C because of the linearity of both the compensators and the contrasts. Consider the case where there is an interaction between V and C;

$$dY_t = (\beta_0 + \beta_1 V_t + \beta_2 C_t + \beta_3 V_t C_t)dt + dM_t. \tag{9.6}$$

Then it can be easily computed that our second contrast is equal to:

$$
\begin{aligned}
CE_2(v', v|C) &= E_{v'}(Y_{t_f}|\bar{C}_{t_f}) - E_v(Y_{t_f}|\bar{C}_{t_f}) \\
&= \beta_1 \int_0^{t_f} (v'_t - v_t)dt + \beta_3 \int_0^{t_f} (v'_t - v_t)C_t dt, \tag{9.7}
\end{aligned}
$$

which depends on C.

As a second example, consider the case where the event of interest Y is the occurrence of a disease; the process of interest is a $0-1$ counting process (a survival analysis context). It is natural to assess the causal effect on the horizon t_f, where t_f is the time of occurrence of the disease which is a random stopping time: $t_f = \min\{t : Y_t = 1\}$. After t_f by definition the process does not change, so no process can influence it. For $t \leq t_f$, the compensator is equal to the cumulative hazard function, and its derivative (the intensity) is equal to the hazard function $\alpha(t; V_t, C_t)$. A possible contrast in this context is the ratio of the intensities, which for $t \leq t_f$ is equal to the ratio of the hazards:

$$CE_1(v', v|C) = \frac{\frac{\partial \Lambda^{v'}_{Y,t}}{\partial t}}{\frac{\partial \Lambda^{v}_{Y,t}}{\partial t}} = \frac{\alpha(t; v'_t, C_t)}{\alpha(t; v_t, C_t)}.$$

In the case of a proportional hazard form, we have:

$$\alpha(t; V_t, C_t) = \alpha_0(t)e^{\beta_1 V_t + \beta_2 C_t}. \tag{9.8}$$

So, we obtain $CE_1(v', v|C) = e^{\beta_1(v'_t - v_t)}$; e^{β_1}, the value of the contrast for a difference of one unit between v'_t and v_t, is the conventional hazard ratio. Because of the multiplicative feature of both hazard function and contrast, in this case too, the conditional effect does not depend on C. In general, however, it does depend on C.

Consider a contrast of the compensators in an exponential scale; here for simplicity we assume that C is a fixed (not time-dependent) covariate. This is a contrast on survival functions because $S(t; \bar{v}_t, C) = e^{-A(t;\bar{v}_t,C)}$. Let us consider for a contrast the ratio of the survival functions at time t: $CE_2(v', v|C) = S(t; \bar{v}'_t, C)/S(t; \bar{v}_t, C)$. With the form (9.8) we have that $S(t; \bar{v}_t, C) = e^{-\tilde{A}(t;\bar{v}_t)\tilde{C}}$, with $\tilde{A}(t; \bar{v}_t) = \int_0^t \alpha_0(u)e^{\beta_1 v_u}du$ and $\tilde{C} = e^{\beta_2 C}$. We thus have

$$CE_2(v', v|C) = e^{-\tilde{C}[\tilde{A}(t;\bar{v}'_t) - \tilde{A}(t;\bar{v}_t)]},$$

which depends on C. In case of non-time-dependent v' and v we have $\tilde{A}(t; \bar{v}'_t) - \tilde{A}(t; \bar{v}_t) = A(t; 0)e^{\beta_1(v'_t - v_t)}$, which gives a relation between CE_1 and CE_2.

9.3.2.2 Expected causal effect

The expected causal effect is the expectation of the conditional causal effect:

$$\text{ECE}(v', v) = \text{E}[\text{CE}(v', v|C)].$$

This is a rather straightforward concept, and a rather easy to compute quantity if one knows the law of C.

For example in the model given by Equation (9.6) we find

$$\text{ECE}_2(v', v) = \text{E}_{v'}(Y_{t_f}) - \text{E}_v(Y_{t_f}) = \beta_1 \int_0^{t_f} (v_t' - v_t) dt + \beta_3 \int_0^{t_f} (v_t' - v_t)\text{E}(C_t) dt.$$
$$(9.9)$$

Note that the expectation of C_t is the same under P^v and $\text{P}^{v'}$ and is denoted by $\text{E}(C_t)$. In the survival model given by (9.8), the contrast defined by the ratio of intensities, that is $\text{CE}_1(v', v|C))$, does not depend on C, so conditional and expected effects are the same. For the contrast defined by the ratio of survival functions at t, that is $\text{CE}_2(v', v|C)$, we obtain:

$$\text{ECE}_2(v', v) = \text{E}\{e^{-\tilde{C}[\tilde{A}(t;\bar{v}_t') - \tilde{A}(t;\bar{v}_t)]}\}.$$

The computation is the same as computing the marginal survival in a frailty model (see Aalen et al., 2008, Chapter 6). Writing $\mathcal{L}(x) = \text{E}_v[e^{-x\tilde{C}}]$ the Laplace transform of the distribution of $\tilde{C}$, we obtain:

$$\text{ECE}_2(v', v) = \mathcal{L}[\tilde{A}(t; \bar{v}_t') - \tilde{A}(t; \bar{v}_t)].$$

In the case where $\tilde{C}$ has a Gamma distribution of expectation 1 and variance δ, this gives: $\text{ECE}_2(v', v) = \{1 + \delta[\tilde{A}(t; \bar{v}_t', C) - \tilde{A}(t; \bar{v}_t, C)]\}^{-1/\delta}$.

9.3.2.3 Marginal causal effect

The marginal causal effect is defined by contrasts between $\text{P}^{v'}$- and P^v-compensators in the system $\boldsymbol{X}' = (V, Y)$. The P^v-intensity of the process Y in $\boldsymbol{X}'$, $\lambda_{Y,t}^{'v}$, can be derived from that in $\boldsymbol{X}$ by the innovation theorem:

$$\lambda_{Y,t}^{'v} = \text{E}_v[\lambda_{Y,t}|\bar{Y}_{t-}, \bar{V}_{t-}].$$

This amounts to integrating $\lambda_{Y,t}^v$ with the kernel $[C_{t-}|\bar{Y}_{t-}, \bar{V}_{t-}]$. So in principle we can compute any contrast after having done this computation; however, this becomes rapidly complicated. In simple cases (discrete time, fixed covariate C) computation may be feasible. When an analytical solution is not possible, one can resort to simulation.

Contrasts bearing on $\text{E}_v(Y_t)$ are easier to compute. We can first compute the conditional expectation of Y_t, $\text{E}_v(Y_t|\bar{C}_t)$ and then the marginal expectation $\text{E}_v(Y_t) = \text{E}[\text{E}_v(Y_t|\bar{C}_t)$ (here the law of C does not depend on v). In the first example, starting form Equation (9.7) we obtain the same result as for the expected causal effect given in (9.9), so we have $\text{MCE}_2(v', v) = \text{ECE}_2(v', v)$.

In the second example, it is also relatively easy to compute the marginal expectation of Y_t: $E_v(Y_t) = P^v(Y_t = 1) = 1 - S(t; \bar{v}_t)$. So, we can compute the contrast:

$$\text{MCE}_2(v', v) = \frac{S(t; \bar{v}'_t)}{S(t; \bar{v}_t)}.$$

By a computation similar as in Aalen et al. (2008, chapter 6), still for the case where $\tilde{C}$ has a Gamma distribution with expectation 1 and variance δ, we obtain that the marginal survival is: $S(t; \bar{v}_t) = [1 + \delta \tilde{A}(t; \bar{v}_t)]^{-1/\delta}$. Hence the contrast:

$$\text{MCE}_2(v', v) = \{\frac{1 + \delta \tilde{A}(t; \bar{v}_t)}{1 + \delta \tilde{A}(t; \bar{v}'_t)}\}^{1/\delta}.$$

From the expression of the marginal survival we can compute the marginal hazard $\alpha'(t; \bar{v}_t) = \frac{\tilde{\alpha}(t; \bar{v}_t)}{1 + \delta \tilde{A}(t; \bar{v}_t)}$. Hence we can compute the contrast based on the ratio of the marginal hazards; in the case where v' and v are time-constant we have:

$$\text{MCE}_1(v', v) = e^{\beta_1 (v' - v)} \frac{1 + \delta \tilde{A}(t; v)}{1 + \delta \tilde{A}(t; v')}.$$

It is to be noted that the ratio of the marginal hazards decreases with t, while in this model, the conditional hazard ratio is constant. This is a well known fact and this shows that we have to be cautious to interpret this type of contrast.

9.3.3   Systems with no unmeasured confounders

Hoping to construct a perfect system for the process of interest may be too ambitious. To get marginal causal effects correct, it is sufficient that there is no unmeasured confounders. Consider a case where X is not perfect for Y but there is another process U which influences Y; a perfect system would be $X'' = (Y, V, C, U)$. If U does not influence V, this is not a confounder. So X is a system with "no unmeasured confounder" (NUC). In this case it has been proven in some contexts (Arjas and Parner, 2004; Commenges and Gégout-Petit, 2015) although not in complete generality, that one can still compute marginal effects from observational studies using X. We can compute causal effects marginal with respect to U but conditional on C, or marginal with respect to both U and C.

9.3.4   Assumptions for causal interpretation

Most often in epidemiology and more generally in life sciences, we have observations of a sample of subjects. Each subject corresponds to a "physical system." The simplest assumption (not always tenable) is that the systems do not interact, that is the events pertaining to different subjects are independent. Then there is the assumption of *stability*, which derives from physical laws. Assuming that "smoking" and "lung cancer" mean the same thing for different subjects, we also assume that the effect of smoking on lung cancer is the same across subjects. This concept is formalized for a simple system in Section 9.6.2. Stability takes its full meaning in a perfect system but makes also sense in a NUC system. If there is a genetic factor (an attribute) which modifies the effect of smoking on lung cancer, we cannot say that smoking has the same effect conditionally on this factor; we could still assert this marginally in a NUC system. It implies that the exposure has the same effect in an observational and in an intervention situation (Berzuini et al., 2012).

9.3.5 Observations

It must be clear that up to now we have seen how to define influences (or absence of influence) of one process on another, and in which cases these influences could be labelled as causal. This was defined assuming the true probability law was known. Inference is another issue, and this is the typical *statistical* problem: the true probability law is unknown and the task is to find probability laws that are close to the true one. This is possible based on observations that are realizations under the true probability law of the processes included in the system. So in principle we must design a model for the system and a model for the observations. This distinction is particularly clear when dealing with mechanistic models, as in Section 9.5, but is however also relevant in more conventional epidemiological analysis.

Most of the time we have "incomplete data"; this term encompasses the selection of the sample and the fact that for selected individuals we do not observe all the relevant events. In survival problems, selection is most often truncation and we do not observe all the relevant events due to censoring (right- left- or interval-censoring). In this section we put aside the selection problem and will speak about incomplete observations of selected subjects. There are generalizations of censoring to more general multivariate stochastic processes. A general definition of incomplete data is that the observed sigma-field $\mathcal{O}$ is smaller that the sigma-field generated by the process of interest $\mathcal{F}_\tau$ on the horizon τ of interest. This generalizes the concept of censoring for survival processes and can also be applied to continuous state-space processes. The term of coarsening has been introduced by Heitjan and Rubin (1991) to describe more general schemes of incomplete data than "missing variables." This has been further extended by Jacobsen and Keiding (1995); Gill et al. (1997); Commenges and Gégout-Petit (2005, 2007). The term *coarsening* is well adapted to these generalizations because one can say that the sigma-field $\mathcal{O}$ is coarser than $\mathcal{F}_\tau$ if $\mathcal{O} \subset \mathcal{F}_\tau$. All authors were interested to study the issue of *ignorability*; the condition of *coarsening at random* (CAR) can be viewed as an extension of independent censoring, and leads to ignorability. Concretely, if the mechanism leading to incomplete observations is ignorable we do not have to model it. For instance when a process is observed at discrete times, if the mechanism is ignorable we do not have to model the distribution of the observation times.

The term (and the concept as well) "coarsening" has rarely been used to characterize quantitative longitudinal data; in our approach this type of data is discrete-time observations of a continuous-time process and in this sense, even if all the variables that were planned to be observed have indeed been observed, this observation scheme really produces a coarsening of the sigma-field of interest, and the question here also arises whether this coarsening is ignorable or not.

9.4 The dynamic approach to causal reasoning in ageing studies

9.4.1 The particular significance of death

In ageing studies, one of the most important events that we have to consider is death. This is why the illness-death model studied in Chapter 7 is important in such studies. But death is not an event which is on the same footing as other events that can happen to subjects. Even if the vital status is part of the state X associated to each subject, this part of the state has a very special meaning, in that all the other components of the state are defined only for a living subject. The consequence is that causal influences must be defined on a maximum horizon T_D, where T_D is the time of death. We do not say that death has an influence on the other components of the state, but that these other components are not defined after death. For instance if we are interested in dementia, the state can be represented by a bivariate counting process $X = (Y, D)$, respectively counting dementia and death as in Section 7.8. However, dementia is defined only for a living subject: after death the subject does not exist anymore (at least on this earth) and cannot be qualified as demented or not demented. When we investigate the causal influence of a factor, we should first look at its causal influence on death, then on its influences on other processes. This has a consequence for the graph representation of the system; we will represent influences of the components of the state on the death process, but not influences of the death process on other components. Since the death process is a special process, we may represent it by a special symbol, for instance a star: ★.

9.4.2 Examples of causal reasoning in ageing studies

Let us start with a study of dementia. In the simplest system, there are two processes, dementia and death, so that the state process is a bivariate counting process $X = (Y, D)$. This can also be represented by an illness-death process.

The only possible causal influence is that of dementia on death. With the Markov property, the intensity of the death process is:

$$\lambda_{Dt} = 1_{\{D_{t-}=0\}}[1_{\{Y_{t-}=0\}}\alpha_{02}(t) + 1_{\{Y_{t-}=1\}}\alpha_{12}(t)]. \qquad (9.10)$$

Dementia influences death if the transition intensities α_{02} and α_{12} (resp. death rates for non-demented and demented) are different, which, returning to the lighter notation referring the system to $\boldsymbol{X}$, is symbolized by $Y \longrightarrow_{\boldsymbol{X}} D$. The graph reduces to two nodes (dementia and death) and one arrow from dementia to death. This simplified form of the graph allows representing influences in more complex models, which cannot be done with the conventional graphs for multistate models. In fact, to approach causal inference, we must introduce other important factors, generally considered as explanatory variables in a multistate model. In this framework, fixed variables are called attributes, while internal time-dependent variables are components of the state process. There may also be external time-dependent variables, that is external processes. External processes by definition can influence the processes of interest but cannot be influenced by them. An example of external process would be air temperature; for instance, death rates are higher when there is a heat wave. In the study of dementia, gender, known genetic factors such as APOE-4, and unknown genetic factors would be attributes. Of course unknown genetic factors would not be observed and would be represented by random effects in a statistical model. An example of a factor that could be added to the state is the blood pressure. This can be represented in a graph as in Figure 9.3.

This is particularly interesting because we can consider blood pressure as a modifiable factor since there are anti-hypertensive treatments. So, the question of the possible causal influence of high blood pressure on dementia is of practical importance in public health because we may expect that anti-hypertensive treatment could decrease the risk of dementia. We cannot, however, dissociate the issue of causal influence of high blood pressure on death and on dementia. Anti-hypertensive treatments may also decrease the risk of death but we have also to consider the theoretical possibility that treating hypertension increases the risk of death. So the parameters of importance are both the effect on the intensity of death and the effect on the intensity of dementia.

Assume $\boldsymbol{X} = (G, Y, V, D)$ is a perfect system, or more realistically a NUC system (see Section 9.3.3); in our example, V represent the blood pressure process and G fixed variables (attributes) like genetic factors. That is, we cannot find a factor C that, if included in the filtration, would change the intensities of the process of interest Y (perfect system), or if we can find such U, U does not influence V and thus is not a confounder: in that case, the causal effect of V in system $\boldsymbol{X}$ is marginal with respect to U. For instance if G does not include educational level, the system is not perfect for Y because it has been shown that educational level influences dementia; if we assume that educational level does not influence blood pressure, the system would still a NUC system. Assume in addition that we know the law of (G, Y, V, D); then we can compute the probability of being alive non-demented, alive demented

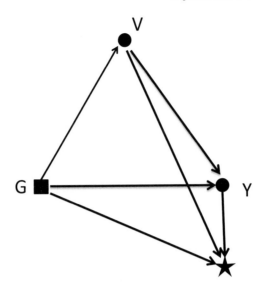

FIGURE 9.3
Influence graph for dementia. Y (dementia) and D (death, represented by a star) are the processes of interest, V represents a modifiable factor (blood pressure) and G represents the attributes (gender, genetic factors).

and dead for any time (age) t for any given value of $V = v$. If the probability of being dead and the probability of being demented are both lower for value v_1 compared to value v_2, v_1 is clearly preferable to v_2. The computation can be done for given $G = g$ or marginally to G.

Definition 15 (*Preferable* partial order) *Let* $\boldsymbol{X} = (G, Y, V, D)$ *a NUC system and note* P^{*v_1} *the true probability for value* v_1 *and* $\mathrm{E}^*_{v_1}$ *the expectation under this true probability:* v_1 *is* preferable *to* v_2 *if* $\mathrm{P}^{*v_1}(D_t = 1) \leq \mathrm{P}^{*v_2}(D_t = 1)$ *and* $\mathrm{E}^*_{v_1}(Y_t) \leq \mathrm{E}^*_{v_2}(Y_t)$, *with strict inequality holding for some* t.

If this is not the case, the comparison of the benefits of v_1 and v_2 will be less clear, and a utility function must be chosen. If Y is a $0-1$ process, $\mathrm{E}^*_{v_1}(Y_t) = \mathrm{P}^{*v_1}(Y_t = 1)$; the definition also applies to a quantitative Y when high values of Y_t are detrimental.

To fix the ideas, let us assume that the true law of Y and D given G, is specified by the intensities:

$$\lambda_{Yt} = 1_{\{Y_{t-}=0\}}\alpha_Y(t), \text{ where } \alpha_Y(t) = \alpha_{0Y}^*(t)e^{\beta_1^*G+\beta_2^*V_t} \qquad (9.11)$$

$$\lambda_{Dt} = 1_{\{D_{t-}=0\}}\alpha_D(t), \text{ where } \alpha_D(t) = \alpha_{0D}^*(t)e^{\gamma_1^*G+\gamma_2^*V_t+\gamma_3^*Y_t} \quad (9.12)$$

The intensity for Y is defined only on $[0, T_D]$. These equations describe the true law of our processes and not a model (that is a family of laws), and this is the meaning of putting a * in superscript of the symbols. The aim here is to eliminate the inference problem; we have a perfect system and we know the law; in this ideal situation what will we do?

If both β_1^* and γ_2^* are positive, a sufficient condition for "v_1 preferable to v_2" is that $v_1(t) \leq v_2(t)$ for all t, with strict inequality for some t. If this model with positive β_1^* and γ_2^* was correct for our example, we could deduce that lowering blood pressure from $v_2(t)$ to $v_1(t)$ would lead to a preferable situation.

As a second example, we consider the case where the process of interest Y is the global cognitive ability. The system can be represented by the same graph 9.3. The true law could be that Y is a diffusion process: $dY_t = \lambda_{Yt}dt + dB_t$, where B is a Brownian motion.

Let us assume that the true law given G, is specified by the intensities:

$$\lambda_{Yt} = \beta_0^*(t) + \beta_1^*G + \beta_2^*V_t \qquad (9.13)$$

$$\lambda_{Dt} = 1_{\{D_{t-}=0\}}\alpha_{0D}^*(t)e^{\gamma_1^*G+\gamma_2^*V_t+\gamma_3^*Y_t}, \qquad (9.14)$$

where $\beta_0^*(\cdot)$ and $\alpha_{0D}^*(\cdot)$ are baseline functions. As before, λ_{Yt} is defined only on $[0, T_D]$. Here, Y (cognitive ability) is clearly a construct and cannot be observed in continuous time. It is indirectly measured by cognitive tests such as the MMSE or Isaacs set test, necessarily at discrete times. As for dementia, if the system is perfect, we can make computation that can be used for choosing the best value of V, in the case where V can be manipulated. For each value $V = v$, we can compute the probability of being alive at any t, then given alive at t, the distribution of Y_t. If the probability of being dead is lower and the mean value of the cognitive ability is higher for value v_1 compared to value v_2, v_1 is clearly preferable to v_2.

If it is possible to choose the trajectory v_1 or v_2, it is rational to choose v_1 if v_1 is *preferable* to v_2. When v_1 and v_2 cannot be ordered this way, a utility function $U(v)$ has to be constructed. If V can be manipulated, one can choose the trajectory v which maximizes $U(v)$.

9.4.3 Observation and inference

Observing the processes in continuous time until T_D, we have complete information. It often happens that we have incomplete observations (the observed sigma-field is smaller than the sigma-field generated by X). Assuming a well specified model, we can consistently estimate the parameters from observations.

In our first example where Y is dementia, if all attributes and processes are observed in continuous time, with possible right-censoring, maximum likelihood estimation can easily be done by splitting the problem into several conventional survival problems, using the technical trick described in Section 7.5.1. This will not be possible either if some attributes which have an influence on both dementia and death are not observed, of if V or Y are observed in discrete time (inducing interval-censoring). In both cases one can write the likelihood conditional on the complete data, and obtain the observed likelihood by taking the expectation. This leads to the computations of numerical integrals.

As for our second example where Y represents cognitive ability, it is tempting to analyze this process without taking death into account (using ordinary models for quantitative longitudinal data) for estimating the $\beta_0(\cdot)$ and β_1: we would just analyze the observations of Y that we have. Let us assume for simplicity that the sequence of observations is interrupted by death and there is no loss of follow-up. Because of the discrete-time observation scheme, if γ_3^* is different from zero, death cannot in fact be considered as coarsening at random (see Section 9.3.5) for estimating the law of Y (because the stopping of the sequence gives us information on the values of Y). Fitting a joint model for cognitive ability and death is necessary. If the frequency of observations is high, we may expect however that the bias due to treating death as noninformative is small; this was implicitly assumed by Jacqmin-Gadda et al. (1997) who studied the evolution of Mini Mental State Examination (MMSE) score with age.

9.5 Mechanistic models

9.5.1 Generalities

The models that we can propose for dementia or cognitive ability most often describe the influences as linear function in a certain scale. In some cases we have biological knowledge which helps us in constructing a model. This is the case when the system is at the level of populations of entities, and the state of the system is the number, or the proportion, of some sub-populations which are in interaction. These interactions are modeled by systems of differential equations which can be deterministic or stochastic. One of the first models based on differential equation in the life sciences was the Predator-Prey model proposed by Voltera, which describes the interaction between two species, one being the prey of the other. Since then, mathematical modeling has played an important role in ecology and more generally in mathematical biology (Murray, 2002). In epidemiology, models based on differential equations have been used for developing epidemics models. Here the system is a given population of subjects and the state of the system includes the numbers, or the prevalences, of susceptible, infected and resistant (SIR) subjects. Deterministic and stochastic models have been developed (Bailey, 1975; Dietz, 1993; Britton, 2010). In pharmacokinetics, models for the diffusion and elimination of drugs in the organisms are based on Fick's law which expresses as an ordinary differential equation (Rosenbaum, 2011). Here the state process is the concentration of molecules of the drug; the number of molecules is so large that there is no point to use stochastic differential equations. Finally, it may be useful to develop models of host-pathogen interaction; here the interest lies in the interaction between the population of pathogens cells and the populations of host cells. The system is this set of populations and the state is the number or the concentrations of these different populations of cells. This modeling has been particularly developed in the field of HIV infection. Ho et al. (1995) and Perelson et al. (1996) developed a simple model of virus dynamics which showed that the turnover of HIV in an infected subject was very high and this had a profound influence on the understanding of HIV infection. Since then, many other models have been proposed (Nowak and May, 2000); this will be developed in Section 9.5.5.

9.5.2 The general structure of a mechanistic model

The characteristic feature of mechanistic models is that they are based on a system of differential equations which expresses some physical laws. A large body of literature, as in Murray (2002), is devoted to a completely deterministic account of this topic, which limits the application to real life problem. Stochasticity can be introduced at different levels. The differential equations can be stochastic, there can be random effects on the parameters and there can be measurement errors. An important issue is whether we restrict to Markov processes or not. In ODE systems we implicitly restrict to Markov processes, as argued in Section 9.2.5, although there are some development in delayed differential equations. In fact the Markov assumption is consistent with the expression of physical laws since most physical laws describe how a system changes, given its present state. Therefore, good mechanistic models should be Markov. Another important feature of mechanistic models is that, most of the time, the system lives in continuous time while observations are taken at discrete times. So the basic structure of a mechanistic model for one system is specified by two equations, an equation for the system and an equation for the observation:

$$
\begin{aligned}
\mathrm{d}\boldsymbol{X}_t &= \lambda(\boldsymbol{X}_t; \xi(t)) + \mathrm{d}M_t, t \geq 0, & (9.15)\\
Y_j &= g_j(\boldsymbol{X}_{t_j}) + \varepsilon_j; j = 1, \ldots, m, & (9.16)
\end{aligned}
$$

where $\xi(t)$ is a p-dimensional vector of parameters which may be time-dependent, M_t is a martingale, Y_j is the a K_j-dimensional vector of observation at time t_j, g_j is a known function and ε_j is a K_j-dimensional measurement error; all measurement errors are mutually independent.

Generally Equation (9.15) is a stochastic differential equation. It describes a Markov process. We might expect that the intensity does not directly depend on time; this is what we expect if it expresses a physical law, since physical laws do not change with time. It may however depend on external variables which may depend on time: a typical time-varying variable is a treatment. Often in applications, X represents continuous biomarkers, so that the martingale M can be chosen as a multivariate Brownian motion. In this case, X is a diffusion process. If there is no martingale term, this equation is an ODE system. The behaviour of so-called dynamical systems described by ODE has been well studied (Jones et al., 2011). One of the characteristics of the trajectories that are studied is the existence and stability of equilibrium points (or steady states). Equilibrium points are defined as satisfying $dX_t = 0$. There are different types of equilibrium points and some complex systems may also have a chaotic behaviour. In most applications we are interested in rather simple systems which have a small number of equilibrium points. For instance the target cell system described in Section 9.5.5 has typically two equilibrium points, one stable and one unstable. The equivalent of equilibrium point for stochastic differential equations is a stationary process. For instance, an Ornstein-Ulhenbeck process tends toward the stationary Ornstein-Ulhenbeck process.

Equation (9.16) is a rather general observation equation. At each time t_j one observes a vector Y_j which is a function of the state at time t_j and a measurement error. The g_j's are known functions that account for the fact that we may not observe all the components of X_{t_j} but only a subset, or combinations, of them; the transformation g_j are also used to make the additive measurement error acceptable. The g_j's may depend on j: for instance, one component of X may be observed at one time, another at another time. The observation scheme may be complicated by censoring: in measurement of biomarkers, detection limits may produce left-censoring. Generally the ε_js are assumed normal. The initial condition of the differential equation, X_0, may be known or not. It can sometimes be assumed that it is an equilibrium point for given values of the parameters; otherwise, fixed or random parameters have to be added.

In some applications we have only one system; this is often the case in epidemics models. In other applications, however, several systems are available. This is the case for the host-pathogens models where we have several subjects. It is often unrealistic to assume that the parameter values corresponding to different subjects are the same. On the other hand, the observation on one subject brings often insufficient information to correctly estimate the parameters. A flexible and powerful approach is to introduce random effects on some parameters. So this is another level where stochasticity can be introduced. We assume that we have n systems (most often subjects); system i is described by the equations:

$$
\begin{aligned}
\mathrm{d}\boldsymbol{X}_t^i &= \lambda[\boldsymbol{X}_t^i; \xi^i(Z^i(t))] + \mathrm{d}M_t^i, t \geq 0, \\
Y_{ij} &= g_{ij}(\boldsymbol{X}_{t_{ij}}^i) + \varepsilon_{ij}; j = 1, \ldots, m,
\end{aligned}
$$

where t_{ij} are not necessarily the same for different subjects, and g_{ij} are functions from $\mathbb{R}^p$ to $\mathbb{R}^{K_{ij}}$. With a sample of systems (subjects) we can develop a model for the natural parameters ξ^i. Like in mixed generalized linear models, we assume that there are transformations of the natural parameters (analogous to a link function) for which the natural parameters can be expressed as a linear form of explanatory variables and random effects. For each component l of ξ^i, let ψ_l be this link function and let us denote $\xi_l^i(t) = \psi_l^{-1}(\tilde{\xi}_l^i)$; for most parameters the log-transform is a good choice. Then we have a linear model for $\tilde{\xi}_l^i$:

$$\tilde{\xi}_l^i = \phi_l + \beta_l^\top Z_l^i(t) + u_l^i, \tag{9.17}$$

where ϕ_l and β_l are fixed parameters, Z_l^i are possibly time-dependent explanatory variables and u_l^i is a random effect, usually assumed normal with zero expectation and variance ω_l^2. Let u^i be the vector of random effects for subject i: the u^i's are assumed i.i.d. For given i, the u_l^i may be assumed independent or not, with p.d.f. f_u. Not all natural parameters have a random effect, so that the dimension of u_i is $q \leq p$.

9.5.3 Inference in mechanistic models

We assume that ε_{ijk} have independent normal distributions with zero expectation and variance σ_k^2. The model is indexed by a parameter $\theta = (\phi, \beta, \omega, \sigma)$, where $(\phi, \beta, \omega, \sigma)$ are the vectors of components $(\phi_l, \beta_l, \omega_l, \sigma_k)$, respectively. From the observations, inference for ODE models can be done by maximum likelihood or by a Bayesian approach. In both cases we have to compute the likelihood. If there is no random effect and assuming a normal distribution for the measurement errors the likelihood for a subject i is:

$$\mathcal{L}_{\mathcal{Y}_i}(\theta) = \prod_{j=1}^m \prod_{k=1}^{K_j} \frac{1}{\sqrt{2\pi\sigma_m^2}} \exp\left[-\frac{1}{2}\left\{\frac{Y_{ijk} - g_{jk}(X_{t_{ijk}})}{\sigma_k}\right\}^2\right] \tag{9.18}$$

The likelihood depends on θ through $X_{t_{ijk}}$ which is a deterministic function of $\tilde{\xi}^i$, themselves functions of θ. The computation of the likelihood requires to compute the trajectories (X_t for given $\tilde{\xi}^i$), which can be done by numerical solvers of differential equations. If there are censored observations (due to detection limits), the likelihood has to be modified (Guedj et al., 2007).

If there are random effects, some of the $\tilde{\xi}^i$s are random. The likelihood on the right hand of Equation (9.18) then has to be understood as the likelihood given the random effects and we write it $\mathcal{L}_{y_i|u_i}$. For obtaining the likelihood, we have to integrate over the random effects:

$$\mathcal{L}_{y_i}(\theta) = \int \mathcal{L}_{y_i|u_i=x}\ f_u(x)\mathrm{d}x, \qquad (9.19)$$

Generally f_u is a normal density which has zero expectation and for variance, a diagonal matrix with entries ω_l^2.

From a strict statistical perspective, we are in the framework of mixed non-linear models treated in Section 4.3, and there is nothing special in likelihood inference. In many applications of mechanistic models, however, there are major identifiability issues. These arise because there are often many parameters, the effects of which are not well separated. It is often necessary to add information coming from biological knowledge or previous studies. In the frequentist paradigm, this can be done by fixing some of the parameters to plausible values. The Bayesian paradigm allows a more flexible way of introducing knowledge by eliciting informative priors for the parameters. However, the implementation of a full Bayesian approach may fail in such complex problems (Drylewicz et al., 2012). An alternative approach allowing incorporating prior knowledge is the penalized likelihood approach. It can be viewed either as a variant of the likelihood approach, or as an approximate Bayesian inference, in fact a crude version of the Approximate Bayesian inference proposed by Rue et al. (2009) which cannot be applied here. The penalized log-likelihood is:

$$pL(\theta) = \mathcal{L}(\theta) - J(\theta), \qquad (9.20)$$

where $L(\theta) = \sum_{i=1}^{n} \log \mathcal{L}_{y_i}(\theta)$ is the log-likelihood and $J(\theta)$ is a penalty term. For instance, if we expect values of a component θ_l to be close to some value θ_{0l}, we could put $J(\theta) = \tau(\theta_l - \theta_{0l})^2$, thus penalizing the likelihood for values far from θ_{0l}. This is a very flexible way of introducing prior knowledge in inference. There is a Bayesian interpretation of the penalized likelihood. In a Bayesian approach the parameter θ is considered as random, there is a prior $\pi(\theta)$ which encapsulates the prior knowledge, and what we know about θ after observing a sample $\mathcal{Y}$ is contained in the posterior distribution of θ. By Bayes theorem the posterior is proportional to the product of the likelihood and the prior:

$$p(\theta|\mathcal{Y}) \propto \mathcal{L}(\theta)\pi(\theta). \qquad (9.21)$$

Therefore, the log of the posterior distribution of θ is, up to an additive constant:

$$\log p(\theta|\mathcal{Y}) = L(\theta) + \log \pi(\theta).$$

Thus the mode of the posterior distribution (called the MAP) is the same as the value which maximizes the penalized likelihood for which $J(\theta) = -\log \pi(\theta) = \log \frac{1}{\pi(\theta)}$: values of θ which are in a region of low prior density are strongly penalized. The MAP can be treated as a frequentist estimator. We can, however, stay in the Bayesian paradigm taking the route of approximating the posterior distribution by a normal distribution, which is justified by the Bernstein-von Mises Theorem (Van der Vaart, 2000). This theorem says that under mild conditions, the posterior distribution converges toward a normal distribution. For approximating the posterior distribution, it is natural to take the normal distribution with same mode and curvature at the mode as the posterior distribution, that is $\mathcal{N}(\hat{\theta}_{MAP}, H_{pL}^{-1}(\hat{\theta}_{MAP}))$, where H_{pL} is the Hessian of minus the log of the posterior distribution (or equivalently of the log penalized likelihood).

A rather different approach has been proposed by Ramsay et al. (2007). It is based on finding smooth trajectories that satisfy the differential equations at given time points. The penalized likelihood allows finding compromise between the smoothness of the trajectories and the degree to which these trajectories fit the differential equations. This has the great advantage to avoid solving the system of differential equations. However, with systems of differential equations including random effects, this approach still leads to considerable numerical difficulties.

Inference for SDE models is much more difficult and is still an area of research. The likelihood can be computed by simulation techniques (Delattre et al., 2013; Picchini et al., 2010) and Bayesian approaches are also possible (Roberts and Stramer, 2001).

9.5.4 Computational challenge in mechanistic models

The first computational difficulty is to solve the ODE system. Analytical solutions exist for linear systems but do not exist in general for non-linear ones. So they have to be solved numerically; there exist good solvers, for instance the Livermore solver DLSODE (Hindmarsh, 1983). The direct approach for finding the MLE requires the computation of the likelihood for any value of the parameters. When there is no random effect, the problem is not very difficult. When there are q random effects, the computation of the likelihood involves the numerical computation of q-dimensional integrals. A Laplace approximation of these integrals, first order (FO) or first order conditional estimation (FOCE), proposed by Lindstrom and Bates (1990) and Pinheiro and Bates (1995), leads to relatively fast algorithms; this has been implemented in the NONMEM package; see Wang (2007) for a review. A more accurate computation of the integrals can be done by Gaussian quadrature; adaptive Gaussian quadrature are the most efficient (Genz and Keister, 1996). On top of that we need a maximization algorithm. Newton-like algorithms need the computation of derivatives of the likelihood, which can also be done numerically. This direct approach is implemented in the NIMROD program (Prague et al., 2013). NIMROD uses the RVS algorithm for maximization. The RVS algorithm (Commenges et al., 2006) uses only first derivatives which are computed using a special algorithm based on "sensitivity equations." The sensitivity equations are obtained by differentiating the original ODE system with respect to the parameters. The user has to give the sensitivity equations to the program using MAPPLE. NIMROD can use parallel computing.

Another approach uses the stochastic approximation EM (SAEM) algorithm proposed by Kuhn and Lavielle (2005). This approach has been implemented in the MONOLIX package. Many examples treated with MONOLIX can be found in Lavielle (2014).

9.5.5 Modeling the HIV-immune system interaction

We present here a model for the interaction of a population of viruses and populations of CD4+ T-lymphocytes (CD4) in subjects infected by HIV. Perelson et al. (1996) proposed an ODE model featuring uninfected CD4, infected CD4 and virus concentrations. We present an extension of this model for our mathematical structure, distinguishing between quiescent uninfected CD4 and activated uninfected CD4 which are targets for the virus. To this basic mathematical structure, we join a model for the inter-individual variability and a model for the observations. Finally we show an application on the ALBI trial.

9.5.5.1 The ODE system

The concentrations in the blood of quiescent uninfected, activated uninfected and infected CD4 are denoted by Q, T, T^*, respectively, the concentration of viruses is denoted by V. The instantaneous change of concentrations of these populations at time t, for all real value of $t > 0$, is given by the ODE system:

$$\begin{cases} \frac{dQ_t}{dt} & = \lambda + \rho T_t - \alpha Q_t - \mu_Q Q_t, \\ \frac{dT_t}{dt} & = \alpha Q_t - \gamma T_t V_t - \rho T_t - \mu_T T_t, \\ \frac{dT^*_t}{dt} & = \gamma T_t V_t - \mu_{T^*} T^*_t, \\ \frac{dV_t}{dt} & = \pi T^*_t - \mu_V V_t^i. \end{cases} \tag{9.22}$$

The parameter λ is the production rate of new CD4 cells, the μ's are mortality rates, α and ρ are transition rates between quiescent and activated cells, π is the rate of production of virions by infected cells, and γ is the infectivity parameter. The model assumes that the rate of infection of target T cells is γV_t.

The system is graphically represented in Figure 9.4. It can be seen as an enrichment of the system depicted in Figure 9.1 (omitting Z), where three populations of CD4 T-cells have been distinguished, leading to consider Y as a trivariate process. Also the relationship between the virus concentration and the CD4 T-cells is more complex.

The trivial equilibrium without infection is:

$$\begin{cases} Q_{0_-} & = \frac{(\rho+\mu_T)\lambda}{\alpha\mu_T+\rho\mu_Q+\mu_Q\mu_T}, \\ T_{0_-} & = \frac{\alpha\lambda}{\alpha\mu_T+\rho\mu_Q+\mu_Q\mu_T}, \\ T^*_{0_-} & = 0, \\ V_{0_-} & = 0. \end{cases} \tag{9.23}$$

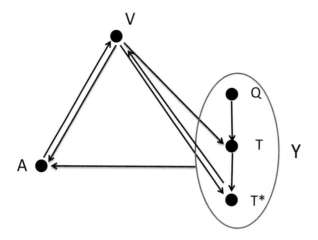

FIGURE 9.4
Influence graph for the target-cells model. Y is the trivariate process of CD4
T-cells concentration; A is the treatment process; V is the viral load process.

The basic reproductive number R_0 is given by:

$$R_0 = \frac{\gamma \pi \alpha \lambda}{\mu_{T^*} \mu_V (\rho \mu_Q + \alpha \mu_T + \mu_Q \mu_T)}. \tag{9.24}$$

If R_0 is higher than or equal to one, after the introduction of virions, the
system stabilizes to a new non-trivial equilibrium:

$$\begin{cases} \bar{Q} = \frac{\lambda \gamma \pi + \rho \mu_{T^*} \mu_v}{\gamma \pi (\alpha + \mu_Q)}, \\ \bar{T} = \frac{\mu_{T^*} \mu_V}{\gamma \pi}, \\ \bar{T}^* = \frac{\lambda \gamma \pi \alpha - \rho \mu_V \mu_{T^*} \mu_Q - \alpha \mu_V \mu_{T^*} \mu_T - \mu_V \mu_{T^*} \mu_Q \mu_T}{\gamma \pi \mu_{T^*} (\alpha + \mu_Q)}, \\ \bar{V} = \frac{\lambda \gamma \pi \alpha - \rho \mu_V \mu_{T^*} \mu_Q - \alpha \mu_V \mu_{T^*} \mu_T - \mu_V \mu_{T^*} \mu_Q \mu_T}{\gamma \mu_{T^*} \mu_V (\alpha + \mu_Q)}. \end{cases}$$

Otherwise the trivial equilibrium (9.23) is the only equilibrium point and
is asymptotically reached.

The equilibrium point is often taken as the initial condition of the ODE
system. When the model is applied to the data of a clinical trial, this is the

equilibrium point without treatment. As we shall see in Section 9.5.5.2, the treatment changes the infectivity parameter, defining a new equilibrium point, hopefully the trivial one.

9.5.5.2   Intra- and inter-individual variability

The above equations give the basic mathematical structure, but to complete the model, we have to take into account that the parameters may vary with time and may be different from one subject to another. The model for inter-individual variability of the parameters is a mixed-effects model (9.17) for the log-transformed parameters; several arguments can be given to support the log-transform; the most obvious one is that the natural parameters are biological parameters like death rates, or productions rates, which are positive by definition. The model may include possibly time-dependent explanatory variables and random effects. Normal random effects can be put on some log-transformed parameters (denoted with a tilde): $\log \alpha_i = \tilde{\alpha}^i = \tilde{\alpha}_0 + u^i_\alpha$, $\log \lambda_i = \tilde{\lambda}^i = \tilde{\lambda}_0 + u^i_\lambda$ and $\log \mu^i_{T^*} = \tilde{\mu}^i_{T^*} = \tilde{\mu}_{T^*0} + u^i_{\mu_{T^*}}$, where u^i_α, u^i_λ and $u^i_{\mu_{T^*}}$ are independent normal random effects; natural log is used. The causal effect of treatment can be modeled as an effect on the infectivity parameter γ. The treatment may depend on time and is denoted by $A^i(t)$. This can be a binary variable, a quantitative variable if it is a function of the dose, and can also be a vector. The parameter γ consequently depends on t through A_t, and the model for the log-transformed parameter may be:

$$\tilde{\gamma}^i(t) = \tilde{\gamma}_0 + \beta A^i(t). \tag{9.25}$$

Up to now, the identifiability issue and the numerical difficulty has precluded putting many explanatory variables and many random effects.

9.5.5.3   Observation model

In most clinical trials as well as in cohort studies, we only have observations of total CD4 counts and viral loads at discrete times t_{ij}, $Q^i_{t_{ij}} + T^i_{t_{ij}} + T^{*i}_{t_{ij}}$ and $V^i_j = V^i_{t_{ij}}$ respectively. We also need to model the measurement error. To make an additive model for measurement error acceptable, we use 4th-root and log-transforms for CD4 and viral load, respectively. So our observation model is:

$$(Y^i_j)^{1/4} = [Q^i_{t_{ij}} + T^i_{t_{ij}} + T^{*i}_{t_{ij}}]^{1/4} + \varepsilon^1_{ij} \;\; ; \;\; \log_{10} V_{ij} = V^i_{t_{ij}} + \varepsilon^2_{ij}, \tag{9.26}$$

where ε^1_{ij} and ε^2_{ij} are measurement errors, independently normally distributed.

9.5.5.4   Application on the ALBI trial

The model was fitted on the data of the Albi trial described in Section 1.4.2. These data were first analyzed with a mechanistic model by Guedj et al. (2007). In this work, only the first two arms of the trial were analyzed and the treatment variable was treated as binary and fixed; the treatment effect was found highly significant. The data were reanalyzed by Prague et al. (2012) with a more complex model. In this analysis the treatment variable $A^i(t)$ was computed by a function taking into account the doses taken by each patient, and was a time-varying variable which allowed taking into account the switch from one treatment to the other in the third arm of the trial. It allowed also taking into account information about compliance. So we have $A^i(t) = (A_1^i(t), A_2^i(t))^\top$, where $A_1^i(t)$ and $A_2^i(t)$ are non-linear functions of the doses of the two treatments AZT + 3TC and ddI + d4T, respectively; $A_j^i(t) = 0$ if treatment j was not given at time t. Thus parameters β_1 and β_2 give the effect on infectivity for a standardized dose of treatment 1 and 2, respectively. Priors were chosen for the parameters according to results in the literature, and the penalized likelihood (or approximate posterior distribution) was maximized using NIMROD. Table 9.1 displays the results of this analysis.

One first interest of this result is to look at the effect of treatments. Both effects of treatments (β_1 and β_2) are highly significantly different from zero, with Wald statistics larger than 10. The estimated difference of effects between treatment $\hat{\beta}_2 - \hat{\beta}_1 = -0.07$ is also highly significant; the Wald statistics can be computed taking into account the correlation between these estimators and is found to be equal to 8.22 which is also highly significant.

The second output of this model is the estimation of parameters which have a biological interpretation. For instance we have estimates of death rates of the different types of CD4 cells. From this we can see that uninfected activated CD4 cells have a longer life expectation (13 days) than infected CD4 (1.7 days); the quiescent CD4 cells have a very low death rate in this model. These orders of magnitude are biologically plausible, although we may expect that with different models or with different data set we would find sensibly different results, essentially due to the misspecification of the model.

The third output of a mechanistic model is the predictive ability. Thanks to the switch arm, the ALBI trial offers a very good opportunity to assess this. We can use the first period to estimate the random effects for these patients and then predict their trajectory after treatment switch; 11 patients were selected from the switch arm; after removing these subjects from the sample, the MAP estimates of the fixed parameters were computed. Then, the empirical Bayes estimates of the random effects based on the first 12 weeks were computed for these 11 patients; finally, viral loads and CD4 counts were computed from the model for the values of the fixed and random parameters thus estimated, taking into account the adherence for the remaining 12 weeks. We also computed a 95% "measurement error predictive interval" as $\left[\hat{Y}_{j1}^i \pm 1.96\hat{\sigma}_{VL}\right]$ and $\left[\hat{Y}_{j2}^i \pm 1.96\hat{\sigma}_{CD4}\right]$. Figure 9.5 presents the viral load and the total CD4 count with a fit in the first 12 weeks and the predictions for the last 12 weeks after the treatment switch for one patient. One can see that the model is able to predict quite well the viral load rebound after the treatment change (because the AZT+3TC treatment is less efficient). The predictions were generally good for the 11 patients.

TABLE 9.1

Priors and posteriors for the "activated cells model" parameters estimated from ALBI trial data. A natural log-transform has been used for the biological parameters.

	Priors		Posteriors	
Biological parameter (Normal priors):				
Parameter	mean	sd.	mean	sd.
$\tilde{\alpha}_0$	-4.00	2.00	-3.19	0.14
$\tilde{\mu}_{T^*0}$	-0.05	0.68	-0.52	0.12
$\tilde{\lambda}_0$	2.55	1.90	2.52	0.10
$\tilde{\mu}_T$	-2.59	0.34	-2.57	0.10
$\tilde{\pi}$	4.04	2.66	2.49	0.54
$\tilde{\rho}$	-4.34	1.38	-5.13	0.54
$\tilde{\gamma}_0$	-5.76	4.02	-5.38	0.03
$\tilde{\mu}_Q$	-9.00	1.00	-11.2	0.99
$\tilde{\mu}_V$	2.90	0.68	1.70	0.59
Regressors for treatments doses (Normal priors):				
Parameter	mean	sd.	mean	sd.
β_1	-1.10	1.00	-0.97	0.09
β_2	-1.10	1.00	-1.03	0.09
Standard deviation for random effects (Half-Cauchy priors):				
Parameter	median		mean	sd.
σ_α	0.53	-	0.38	0.03
$\sigma_{\mu_{T^*}}$	0.37	-	0.03	0.01
σ_λ	0.10	-	0.03	0.01
Standard deviation for measurement error (Jeffrey's priors):				
Parameter			mean	sd.
σ_{CV}	-	-	0.45	0.01
σ_{CD4}	-	-	0.20	0.01

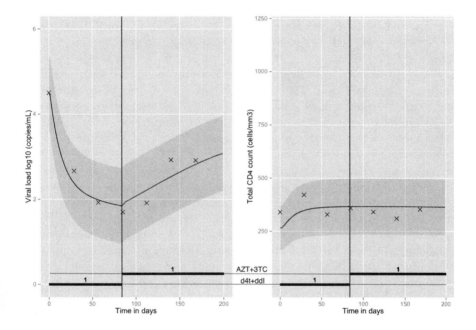

FIGURE 9.5
Predictions of viral load (log10 copies/mL) and CD4 count (cells/mL) for one patient from the switch arm who took full dose of d4T+ddI and then switched after 85 days to full dose AZT+3TC. Triangles are observations. Shaded area represents 95% "measurement error predictive interval." Vertical line materializes when the treatment switch occurred. Left side of the line: fit; right side of the line: predictions.

Finally, a possible use of the model is for treatment monitoring; this was precisely the goal of Prague et al. (2012). The algorithm proposed was based on the characteristic of dynamical models to have equilibrium points which depend on the parameters through the basic reproductive number R_0. As explained in Section 9.5.5.1, the stable equilibrium point of the system is the trivial one without virus if $R_0 < 1$. The problem is thus to find the minimum dose for which $R_0 < 1$. Since $R_0 < 1$ is a combination of parameters, the dose cannot be determined deterministically. Taking into account the information gathered up to time t_k, $\mathcal{F}_{t_k}$, R_0 has a certain distribution that can be computed by a MCMC algorithm. An adaptive algorithm for decreasing the dose was designed, ensuring at each change of the dose at time t_k that $P(R_0 < 1|\mathcal{F}_{t_k}) > 0.95$.

One central question when using mechanistic models is: "Is the model really mechanistic?" Specifically, when we say that μ_T is the death rate of activated CD4, does it have a biological meaning? Maybe a well-designed descriptive model could fit the data as well. The first criterion is the biological plausibility: we know that there are activated cells, that activated cells are more vulnerable to infection than quiescent cells, the estimated death rates are in the good order: $\mu_Q < \mu_T < \mu_{T^*}$. This criterion is rather well satisfied here. A second criterion is the reproducibility. Since the parameters have biological meanings, they should have approximately the same value on different data sets. There have been few analyses of different data sets with the target cells model. The target cell model was fitted in the context of primo-infection, with the added difficulty of unknown time origin (infection date) (Drylewicz et al., 2012). If we compare the estimates of the parameters obtained in Prague et al. (2012) and in Drylewicz et al. (2012), we see that for some parameters the estimates have the same order of magnitude, but that for other parameters they take sensibly different values. The third criterion is the ability of a mechanistic model to predict future values of the markers in complex situations. We have just seen that the target cell model has good predictive ability, which seems difficult to challenge with a descriptive model.

9.6 The issue of dynamic treatment regimes

The effects of treatments are most often assessed in randomized clinical trials. As mentioned in Section 9.1.1.3, such trials however have several limitations. Thus, in spite of the great importance of randomized trials, it remains useful to assess the effects of treatments on observational studies. This is however challenging because most of the time-dependent treatments are given based on the severity of the disease. The result is that treated subjects are generally in a more severe state of the disease than untreated ones. Naive methods which simply regress severity of the disease on treatment can badly underestimate the effect of the treatment, and even find a deleterious effect of treatment.

This is called a "time-dependent confounding" or an "indication bias," and is also an example of inverse causality; subjects receive the treatment because they are in a severe state.

9.6.1   Effect of HAART on CD4 counts: notation and MSM

This problem has been most of the time tackled in discrete time. Marginal structural models (MSM) have been developed to treat this problem; they have been in particular used for estimating the marginal effect of HAART in HIV infected subjects. We will describe the problem of estimating the effect of HAART on CD4 counts. The value of the marker of interest (e.g., CD4 count) Y for subject i at time t is denoted by Y_t^i. The value of a treatment given at time t for subject i is denoted by A_t^i. We drop the superscript i in the first part of the presentation but we will need to restore them later. Assume that there are only two treatment values: $A_t = 0$ when treatment is not given, and $A_t = 1$ when treatment is given at time t, and assume that once initiated, the treatment is not interrupted; generalization with different treatment levels is possible. In fact the treatment is attributed just after observation of the marker, thus if treatment is attributed at time t then $A_t = 1$ and $A_{t-1} = 0$. There may be other covariates V_t, which may represent the viral load or other biological processes linked to the infection. Overbars are used to represent histories of the processes: for instance $\bar{A}_t = (A_0, A_1, \ldots, A_t)$. We denote $\text{cum}(\bar{A}_t)$ the cumulative time under treatment until time t. Since A is binary, we can write $\text{cum}(\bar{A}_t) = \sum_{j=1}^{t} A_j$

In the absence of confounding by indication, a regression of Y_t on the history of treatment would give the effect of treatment on the marker. The simplest model would be to regress Y_t on $\text{cum}(\bar{A}_{t-1})$. It has been noted, however, that a piecewise linear regression model allowing a change of treatment effect after one year was better suited (Cole et al., 2005). Thus, the naive model that we will consider is:

$$E(Y_t|\bar{V}_t, \bar{A}_t) = \beta_0 + \beta_1 \text{cum}(\bar{A}_{t-1}) + \beta_2 \text{cumlag}(\bar{A}_{t-1}) + \beta_4 L_0. \qquad (9.27)$$

where $\text{cumlag}(\bar{A}_t)$ is the cumulative time under treatment up to time t minus one year: $\text{cumlag}(\bar{A}_t) = \max(0, \text{cum}(\bar{A}_t) - 1)$, and L_0 are baseline covariates. The β's are estimated by GEE because it is very likely that the Y_t are positively correlated and because these authors are interested in the population average effect (Hubbard et al., 2010). A working correlation structure has to be chosen and the choice may have an impact, not on the bias, but on the efficiency of the estimators (Liang and Zeger, 1986). However, in the presence of time-varying covariates, the independence working correlation structure should be chosen, otherwise results could be seriously biased, as shown by Pepe and Anderson (1994).

In the MSM, it is assumed that for each particular value $\bar{a}_t$ of $\bar{A}_t$ (or treatment regime), a potential outcome $\bar{Y}_t(\bar{a})$ is associated to each subject. This means that if a subject had treatment trajectory $\bar{a}_t$, possibly contrary to the fact, his outcome would have been $\bar{Y}_t(\bar{a})$. A model is postulated to describe how the potential outcomes vary as a function of the different treatment regimes:

$$E(Y_t(\bar{a})) = \beta_0 + \beta_1 \text{cum}(\bar{a}_{t-1}) + \beta_2 \text{cumlag}(\bar{a}_{t-1}) + \beta_4 L_0. \qquad (9.28)$$

Then it has been shown that the parameters of this model, called "causal parameters," can be estimated with a suitably weighted GEE. The weights are called "inverse-probability-of-treatment" (IPT) weights; an extension to the case with censoring has also been developed (Cole and Hernán, 2008), leading to inverse-probability-of-treatment and censoring (IPTC) weights. The weights are generally estimated using logistic regression models for each time and are the product of weights deriving from a model of treatment attribution and for censoring. The causal parameters can be estimated consistently if all the confounders (factors influencing both the outcome of interest and treatment attribution) have been taken into account.

Cole et al. (2005) used this approach for estimating the effect of HAART on CD4 from data of the Multi-center Cohort study (MACS) and the Women's Interagency HIV study. The sample included 1763 HIV-positive subjects under follow-up in April 1996 (when HAART became available). CD4 counts and other variables were collected every six months. An unweighted GEE for model (9.27) yielded an effect of one year of treatment (parameter β_1) equal to 21.5 and an effect for each subsequent year ($\beta_1 + \beta_2$) equal to 33. For applying the MSM, the weights were computed by logistic models including baseline covariates (gender, type of treatment, initial CD4 counts and viral load in categories) and time varying covariates (CD4 counts, viral load, indicators of undetectable viral load, non-HAART retroviral therapy). The estimates of the weighted GEE were 71 for the first year and 29 for the subsequent years. Thus the MSM corrected a bias of the naive regression model which appeared to be large for the first year.

9.6.2 Assumptions and inference for the dynamic approach

9.6.2.1 Assumptions

It was suggested by Aalen et al. (2012) that discrete time dynamic models could be used for this problem. The dynamic approach can be cast in the general theory of causality based on the Doob-Meyer decomposition (in discrete time, the "Doob decomposition") developed in Sections 9.2 and 9.3. We give here a precise description of this approach, using the perfect system assumption and formulating the yet implicit assumption of *stability* which is necessary when working with a population (see Section 9.3.4). The presentation is for simple perfect systems; a development for NUC systems can be found in Commenges and Gégout-Petit (2015).

The events of interest for subject i are represented by the process $X^i = (Y^i, A^i)$, which generates the filtration $\{\mathcal{F}_i\}$, and Y^i has a Doob decomposition in this filtration under probability P^{*i} (the true probability law for subject i):

$$Y_t^i = Y_0^i + \Lambda_{Y^i,t} + M_{Y^i,t} = Y_0^i + \phi_t^i(\bar{Y}_{t-1}^i, \bar{A}_{t-1}^i) + M_{Y^i,t},$$

where for all t, ϕ_t is a measurable functional. We assume that the martingales for different subjects i and i' are independent. Treatment attribution at time t may depend on information available just before t. The way treatment attribution is made is the treatment regime, or treatment strategy, and this may be different for different patients.

It is illuminating to look at the difference equation which gives the evolution of Y between $t-1$ and t:

$$Z_t^i = Y_t^i - Y_{t-1}^i = \Lambda_{Y^i,t} - \Lambda_{Y^i,t-1} + M_{Y^i,t} - M_{Y^i,t-1}. \tag{9.29}$$

Because of the martingale property, we have that $E(M_{Y^i,t} - M_{Y^i,t-1}|\mathcal{F}_{t-1}^i) = 0$ and thus, because of the previsibility of Λ_{Y^i},

$$E(Z_t^i|\mathcal{F}_{t-1}^i) = E(\Lambda_{Y^i,t} - \Lambda_{Y^i,t-1}|\mathcal{F}_{t-1}^i) = \Lambda_{Y^i,t} - \Lambda_{Y^i,t-1}. \tag{9.30}$$

That is, if we know Λ_{Y^i}, we can compute the expectation of the evolution of Y^i between $t-1$ and t; or in other terms, the evolution is equal to something which can be computed from information at $t-1$ plus a random term of null expectation. We make the following additional assumptions.

Perfect system assumption: The system represented by the filtration $\{\mathcal{F}_i\}$ is perfect for Y^i, for all i.

Stability assumption: Under P^*, $\phi_t^i(.,.) = \phi_t(.,.)$ for all t and i; the martingales M_{Y^i}, for all i, have the same law denoted $P_{M_Y}^*$; the Y_{0i} have the same law for all i.

The perfect system assumption implies here that Y^i does not influence $Y^{i'}$, so that with the additional assumption that Y_0^i and $Y_0^{i'}$ and A^i and $A^{i'}$ are independent, the processes Y^i and $Y^{i'}$ are independent; the proof is analogous to that of Lemma 4 of Commenges and Gégout-Petit (2009).

Remark about the stability assumption: We cannot say of course that $\Lambda_{Y^i,t}$ and $\Lambda_{Y^{i'},t}$ for $i \neq i'$ are the same process, not even that they have the same law; what is invariant is the function $\phi_t(.,.)$. Also the Y^i do not have the same law because the A^i may have different laws for different i's. The definition of the stability assumption is not the same as in Berzuini et al. (2012), but the conjunction of the perfect system assumption and our stability assumption implies stability in their sense, that is stability across different regimes, as developed below.

The conjunction of the perfect system and the stability assumptions is called the **physical law assumption** for Y. To completely specify the probability law for Y on horizon t_f one must specify the law of Y_0^i, $\phi_t(.,.)$ for $t \leq t_f$, and the law of the martingale $P_{M_Y}^*$. The laws of X^i, P^{*i}, may be different because the treatment regimes may be different. Finally, the law of $X^i = (Y^i, A^i)$, P^{*i}, is completely specified by the law of Y_0^i, the physical law for Y and the treatment regime.

The treatment regimes may differ, in particular between subjects who are part of an observational study and subjects enrolled in a randomized study. If one knows the physical law for Y, one knows the causal effect of A on Y. For instance if by an intervention on subject i, we give the treatment regime $A^i = a$ (that is, $A_t^i = a_t, t = 0, \ldots, t_f$ where the a_t are fixed values), the law of X^i is completely specified if we know the specific physical law for Y; we denote it by P^{*a}. More generally, if we know the physical law, including the law of the martingale, and the law of Y_0^i, we know the probability law of Y^i for any treatment regime.

As an example, suppose that the physical law is such that the compensator of Y is specified by the difference equation:

$$\Delta \phi_t(\bar{Y}_{t-1}, \bar{A}_{t-1}) = \beta_1^* A_{t-1} + \beta_2^* A_{t-1} + \beta_3^*. \tag{9.31}$$

Summing Equations (9.31) for $t = 1$ to t_f, we obtain $\phi_{t_f}(\bar{Y}_{t_f-1}, \bar{A}_{t_f-1}) = \beta_1^* \mathrm{cum}(\bar{A}_{t_f-1}) + \beta_2^* \mathrm{cumlag}(\bar{A}_{t_f-1}) + \beta_3^* t_f$ and thus

$$Y_{t_f} = Y_0 + \beta_1^* \mathrm{cum}(\bar{A}_{t_f-1}) + \beta_2^* \mathrm{cumlag}(\bar{A}_{t_f-1}) + \beta_3^* t_f + M_{Y,t_f}, \tag{9.32}$$

We can assess the causal effect between two treatment regimes a and a' at horizon t_f by: $\mathrm{CE}(a, a') = \mathrm{E}_a(Y_{t_f}) - \mathrm{E}_{a'}(Y_{t_f}) = \beta_1^*[\mathrm{cum}(\bar{a}_{t_f-1}) - \mathrm{cum}(\bar{a}'_{t_f-1})] + \beta_2^*[\mathrm{cumlag}(\bar{a}_{t_f-1}) - \mathrm{cum}(\bar{a}'_{t_f-1})]$.

Remark 1 (Equivalence between a dynamic model and a MSM): In the MSM, it is assumed that each subject has potential responses for trajectories $\bar{a}$, $Y_{\bar{a}}(t)$. If we assume the potential outcome model of Cole et al. (2005), there are true values for the β_k's, β_k^*, $k = 0, 1, 2$, for which Equation (9.28) holds. From Equation (9.32), taking the expectation under P^{*a} we have $\mathrm{E}_a(Y_{t_f}) = Y_0 + \beta_1^* \mathrm{cum}(\bar{a}_{t_f-1}) + \beta_2 \mathrm{cumlag}(\bar{a}_{t-1}) + \beta_3^* t_f$. We see that if $\beta_3 = \beta_4 = 0$ the expectations as well as the causal effects are the same in both models, although the meaning of the expectation is somewhat different.

9.6.2.2 Inference

Suppose that we observe $(\bar{Y}_{t_f}^i, \bar{A}_{t_f-1}^i), i = 1, \ldots, n$. One important fact is that we can infer causal effects without knowing the law of A_i. Indeed, if there was a very large number of observations and both $\bar{A}_{t-1}^i, \bar{Y}_{t-1}^i$ took a finite number of values we could estimate $\Delta \phi_t(\bar{A}_{t-1}^i, \bar{Y}_{t-1}^i)$ by a simple mean of the observations Z_t^i (see Equation (9.29)). An interesting factorization of the likelihood also shows that the distribution of A^i is not needed, a fact already noted by Arjas and Parner (2004). We use light notations writing the likelihood for variable X as $f(X)$ rather than the more rigorous $f_X(X)$, where $f_X(.)$ is the probability density function of X. The likelihood of observation

$(\bar{Y}_{t_f}^i, \bar{A}_{t_f-1}^i)$, factors in

$$f(\bar{Y}_{t_f}^i, \bar{A}_{t_f-1}^i) = \prod_{t=1}^{t_f} f(Y_t^i | \bar{Y}_{t-1}^i, \bar{A}_{t-1}^i) \prod_{t=1}^{t_f} f(A_t^i | \bar{Y}_t^i, \bar{A}_{t-1}^i). \tag{9.33}$$

This factorization always holds and can be easily checked. For inference, provided the same parameters are not involved in both $f(Y_t^i | \bar{Y}_{t-1}^i, \bar{A}_{t-1}^i)$ and $f(A_t^i | \bar{Y}_t^i, \bar{A}_{t-1}^i)$, we can use the partial likelihood (in the sense of Andersen et al. (1993)):

$$\prod_{t=1}^{t_f} f(Y_t^i | \bar{Y}_{t-1}^i, \bar{A}_{t-1}^i). \tag{9.34}$$

It is clear that we do not need to model treatment attribution. The term $f(Y_t^i | \bar{Y}_{t-1}^i, \bar{A}_{t-1}^i)$ gives the "physical law" of the dynamics of Y^i and can be expressed in terms of $\phi_t(.,.)$ and the law of the martingale M_{Y^i}. Specifically, the contribution to the likelihood of subject i is $\prod_{t=1}^{t_f} f_{\Delta M_{Y,t} | \bar{Y}_{t-1}^i, \bar{A}_{t-1}^i}[Z_t^i - \Delta\phi_t(\bar{Y}_{t-1}^i, \bar{A}_{t-1}^i)]$.

In practice we must make assumptions to obtain good estimates with a moderate number of observations. First, a Markov assumption leads to $\phi_t(\bar{A}_{t-1}^i, \bar{Y}_{t-1}^i) = \phi_t(A_{t-1}^i, Y_{t-1}^i)$. A very simple parametric form is

$$\Delta\phi_t(A_{t-1}^i, Y_{t-1}^i) = \beta_1 A_{t-1}^i + \beta_2 A_{t-2}^i + \beta_3, \tag{9.35}$$

with $(\beta_1, \beta_2) \in \mathbb{R}^2$. Note that here we are describing a model while Equation (9.31) described the true physical law. This gives $\phi_t(A_{t-1}^i, Y_{t-1}^i) = \beta_1 \mathrm{cum}(\bar{A}_{t-1}^i) + \beta_2 \mathrm{cumlag}(\bar{A}_{t-1}^i) + \beta_3 t$. In terms of Y_t^i this model implies that:

$$\mathrm{E}_a(Y_t^i) = Y_0^i + \beta_1 \mathrm{cum}(\bar{a}_{t-1}) + \beta_2 \mathrm{cumlag}(\bar{a}_{t-1}) + \beta_3 t,$$

which is the same model as in Cole et al. (2005) if $\beta_3 = \beta_4 = 0$ as discussed in Remark 1. If one makes the assumption that all the martingale increments are independent (both in t and i), all the Z_t^i are independent; we may in addition make a distribution assumption for the martingale increments, for instance assume they are distributed as $\mathcal{N}(0, \sigma^2)$: this completes the model, up to the law of A^i.

9.6.2.3 Dynamic treatment regimes and mechanistic models

The effect of treatment on CD4 counts can also be estimated using mechanistic models such as presented in Section 9.5.5. If we assume that there are no unmeasured confounders, inference can be conditional on treatment attribution as shown in Section 9.6.2.2 for discrete time models. Mechanistic models have been fitted in the past on data from clinical trials; fitting such models on large observational studies is even more challenging numerically because the amount of computations is proportional to the number of subjects, and also because there is more heterogeneity in a large cohort than in a clinical trial. One obvious heterogeneity is due to the variety of treatments that can be given, even if we restrict to HAART. One possibility is to represent the effect of different treatments by different parameters, but this leads to increase the number of parameters, and thus the numerical difficulty. One can also attempt to model the effect of a treatment which is a combination of several drugs by attributing an effect to each drug and constructing a model for the effect of the combination of drugs. A simpler and less ambitious approach is to ignore this variety and consider the HAART treatment as a binary variable.

9.6.3 Effect of HAART on CD4 counts: results from the dynamic models

The dynamic models were fitted using the data of the Aquitaine cohort by Prague et al. (2015); we give here a brief summary of the results. The raw data set is composed of 4541 patients for a total of 110,663 observations. Similarly to Cole et al. (2005) the sample included HIV positive patients yet untreated and under follow-up in April 1996. Once a patient was on any therapy, we assumed he or she remained on it. For each of them, the follow-up began with the first visit after April 1996 and ended with (1) the last visit at which he or she was seen alive, (2) the last visit before patient discontinued the study, or (3) April 2005, whichever came first. The resulting sample included 1591 patients (19,597 observations).

The naive model (9.27) was fitted. A version of the discrete-time dynamic model (9.35) including a random effect on the intercept was also fitted. This has been done with the linear mixed-effect package lme4 (Bates et al., 2014). The mechanistic model described in Section 9.5.5 was also fitted; the treatment is represented by a binary variable indicating whether the subject received HAART at time t or not.

The results are shown in Table 9.2. The naive model indicated a deleterious effect of treatment for the first year. A MSM model with similar weights as in Cole et al. (2005) gave positive effects of the treatment, but with the strange feature that the increase was smaller for the first year compared to subsequent years. Both discrete-time dynamic and mechanistic models gave positive effects, with a larger effect for the first year, but the former model gives larger estimates than the latter. The statistics for testing the null hypothesis of no-effect are large for the dynamic and the mechanistic models. In the mechanistic model, this is the effect on the infectivity parameter which is tested. The Wald statistic reaches the impressive value of -85.8. One may be skeptical with such large absolute values and it is not necessary to compute an exact p-value in that case. However, this can be interpreted as a near certainty that there is an effect. This can be confirmed by a likelihood ratio statistic which takes also a very high value. Thus, the mechanistic model has the potential to lead to very powerful analyses. Moreover, the mechanistic model can treat unequally spaced observations and thus could benefit of more information and incur less bias due to selection of observations. Finally, most dynamic models have an equilibrium point, which makes sense from biological point of view. Fitting the target cell model is however computationally demanding; it takes several hours using parallel computing. The discrete-time models are very fast. Moreover, biological knowledge must be available to construct a mechanistic model, and this is not the case in all the diseases.

TABLE 9.2
Estimated treatment effect on CD4 count from data of the Aquitaine cohort: Naive regression, MSM, discrete-time dynamic model and mechanistic model.

Model	β treatment	Aquitaine Cohort		
		Effect	Sd.	Z-stat
Naive model	< 1 yr	-94	12	-7.55
	> 1 yr	30	19	2.4
MSM	< 1 yr	36	20	1.87
	> 1 yr	53	31	2.7
Discrete-time dynamic	< 1 yr	109	9	12.03
	> 1 yr	55	13	4.28
Mechanistic	< 1 yr	71	-	-
	> 1 yr	9	-	-
	Param. γ	-0.89	0.01	-85.77

10

Appendix: software

10.1 Appendix for Chapter 3: survival analysis

10.1.1 SAS and R softwares

For survival analysis using SAS software (Allison, 2012), there are mainly three procedures: the LIFETEST procedure, which, among other things, is designed to produce non-parametric estimator of the survival function, the LIFEREG procedure, to estimate survival function and regression model with parametric approach, and the PHREG procedure for Cox's model.

An alternative to the LIFEREG procedure is the NLMIXED procedure. The use of the latter is a little bit more complex because you have to "write" the likelihood. It is thus possible, to a little programming cost, to use parametric models taking into account cases a little bit more complex than those offered routinely by SAS. It is possible, for example, to estimate frailty models with random effects.

Regarding R software, it is mainly the packages survival and SmoothHazard that are used in this chapter. The package survival allows, among other things, to produce non-parametric estimator of the survival function and Cox's proportional hazard regression model. The package SmoothHazard allows to take into account interval-censored data with a Weibull model or with a penalized likelihood approach. This package allows also to make an estimation with the "Illness-death model."

This two softwares treat data with the same basic structure.

10.1.2 PROC LIFETEST

The Kaplan-Meier estimator is the default in the LIFETEST procedure. There are many options in this procedure. We will give just one example and refer to the book of Allison (2012) for more details.

```
proc lifetest data=ech_livre plots=survival (nocensor atrisk=0 to
12 by 1) timelist = 0 to 12 by 1;
time delai_ins*indic_dc(0);
```

```
run ;
```

In this example, the statement `atrisk` allows displaying on the graph the number of subjects at risk and the `timelist` statement allows specifying the times where the values of the estimator are given (default is values for all subjects).

To have several tables and several curves of the survival functions (or $\ln[-\ln(\hat{S}(t))]$) superimposed on the same graph for each stratum of a covariate the `strata` statement should be used. Likewise, with `strata` statement, this procedure tests whether survival curves are the same in several groups. The `LIFETEST` procedure does not take into account left-truncated data. For this purpose, it is possible to use the R package `survival` or the `PHREG` procedure with a Breslow estimator.

10.1.3   PROC PHREG

The `PHREG` procedure implements the proportional hazards regression model proposed by D. Cox. It is a very comprehensive procedure (Allison, 2012), taking into account right-censored and left-truncated survival time. This procedure handles time-dependent covariates and covariates with time-dependent effect and it allows stratification.

For example, to obtain the results presented in Table 3.1, the syntax is:

```
proc phreg data=ech_livre;
model delai_ins*indic_dc(0) = age_ins niv2 niv3 sexe / rl;
test niv2, niv3;
run ;
```

Here, the statement `test` allows to test the null hypothesis "$H_0 : \beta_{niv2} = \beta_{niv3} = 0$" with a Wald test. The model includes two dummy variables previously coded for the educational level. The statement `class` (not used here) allows constructing dummy variables.

To take into account left-truncation, we can specify it in the following way:
```
proc phreg data=ech_livre;
model (age_ins,age_dc)*indic_dc(0) = niv2 niv3 sexe / rl ;
test niv2, niv3;
run ;
```

where `age_ins` is the age of entry into institution (i.e., into the risk set) and `age_dc` is age at death or at right-censoring. Another way to deal with delayed entry is to use the option `entry=` like in the following syntax equivalent to the previous one:

```
proc phreg data=ech_livre;
model age_dc*indic_dc(0) = niv2 niv3 sexe / rl entry=age_ins;
test niv2, niv3;
run ;
```

10.1.3.1 Testing the proportionality assumption with residuals

Martingale and Schoenfeld residuals are presented in Section 3.5.8. Martingale residuals can be used to test for non-proportionality using the ASSESS PH statement:

```
proc phreg data=ech_livre;
model delai_ins*indic_dc(0) = age_ins niv2 niv3 sexe / rl;
assess ph / resample ;
test niv2, niv3;
run ;
```

For each covariate, the ASSESS PH statement produces a graphical display and give a p-value produced by the RESAMPLE option. With the statement ASSESS VAR= we can also check the functional form (log-linearity) for a covariate (age_ins in the following example):

```
proc phreg data=ech_livre;
model delai_ins*indic_dc(0) = age_ins niv2 niv3 sexe / rl;
test niv2, niv3;
assess var=(age_ins) / resample ;
run ;
```

To detect possible departures from the proportional hazards assumption with Schoenfeld residuals, correlation between time and residuals should be tested. There should not be any correlation between time and Schoenfeld residuals. First, data set containing the Schoenfeld residuals must be created using these statements:

```
proc phreg data=ech_livre;
model delai_ins*indic_dc(0) = age_ins niv2 niv3 sexe / rl;
output out=table_res ressch = schage_ins schniv2 schniv3 schsexe ;
test niv2, niv3;
run ;
```

Here the data set with residuals is table_res with the residuals for the four covariates: schage_ins schniv2 schniv3 schsexe. Then, with the CORR procedure a correlation between time and residuals should be tested.

10.1.3.2 Testing the proportionality assumption with interaction with time

With SAS you can easily estimate a model with a time-dependent covariate and include an interaction between it and a covariate. For example, to include an interaction between the covariate sexe and the logarithm of the time:

```
proc phreg data=ech_livre;
model delai_ins*indic_dc(0) = age_ins niv2 niv3 sexe int / rl;
int = sexe*log(delai_ins);
test niv2, niv3;
run ;
```

Here, for the covariate sexe there are two regression parameters: β_4 and β_5. The hazard ratio for the gender is equal to $\exp(\beta_4 + \beta_5 \times log(delai\_ins))$. To test the proportional hazards assumption the parameter β_5 must be tested to 0.

10.1.3.3 Time-dependent covariates

The following syntax is an example of a time-dependent covariate (the season) coded with three dummies variable. In the PHREG procedure a lot of statements like IF, DO, ARRAY can be used allowing to incorporate in the model more or less complex time-dependent covariate.

```
proc phreg data=season;
model age_dc*indic_dc(0) = spring summer autumn / rl entry=ageentre;
array age{89} age1-age89;
array a_autumn{89} autumn1-autumn89;
array a_spring{89} spring1-spring89;
array a_summer{89} summer1-summer89;
do i=1 to 88;
   if (age{i} le age_dc) and age{i} ne . then do;
      spring = a_spring{i};
      summer = a_summer{i};
      autumn = a_autumn{i};
   end;
end;
test spring, summer, autumn;
run;
```

10.1.4 The R package `survival`

The function `Surv` of the package creates an object which is used by the functions `survfit`, `survdiff` and `coxph`. The function `Surv` takes into account left-censoring by adding an argument to specify the entry time.

The function `survfit` allows estimation of survival function by Kaplan-Meier estimator:

```
km1 <- survfit(Surv(delai_ins,indic_dc)~1,data=ech_livre,
type="kaplan-meier")
```

With left-truncated data, an entry time must be specified (`age_ins` in the following example):

```
km2 <- survfit(Surv(age_ins,age_dc,indic_dc)~1,data=ech_livre,
type="kaplan-meier")
```

The function `survdiff` test whether survival curves are the same in several groups by a log-rank test. In the following example, we test if the survival since entry in institution of women and men is different:

```
lg1 <- survdiff(Surv(delai_ins,indic_dc)~SEXE,data=ech_livre)
```

The `coxph` function implements the Cox proportional hazards regression model. This function takes into account right-censored and left-truncated survival time. To obtain the results presented in Table 3.1, the syntax is:

```
coxph(Surv(delai_ins,indic_dc)~SEXE+niv1+niv2+age_ins,data=ech_livre)
```

The statement `factor` (not used here) makes easy to create dummies variables and the function allows stratification with the statement `strata`. But it is difficult to handle interaction between time and covariates.

The function `cox.zph` allows to use Schoenfeld residual in order to check proportionality. For the example of Section 3.5.8 the syntax is:

```
ex1 <- coxph(Surv(delai_ins,indic_dc)~SEXE+niv1+niv2+age_ins,
data=ech_livre)
prop <- cox.zph(ex1,transform='identity')
print(prop)
plot(prop)
```

Here the statement `'identity'` states that the function of time used is the identity. To have the logarithm the statement should be `'log'`. The function `'plot'` makes a graph of the Schoenfeld residual.

10.1.5   The package `SmoothHazard`

The `SmoothHazard` package for R implements algorithms for fitting regression model and hazard function for interval-censored data with a penalized likelihood approach or with a parametric Weibull model. In this package, survival model and illness-death model are proposed.

For survival model, the function to use is `shr`. For example, to have an estimator of the hazard function with a penalized likelihood approach the syntax is:

```
hz1 <- shr(Hist(time=age_dc,indic_dc,entry=age_ins)~1,\\
method='Splines',CV=1,data=ech_livre)\\
plot(hz1$time,hz1$hazard,xlab="Age",ylab="Hazard",xlim=c(65,100),
    ylim=c(0,0.5),type="l")
```

Here, the penalized likelihood approach is specified by `method='Splines'`, no covariates are specified by the statement $\sim$ 1 and the smoothing parameter is estimated by cross-validation (statement `CV=1`). The data are left-truncated as specified by the statement `entry=`.

To obtain with `SmoothHazard` results similar to those presented in Table 3.1, the syntax is:

```
shr(Hist(time=delai_ins,indic_dc)~SEXE+niv1+niv2+age_ins,\\
data=ech_livre)
```

Here, a Weibull parametrization for the baseline hazard function is used (by default if the statement `method` is not specified).

10.2   Appendix for Chapter 4: models for longitudinal data

10.2.1   Linear mixed models

Linear mixed models can be fitted in SAS with procedure `MIXED` and in R with different functions, the most well-known being `lmer` of package `lme4` and `lme` of package `nlme`. Note that function `hlme` of package R `lcmm` described below for the analysis of latent class mixed model also estimates linear mixed models.

Estimated model

In Application 4.1.10, the linear model with random intercept and slope is:

$$\text{CD4t}_{ij} = \beta_0 + \beta_1 \text{Time}_{ij} + \beta_2 \text{RAN\_GRP}_{2i} + \beta_3 \text{RAN\_GRP}_{3i} + \beta_4 \text{RAN\_GRP}_{2i}\text{Time}_{ij}$$
$$+ \beta_5 \text{RAN\_GRP}_{3i}\text{Time}_{ij} + b_{0i} + b_{1i}\text{Time}_{ij} + \epsilon_{ij}$$

with $(b_{0i}, b_{1i})^{\top} \sim \mathcal{N}\left(0, B = \begin{bmatrix} \sigma_0^2 & \sigma_{01} \\ \sigma_{01} & \sigma_1^2 \end{bmatrix}\right)$ and $\epsilon_{ij} \sim \mathcal{N}(0, \sigma_\epsilon^2)$.

Translation in R

This model can be fitted with function `lmer` of package R `lme4` by calling:

```
library(lme4)
mlmer <- lmer(CD4t ~ Time + factor(RAN_GRP) * Time +
        (1 + Time | NUM_PAT), data = albi, REML = F)
summary(mlmer)
```

or

```
mlmer <- lmer(CD4t ~ Time + RAN_GRP2 * Time + RAN_GRP3 * Time +
        (1 + Time | NUM_PAT), data = albi, REML = F)
```

if binary indicators for treatment RAN_GRP are used.

In these calls, the linear mixed model is defined in one block with the dependent variable CD4t on the left side of $\sim$, and all the covariates that intervene either with fixed effects (`Time + factor(RAN_GRP) * Time`) or with the random effects (`1 + Time | NUM_PAT`) on the right side of $\sim$. For the latter, `| NUM_PAT` specifies the unit on which the random effects are defined. With this call, the random effects are assumed to be correlated. In order to assume independent random effects, one should specify `(1 | NUM_PAT) + (-1 + Time | NUM_PAT)`.

In this call `data=` gives the data frame to use and option `REML=F` means that parameters are estimated by maximum of likelihood rather than by maximum of restricted likelihood (`REML=T`).

From this model which estimation is recorded in object `mlmer`, several functions can be used, such as `summary` or `plot` in order to display the estimates of the model or a graph of the model residuals.

Function `lme` of the R package `nlme` can fit this model too. The syntax is a little bit different:

```
library(nlme)
mlme <- lme(CD4t ~ Time + factor(RAN_GRP) * Time,
        random=~ 1 + Time | NUM_PAT,
        data = albi, na.action = na.omit, method = "ML")
summary(mlme)
```

With function `lme`, the regression at the population level (with fixed effects) (`CD4t ~ Time + factor(RAN_GRP)*Time`) and the regression at the individual level (with random effects) (`random =~ 1 + Time | NUM_PAT`) are specified separately. As in `lmer`, the default estimation technique is REML so that `method = "ML"` has to be specified to obtain maximum likelihood estimates. Note that in case of missing data, their management has to be specified in option `na.action=`. This can consist in removing the observations with missing data (`na.action = na.omit`), which is the usual default option in other functions described in this paragraph.

Again, many options can be added in order to estimate more sophisticated linear mixed models, and objects containing the estimated models, here `mlme`, can be used in other functions including `summary` and `plot`.

Function `hlme` (that will be detailed for the latent class mixed models) also fits standard linear mixed models. One of its assets is that it is very easy to add correlated errors in addition to the measurement independent errors in (4.8) while it is not necessarily feasible with functions `lme` and `lmer`. The estimation of the application model is done by the following call and its variation to include additional correlated errors:

```
library(lcmm)
# standard linear mixed model (independent measurement errors)
mhlme <- hlme(CD4t ~ Time + factor(RAN_GRP) * Time,
        random=~ 1 + Time, subject = "NUM_PAT", data = albi)
# linear mixed model with independent measurement errors and
# autoregressive errors
mhlme <- hlme(CD4t ~ Time + factor(RAN_GRP) * Time,
        random =~ 1 + Time, subject = "NUM_PAT", data = albi,
        cor = AR(Time))
summary(mhlme)
```

As for `lme`, the model specification is divided in two parts with the regression at the population level (`CD4t ~ Time + factor(RAN_GRP) * Time`) and the regression at the individual level (`random =~ 1 + Time`). However, in contrast with `lme`, the grouping variable is defined separately with attribute `subject`. By default, an unstructured variance-covariance matrix is assumed for the random effects. They can be considered independent with option `idiag = T`.

In the second call, `cor = AR(Time)` specifies that there is an autocorrelated process w with covariance between times s and t: $\mathrm{cov}(w(s), w(t)) = \sigma_w^2 \exp(\rho|t - s|)$. Option `cor = BM(Time)` would have specified a Brownian process w in addition to the independent measurement errors with covariance between times s and t: $\mathrm{cov}(w(s), w(t)) = \sigma_w^2 \min(s, t)$.

Translation in SAS

The model is fitted with `MIXED` procedure by calling:

```
Proc MIXED data = ALBI method = ml;
class NUM_PAT;
```

```
model CD4t = Time RAN_GRP2 RAN_GRP3 RAN_GRP2 * Time
            RAN_GRP3 * Time / s;
random intercept Time / type = UN subject = NUM_PAT G;
run;
```

Statement `model` defines the linear regression at the population level with the dependent variable `CD4t` on the left, and the covariates defining the linear predictor (`Time RAN_GRP2 RAN_GRP3 RAN_GRP2*Time RAN_GRP3*Time`) on the right. Options can be added to the statement on the right side of symbol `/`, the main one being `solution` or `s` to obtain the estimated fixed parameters. Statement `random` specifies the list of covariates associated to a random effect. This includes the intercept noted `intercept` or `int`. Options can again be specified after symbol `/`, including the grouping variable (statistical unit on which random effects are defined) with option `subject=` or `sub=`, and the type of structure for the covariance matrix of the random effects with `type`. For example, `type=UN` specifies an unstructured variance-covariance matrix while `type=VC` specifies a diagonal variance-covariance matrix. Other options include `G` and `Gcorr` in order to obtain respectively the estimated variance-covariance matrix and the estimated correlation matrix in output.

The first statement (`Proc MIXED`) provides the data set to use with option `data` as well as many options related for instance to the estimation process and the output. In particular, REML is the default estimation technique; ML technique is performed with option `method=ml`.

Statement `class` is used to define the categorical covariates, and most often the grouping variable is specified in `class`. Indeed, when indicated in `class`, the data do not need to be sorted by the grouping variable while it needs to be done otherwise. Categorical covariates can also be specified like `RAN_GRP`, a three-level covariate. In the syntax above, however, the same model could be estimated with the following syntax, and the use of the categorical covariate directly

```
Proc MIXED data = ALBI method = ml;
class NUM_PAT RAN_GRP;
model CD4t = Time RAN_GRP RAN_GRP * Time / s;
random intercept Time / type = UN subject = NUM_PAT G;
run;
```

Finally, in the two preceding syntaxes, the errors were assumed to be independent. A statement `repeated` can be added to specify a correlation structure for the errors. Here is an example:

```
Proc MIXED data = ALBI method = ml;
class NUM_PAT RAN_GRP;
model CD4t = Time RAN_GRP RAN_GRP * Time  / s;
random intercept Time / type = UN subject = NUM_PAT G;
repeated / subject = NUM_PAT type = SP(POW)(Time) local;
run;
```

This statement adds an autocorrelated process to the measurement errors in order to further take into account the correlation between the repeated measures of a same subject. The autocorrelation process is defined by option `type=` which specifies the structure of the covariance matrix. Here, `type=SP(POW)(Time)` specifies a process w with covariance structure between s and t: $\mathrm{cov}(w(s), w(t)) = \sigma_w^2 \rho|t-s|$. Option `local` is essential here. It specifies that there are independent measurement errors in addition to the autocorrelated errors defined in `repeated`, as it was in Equation (4.8). Without option `local`, only correlated errors would be assumed.

Other statements can be added, for example `estimate` that computes *a posteriori* mean quantities derived from the estimated linear mixed model.

10.2.2 Generalized linear mixed models

Generalized linear mixed models can be fitted in SAS with procedure NLMIXED and more recently with procedure GLIMMIX available in version 9.2 and later. We note that a macro (called ORDINAL and derived from NLMIXED) is also available on the website http://www.isped.u-bordeaux.fr/BIOSTAT to estimate proportional odds logistic mixed models and cumulative probit mixed models.

Generalized linear mixed model can be fitted in R with function `glmer` of package lme4. There exist other more specific functions such as function `clmm` of package `ordinal` to estimate logistic and probit cumulative mixed models, or function `lcmm` of package `lcmm` to estimate cumulative probit mixed models (see Section 10.3.1 for further details).

Estimated model

In Application 4.2.8, the logistic model with a random intercept is:

$$\mathrm{logit}(P(\texttt{cesd16}_{ij} = 1)) = \beta_0 + \beta_1\,\texttt{age65}_{ij} + \beta_2\,\texttt{male}_i + \beta_3\,\texttt{male}_i \times \texttt{age65}_{ij} + b_{0i}$$

with $b_{0i} \sim \mathcal{N}\left(0, \sigma_0^2\right)$.

Translation in R

The model is fitted with function `glmer` by calling:

```
# loading of the dataset
library(lcmm)
data(paquid)
#  loading of lme4 and call of glmer
library(lme4)
mglmm <- glmer(cesd16 ~ male * age65 + (1 | ID), data = paquid,
```

```
family = binomial)
```

The first part of **glmer** call gives the regression with the dependent variable cesd16 on the left and the fixed effects **male** * **age65** (or equivalently 1 + male + age65 + male:age65) as well as the random intercept (1 | ID) for which the grouping variable ID is specified on the right. Here (1 + age65 | ID) could have been written to estimate a logistic model with correlated random intercept and slope. Then, **data** gives the date frame and **family** specifies the type of generalized linear mixed model. For example, **family=binomial** fits a logistic model and **family=poisson** a Poisson model.

An essential point in the estimation of generalized linear mixed models is the numerical integration over the random-effect distribution. With **glmer**, a Laplace approximation is used by default, which corresponds to an adaptive Gaussian quadrature with 1 quadrature point. More points can be specified with option **nAGQ** to use adaptive Gauss-Hermite quadrature (for example, nAGQ=9 specifies 9 points). The more the number of quadrature points, the longer the estimation process but also the more accurate the estimates.

Translation in SAS

The model can be fitted with **GLIMMIX** procedure by calling:

```
proc GLIMMIX data = paquid METHOD = QUAD;
class ID;
model cesd16(descending) = age65 male age65 * male
                 /dist = binary link = logit solution;
random int / subject = ID;
run;
```

The call of **GLIMMIX** procedure is similar to that of **MIXED** procedure with statement **model** that specifies the dependent variable on the left, and the linear predictor at the population level on the right. The difference is that the type of generalized linear mixed model has to be defined along with other options such as **solution** (to obtain parameter estimates). The type of model is defined by the distribution and the link function used, for example **dist=binary** and **link=logit** in the case of a logistic mixed model.

Statement **random** that defines the random effects is exactly the same as in **MIXED** procedure. Here **random int / subject=ID** specifies a random intercept for each level of the grouping variable ID.

Again, an essential point when using **GLIMMIX** procedure is the specification of the technique used for the numerical integration over the random-effect distribution. In contrast with **glmer**, **GLIMMIX** procedure does not use by default a Laplace approximation. It favors a linearization of the model which is very fast but may induce substantial biases in the estimates. It is thus recommended to systematically specify the type of numerical technique, that is either a Laplace approximation with option METHOD=LAPLACE or an adaptive Gauss-Hermite quadrature with METHOD=QUAD, the number of quadrature points being defined with option qpoints.

The general NLMIXED procedure can fit a logistic mixed model too, either by specifying a logistic distribution for cesd16:

```
proc NLMIXED data = paquid;
mu = beta0 + beta1*age65 + beta2*male + beta3*age65*male + b0i;
p = exp(mu) / (1 + exp(mu));
model cesd16 ~ binary(p);
random b0i ~ normal(0, s0 * s0) subject = ID;
run;
```

or by writting the complete individual contribution to the log-likelihood conditional to the random effects:

```
proc NLMIXED data = paquid;
mu = beta0 + beta1*age65 + beta2*male + beta3*age65*male + b0i;
p = exp(mu) / (1 + exp(mu));
ll = log(p) * cesd16 + log(1-p) * (1-cesd16);
model cesd16 ~ general(ll);
random b0i ~ normal(0, s0 * s0) subject = ID;
run;
```

In both cases, the linear predictor conditional to the random effects mu must be completely specified according to covariates, fixed effects and random effects. The distribution of the random effects (here a random intercept b0i) is defined in statement random. In both cases, the intercept has a Gaussian distribution with zero mean and standard deviation |s0|. The grouping variable is specified with option subject=.

From this linear predictor, in the first call, the probability of cesd16=1 is computed in the local variable p and the distribution of cesd16 is defined in statement model by binary(p), that is a Bernoulli with success probability p. In the second call, the distribution of cesd16 in statement model is not explicitly given. Instead, general(loglik) means that the local variable loglik contains the individual contribution to the log-likelihood conditional to the random effects.

NLMIXED procedure includes many possible options relative to the integration method and the optimization algorithm. These options are important because convergence is very sensitive to them. We also highly recommend to specify the initial values for the optimization algorithm by adding statement parms which would be for the example above:

parms beta0=-2.0 beta1=0.4 beta2=-1.5 beta3=0.2 s0=2;

This may help reach a good convergence and the maximum of log-likelihood.

10.2.3 Non-linear mixed models

Non-linear mixed models are complex to estimate, and were not detailed in this book. We note that in SAS, the procedure that can fit any model (linear or not) with Gaussian random effects is NLMIXED procedure. As illustrated for the logistic mixed model, any contribution to the log-likelihood conditional to the random effects (noted loglik in the example) can be specified along with the Gaussian random-effect distribution in statement random, and the corresponding model be fitted with general(loglik).

In R, general functions for non-linear mixed models are nlme of package nlme and nlmer of package lme4.

10.2.4 Marginal models

Marginal models can be fitted in SAS with GENMOD procedure and in R with for instance gee function of package gee.

Estimated model

In application 4.4.3, the marginal logistic model is written:

$$\text{logit}(P(\texttt{cesd16}_{ij} = 1)) = \beta_0 + \beta_1\,\texttt{age65}_{ij} + \beta_2\,\texttt{male}_i + \beta_3\,\texttt{male}_i \times \texttt{age65}_{ij}$$

Translation in R

The model can be fitted with gee function by calling:

```
# load of lcmm for the dataset
library(lcmm)
data(paquid)
# load and call of gee
require(gee)
mgee <- gee(cesd16 ~ male * age65, id = ID, data = paquid,
        corstr = "unstructured", family = binomial)
```

The first formula specifies that regression with the dependent variable cesd16 on the left side of ∼ and the fixed effects male * age65 (or equivalently 1 + male + age65 + male:age65) on the right side of ∼. The grouping variable is indicated with argument id. The correlation structure for the working matrix is specified in corstr. The possible specifications are "unstructured" for an unstructured working matrix, "exchangeable" for an exchangeable working matrix (uniform correlation) and "independence" for a diagonal working matrix. As previously with function glmer, family is used to specify the type of link function. Finally, data gives the data frame.

Translation in SAS

The model can be fitted with `GENMOD` procedure by calling:

```
proc GENMOD data = paquid descending;
class  ID;
model cesd16 = age65 male age65 * male / dist = bin;
repeated subject = ID / corr = cs;
run;
```

Statement `model` defines the regression with the dependent variable `cesd` on the left side of = and the covariates `age65 male age65*male` on the right side of =. Option `dist` gives the family of the model, here a logistic model with the binomial distribution. Statement `repeated` gives the grouping variable with option `subject` and the structure of the correlation working matrix with option `corr`. It can be for instance `corr=un` for a unstructured working matrix, `corr=cs` for an exchangeable working matrix (uniform correlations) or `corr=vc` for a diagonal working matrix (independent). Statement `class` that contains the categorical variables also contains the grouping variable.

10.3   Appendix for Chapter 5: extensions of mixed models

10.3.1   Mixed models for curvilinear data

Mixed models for curvilinear data and cumulative probit mixed models can be fitted in `R` with function `lcmm` of package `lcmm`.

Estimated model

The latent process mixed model described in illustration of Chapter 5, Section 5.1 is:

$$H(\texttt{cesd}_{ij};\eta) = \beta_1\ \texttt{age65}_{ij} + \beta_2\ \texttt{male}_i + \beta_3\ \texttt{male}i \times \texttt{age65}ij +$$
$$b_{0i} + b_{1i}\ \texttt{age65}ij + \epsilon_{ij}$$

with $b_i = \begin{pmatrix} b_{0i} \\ b_{1i} \end{pmatrix} \sim \mathcal{N}\left(\begin{pmatrix} 0 \\ 0 \end{pmatrix}, \begin{pmatrix} \sigma_0^2 & \sigma_{01} \\ \sigma_{01} & \sigma_1^2 \end{pmatrix} \right)$ et $\epsilon_{ij} \sim \mathcal{N}(0,1)$.

Translation in R

The model can be fitted in R with function `lcmm` by calling:

```
library(lcmm)
data(paquid)
mspl <- lcmm(CESD ~ male * age65, random =~ age65,
             subject = "ID", data = paquid, link = "splines")
```

The first part of this call indicates the structure of the regression at the population level with the dependent variable on the left side of ~ and the covariates with a fixed effect on the right side of ~. Argument `random` specifies the covariates with a random effect (correlated by default) and `subject` provides the name of the grouping variable. Finally `link` specifies the type of link function. By default, the link function is linear (`link="linear"`) which reduces to a standard linear mixed model (with the parameterization described in the paragraph on identifiability in Section 5.1). Other possible link functions are the rescaled Beta cumulative distribution function with `link="beta"`, the thresholds link function with `link="thresholds"` which provides a cumulative probit mixed model, and the link function modelled by splines with `link="splines"`. It defines by default a basis of quadratic I-splines with 5 equidistant knots but the number and place of the knots can be given (equidistant, at percentiles or entered manually). For example, `link="7-manual-splines"` defines a Splines link function with 7 knots entered manually in option `intnodes` (the 5 internal knots should be given in a vector, the external knots being placed at the minimum and maximum value of the dependent variable by default). This function takes into account a possible autocorrelated process in addition to the random effects and the independent measurement errors with option `cor=`. Specifically, `cor=BM(age65)` adds a Brownian process and `cor=AR(age65)` adds an autoregressive type of process.

Several functions can be used on an estimated model: `summary(mspl)` summarizes the estimation and the estimated parameters; `plot(mspl)` gives a series of plots including residuals (by default), estimated link functions with option `which="link"`, comparison of observed and predicted trajectories with `which="fit"`, etc. Predicted trajectories can also be computed from any covariate profile with functions `predictL(mspl,...)` for computations in the latent process scale, and `predictY(mspl,...)` for computations directly in the outcome scale. Plots of these trajectories are displayed when using `plot` on these objects. Finally, output `mspl$pred` contains the individual predictions (marginal and conditional).

We note that this function can also fit models in the presence of heterogeneous population as described in Section 5.3. In this case, arguments `mixture` and `ng` explained below with function `hlme` are added.

Further examples and details are given in the package companion paper (Proust-Lima et al., 2015).

10.3.2 Multivariate linear mixed models

Multivariate linear mixed models can be fitted with the standard procedure MIXED in SAS and the standard function lme in R.

Estimated model

The bivariate linear mixed model fitted in the illustration (with k=1 for CD4 and k=2 for viral load (LCV)) is:

$$Y'_{kij} = \beta_{1k} \min(t_{ij}, t_1) + \beta_{2k}(t_{ij} - t_1)\mathbb{1}_{t_{ij}>t_1} + b_{1ik} \min(t_{ij}, t_1) + b_{2ik}(t_{ij} - t_1)\mathbb{1}_{t_{ij}>t_1} + \epsilon_{ijk}$$

where $Y'_{kij} = Y_{kij} - Y_{ki0}$, $\epsilon_{ijk} \sim \mathcal{N}(0, \sigma^2_{\epsilon_k})$ and

$$(b_{1i1}, b_{2i1}, b_{1i2}, b_{2i2})^\top \sim \mathcal{N}\left(0, B = \begin{bmatrix} \sigma^2_1 & \sigma_{12} & \sigma_{13} & \sigma_{14} \\ \sigma_{12} & \sigma^2_2 & \sigma_{23} & \sigma_{24} \\ \sigma_{13} & \sigma_{23} & \sigma^2_3 & \sigma_{34} \\ \sigma_{14} & \sigma_{24} & \sigma_{34} & \sigma^2_4 \end{bmatrix}\right).$$

Whatever the software, the trick is to organize the data so that the two dependent variables CD4t et LCV become a unique dependent variable (Y for example below) with binary indicators indicating the nature of the variable (indCD4 and indLCV below). With this unique dependent variable, the bivariate linear mixed model becomes a standard linear mixed model stratified on these indicators for the fixed effects, random effects and marker-specific errors.

Translation in R

The model is fitted with function lme by calling:

```
# creation of two data frames for CD4 and LCV
# and of a unique dependent variable named Y
CD4 <- aids[ , c("NUM_PAT", "Time")]
CD4$Y <- aids$CD4t
CD4$indCD4 <- 1
CD4$indLCV <- 0
LCV <- aids[ , c("NUM_PAT", "Time")]
LCV$Y <- aids$LCV
LCV$indCD4 <- 0
LCV$indLCV <- 1
```

```
# The two tables are stacked
aidsBiv <- rbind(CD4, LCV)
aidsBiv  <- aidsBiv[order(aidsBiv$NUM_PAT), ]
head(aidsBiv)

# caution with missing data since the model is fitted with lme
aidsBiv <- aidsBiv[!is.na(aidsBiv$Y) & !is.na(aidsBiv$Time), ]
aidsBiv$T1 <- pmin(aidsBiv$Time, 30 / 100)
aidsBiv$T2 <- pmax(aidsBiv$Time - 30 / 100, 0)

# estimation of the bivariate linear mixed model
library(nlme)
Bivariate <- lme(Y ~ -1 + T1:indCD4 + T2:indCD4 + T1:indLCV
            + T2:indLCV, random =~ -1 + T1:indCD4 + T2:indCD4
            + T1:indLCV + T2:indLCV | NUM_PAT, data = aidsBiv,
            method = "ML", weights = varIdent(form =~ 1 | indLCV))
summary(Bivariate)
```

Option `weights = varIdent(form =~ 1 | indLCV)` allows to define variances for the independent errors that differ according to the levels of the variable indLCV that is depending on whether Y corresponds to CD4 or to LCV. One has to be careful and not include any intercept (with indicators -1 in the fixed-effect and random-effect parts). Indeed, first this application works with differences in CD4 and LCV so there is no effect at baseline. Second, even when working on the trajectories of absolute CD4 and LCV, one would add a specific effect for each marker on baseline level rather than a global intercept, that is -1 + indCD4 + indLCV instead of -1 presently.

Translation in SAS

The model is fitted with procedure MIXED by calling:

```
/*creation of two data frames for CD4 and LCV
   and of a unique dependent variable named Y  */
data CD4; set aids;
Y = CD4t; indCD4 = 1; indLCV = 0;
run;
data LCV; set aids ;
Y = LCV; indCD4 = 0; indLCV = 1;
run;

/*  The two tables are stacked */
Data aidsbiv;
```

```
set CD4 LCV;
run;
Proc sort data = aidsbiv;
by NUM_PAT indLCV T;
run;

/* estimation of the bivariate linear mixed model */
Proc mixed data = aidsBiv method = ML covtest;
class NUM_PAT indLCV;
model Y = CD4ind*T1 CD4ind*T2 LCVind*T1 LCVind*T2
        / noint s ddfm = bw;
random CD4ind*T1 CD4ind*T2 LCVind*T1 LCVind*T2
        / type = UN sub = NUM_PAT GCORR;
repeated / type = VC grp = indLCV sub = NUM_PAT;
run;
```

Here, the option `grp` of statement `repeated` is used to specify variances of measurement errors that differ according to the level of the covariate `indLCV`. In addition, option `noint` is used to remove the fixed effect on the intercept.

10.3.3   Multivariate mixed models with latent process

The latent process multivariate mixed models are implemented in function `multlcmm` of package `lcmm`. The function directly extends function `lcmm` described above for curvilinear mixed models and uses the same syntax.

Estimated model

The latent process mixed model estimated in illustration of Chapter 5, Section 5.2.2 is:

$$\Lambda_i(t) = \beta_1\, t + \beta_2\, t^2 + \beta_3\, \mathrm{CEP}_i + \beta_4\, \mathrm{CEP}_i \times t + \beta_5\, \mathrm{CEP}_i \times t^2 + b_{0i} + b_{1i}\, t + b_{2i}\, t^2$$
$$H_1(\mathrm{MMSE}_{ij1}; \eta_1) = \Lambda_i(\mathtt{time}_{ij1}) + \sigma_{\epsilon_1}\epsilon_{ij1}$$
$$H_2(\mathrm{IST}_{ij2}; \eta_2) = \Lambda_i(\mathtt{time}_{ij2}) + \sigma_{\epsilon_2}\epsilon_{ij2}$$
$$H_3(\mathrm{BVRT}_{ij3}; \eta_3) = \Lambda_i(\mathtt{time}_{ij3}) + \sigma_{\epsilon_3}\epsilon_{ij3}$$

$$(10.1)$$

where $b_i = (b_{0i}, b_{1i}, b_{2i}) \sim \mathcal{N}(0, B)$, $\mathrm{var}(b_{0i}) = 1$, $\epsilon_{ijk} \sim \mathcal{N}(0,1)$ with $k \in \{1,2,3\}$ and H_1, H_2, H_3 are the Beta cumulative distribution functions parameterized by vectors η_1, η_2 and η_3.

Translation in R

This model can be fitted in R with function `multlcmm` by calling:

```
library(lcmm)
data(paquid)
mquadCEP <- multlcmm(MMSE + IST + BVRT ~ time + I(time^2/10) +
        CEP + CEP:time + CEP:I(time^2/10),
        random =~ time + I(time^2/10), subject = "ID",
        data = paquid, link = c("beta", "beta", "beta"))
mquadCEP
summary(mquadCEP)
```

In this call, the regressions at the latent process level and at the dependent variables levels are merged in a unique regression with the dependent variables (here MMSE+IST+BVRT) on the left-hand side of ~, and the covariates associated with fixed effects (here `time + I(time^2/10) + CEP * time + CEP * I(time^2/10)`) on the right-hand side of ~. As for other functions of lcmm package, random effects are defined separately in argument `random` that provides the formula with the covariates associated with a random effect (here `time+ I(time^2/10)`). Random effects are correlated by default and can be assumed independent by specifying `idiag=T`. Argument `subject` specifies the name of the grouping variable. For each dependent variable, the link function H should be defined with argument `link`. By default link functions are linear. Alternatives are `"beta"` for beta cumulative distribution functions recentered and rescaled, or `"splines"` for link functions approximated by a basis of quadratic I-splines. The same options as defined for function `lcmm` in Section 10.3.1 can be used with `multlcmm`.

This function can fit models in which correlated errors are specified in the structural equation with option `cor=BM(time)` or `cor=AR(time)` for respectively a Brownian process or an autoregressive process. Marker-specific random intercept can also be assumed in the marker-specific model to take into account the specific variability of each pair (subject× dependent variable) with option `randomY=T`. Finally, different covariate effects from one dependent variable to another can be assumed with function `contrast`. For example:

```
library(lcmm)
data(paquid)
mquadCEP <- multlcmm(MMSE + IST + BVRT ~ time + I(time^2/10) +
        contrast(gender) + CEP + CEP:time + CEP:I(time^2/10),
        random =~ time + I(time^2 / 10), subject = "ID",
        data = paquid, link = c("beta","beta","beta"))
mquadCEP
summary(mquadCEP)
```

fits the same model with in addition an effect of **gender** which is different for each psychometric test MMSE, IST and BVRT.

Several functions exist to analyze the results using similar syntaxes as for function `lcmm` (see Section 10.3.1 for more details and Proust-Lima et al. (2015)).

10.3.4 Latent class mixed models

Latent class mixed models can be fitted in R with package `lcmm`. Function `hlme` fits latent class linear mixed models, function `lcmm` fits latent class mixed models for curvilinear and ordinal data, and function `multlcmm` fits latent class mixed models for multivariate data with a common underlying process.

Estimated model

The latent class linear mixed model described in illustration of Section 5.3 is defined in each latent class g by:

$$\text{IST}_{ij} = b_{0i} + b_{1i}\,\text{age65}_{ij} + b_{2i}\,\text{age65}^2_{ij} + \beta_1\,\text{CEP}_i + \beta_2\,\text{CEP}_i \times \text{age65}_{ij}$$
$$+ \beta_3\,\text{CEP}_i \times \text{age65}^2_{ij} + \epsilon_{ij}$$

with $b_i = (b_{0i}, b_{1i}, b_{2i})^\top \sim \mathcal{N}((\mu_{0g}, \mu_{1g}, \mu_{2g})^\top, B)$ in latent class g and $\epsilon_{ij} \sim \mathcal{N}(0, \sigma^2)$.

Translation in R

This model can be fitted in R with function `hlme` by calling (for 4 latent classes here):

```
library(lcmm)
data(paquid)
m4 <- hlme(IST ~ CEP*age65 + CEP*I(age65^2),
    mixture =~ age65 + I(age65^2), random =~ age65 + I(age65^2),
    ng = 4, subject = "ID", data = paquid)
summary(m4)
```

The first part of the call indicates the global structure of the model with the dependent variable on the left-hand side of $\sim$ and the covariates with a fixed effect (common or specific to the latent classes) on the right-hand side of $\sim$. Covariates with a class-specific effect are also listed in `mixture` formula. Argument `random` specifies the variables with a random effect (correlated by default); `subject` gives the name of the grouping variable. At last, `ng` indicates the number of latent classes. Other options can be used to specify independent random effects, varying variance of the random effects over classes or a vector of initial values. As for function `lcmm`, this function handles autocorrelation processes (Brownian or autoregressive type) in addition to the random effects and the independent measurement errors with option `cor=`.

Several functions analyze the results of a `hlme` object; `summary(m4)` provides a summary of the optimization and the estimated parameters, `postprob(m4)` computes the posterior classification and gives the classification table from the posterior class-membership probabilities contained in `m4$pprob`, `predictY` computes the predicted trajectories in each latent class, object `m4$pred` contains the marginal and subject specific predictions and residuals. Finally, different types of plots can be obtained with function `plot`.

More details and examples can be found online `http://cran.r-project.org/web/packages/lcmm` and in the companion paper of the package (Proust-Lima et al., 2015).

10.4   Appendix for Chapter 6: advanced survival

10.4.1   Relative survival models with the R package `relsurv`

We describe in this example the implementation of a model of the additive relative survival using the R package `relsurv`. The advantage of using R for relative survival is to use the way the data are organized in the tables of mortality. An object class called `ratetable` is dedicated to the tables of mortality. The Human Life Table Database `http://www.lifetable.de/` contains a collection of tables of mortality covering several countries over several years. The function `transrate.hld` from the package `relsurv` transforms data format (such as .txt) into an object `ratetable`. In general an object `ratetable` is a rectangular matrix in dimension 3 according to sex, age and calendar year. Time units are used in days, and the variable `year` is given by year; we transform it into days. In the following example the tables of mortality are provided by the file `slopop` (in the population of Slovenia).

```
#= RELATIVE SURVIVAL according to the model proposed by ESTEVE ==
#==Call of the R package relsurv and the datasets ==
library(relsurv)
data(slopop) # data for the tables of mortality in the population
data(rdata)# dataset to analyze

fit.add <- rsadd(Surv(time,cens)~sex+age+ratetable(age=age*365,
sex=sex,year=year), ratetable=slopop,data=rdata,int=5,method="EM")
```

The excess hazard function (linked to the disease) can be represented on a graph with the smoothing approach and Epanechnikov knots.

```
sm <- epa(fit.add)
plot(sm$times,sm$lambda)
```

10.4.2   Competing risks models with the R packages cmprsk and mstate

This section presents R codes which enable us to produce all the results presented in Section 6.2.

Data could be imported by using:

```
data <- read.csv(file="prostate.csv",header=TRUE,sep="\t")
prostate <- na.omit(data)
```

The last command enables us to get a data frame **prostate** without any missing values. Let us define a new variable **type** representing the type of events: 0 for no even; 1 for death from prostate cancer and 2 for death from other causes.

```
type <- rep(0,483)
type[prostate$status=="dead - prostatic ca"] <- 1
type[prostate$status!="dead - prostatic ca" &
        prostate$status!="alive"] <- 2
prostate <- cbind(prostate,type=type)
```

The variable **dtime** included in **prostate** represents the time to the first event (or until a censored event). The observations for which the time to the first event was equal to 0 month have been replaced by 1 month.

```
prostate$dtime[prostate$dtime==0] <- 1
```

Packages **cmprsk** and **mstate** enable us to get an estimation of the cumulative incidence:

```
require(cmprsk)
Inci.cum <- cuminc(ftime=prostate$dtime, fstatus=prostate$type)
##It is also possible to use mstate package
require(mstate)
inci.cum <- Cuminc(time=prostate$dtime, status=prostate$type)
```

The following instructions enable to obtain and save the plot (pdf format) of the cumulative incidence function.

```
pdf(file="fig2-comp-risq.pdf")
plot(Inci.cum, xlab="Time (Month)", ylab="Probability",
        curvlab=c("Death from prostate cancer", "Death from other caus
dev.off()
```

Let us define the variable `treatment`: 0 for placebo and low dose of estrogen (0 or 0.2 mg) and 1 for high dose of estrogen (1 or 5 mg). This variable is defined from the variable `rx`.

```
treatment <- rep(0,483)
treatment[prostate$rx=="1.0 mg estrogen" |
          prostate$rx=="5.0 mg estrogen"] <- 1
prostate <- cbind(prostate,treatment=treatment)
```

The non-parametric test developed by Gray for testing the treatment effect for each event is obtained by using the function `cuminc`.

```
cuminc(ftime=prostate$dtime,fstatus=prostate$type,
       group=prostate$treatment)
```

To estimate the cause-specific hazards functions, we need to create two indicator variables which we include in the data frame `prostate`:

```
# dc.ca; indicator 1 if death from prostate cancer  0 otherwise
# dc.other; indicator 1 if death from other causes 0 otherwise
dc.ca <- rep(0,483)
dc.ca[type==1] <- 1
dc.other <- rep(0,483)
dc.other[type==2] <- 1
prostate <- cbind(prostate,dc.ca=dc.ca,dc.other=dc.other)
```

We transform the variable `age` into a categorical variable (3 categories: 0 for an age <75; 1 for an age between 75 and 80; 2 for an age ≥80).

```
# 0=[;75[ 1=[75;80[  2=[80;++[
agegrp <- cut(prostate$age,c(0,75,80,999),include.lowest=TRUE,
              right=FALSE)
levels(agegrp) <- c(0,1,2)
prostate <- cbind(prostate,agegrp=agegrp)
```

The cause-specific hazards functions are obtained by using the function `coxph` from the `survival` package,

```
require(survival)
# Cox model when the event of interest is the death
# due to prostate cancer
coxph(Surv(dtime, dc.ca)~treatment+ agegrp, data=prostate)
# Death from others causes
coxph(Surv(dtime, dc.other)~treatment+ agegrp, data=prostate)
```

Similar results could be obtained by using the `mstate` package.

```
require(mstate)
tmat <- trans.comprisk(2, names = c("0", "1", "2"))
prost.long <- msprep(time = c(NA, "dtime", "dtime"),
                     status = c(NA,"dc.ca", "dc.other"),
                     data = prostate, keep = c("treatment","agegrp"
                     trans = tmat)
events(prost.long)


prost.long <- expand.covs(prost.long, covs = c("treatment","agegrp"


coxph(Surv(time,status)~treatment.1+treatment.2+agegrp1.1+agegrp1.2
      +agegrp2.1+agegrp2.2+strata(to),data=prost.long)
```

The joint model is obtained by using the `coxph` function. However, we first need to duplicate the data by using the `duplicate` function which is available in the following link:
`http://cybertim.timone.univ-mrs.fr/Members/rgiorgi/DossierPublic/`
`fonctions-r-s/`.
After saving the file `duplicate.r`, you can use the function `duplicate` by using the following code:

```
source("duplicate.r")
```

You can now duplicate the data:

```
## Creation of the variable status.event indicating
## if the event has been observed.
status.event <- rep(0,483)
status.event[type>0] <- 1
prostate <- cbind(prostate,status.event=status.event)
prostate2 <- duplicate(status=status.event, event=type, data=prosta
```

To produce the result from the table of the joint model analysis, you need to use the following instructions:

```
coxph(Surv(dtime,status.event)~delta.2+treatment+agegrp
      +delta.2:(treatment+agegrp),
      data=prostate2)
```

```
# Pvalues of the treatment effect on the risk of death
#   due to other causes:
coxph(Surv(dtime,status.event)~delta.1+treatment+agegrp
      +delta.1:(treatment+agegrp),
      data=prostate2)
```

Similar results could be obtained by using `mstate` package:

```
coxph(Surv(time,status)~treatment.1+treatment.2+agegrp1.1+agegrp1.2
      +agegrp2.1+agegrp2.2+factor(to),data=prost.long)
```

The joint model with different baseline hazards functions for each event is obtained by:

```
# Cox model  on duplicate data
# stratified on the event type:
coxph(Surv(dtime, status.event)~treatment+agegrp
      +delta.2:(treatment+agegrp)
      +strata(type), data=prostate2)
```

The variable `delta.2` is the indicator variable for the event 2. The instruction `delta.2:(treatment+agegrp)` indicates the interaction between this variable and variables introduced in the model. It enables us to estimate jointly the covariates effect for the event 2.

Finally, the estimation of the subdistribution hazards function (Fine and Gray model) is presented in the following:

```
require(cmprsk)
# Death from prostate cancer
crr(ftime=prostate$dtime,fstatus=prostate$type,
    cov1=cbind(prostate[,c("treatment","agegrp")]), failcode=1)
# Death from other causes
  crr(ftime=prostate$dtime,fstatus=prostate$type,
      cov1=cbind(prostate[,c("treatment","agegrp")]), failcode=2)
```

10.4.3 Shared frailty models with R packages coxph and frailtypack

Packages R `frailtypack` and `coxph` are able to estimate gamma or log-normal frailty models. An estimate of the baseline hazard function can be achieved with the package `frailtypack`, either using a parametric form (Weibull, piecewise constant) or with a semi-parametric approach with splines.

```
#--------------    R Package FRAILTYPACK ---------------------
  library(frailtypack)

### Call of the dataset :
  data(readmission)

### Shared frailty models ##
  fit.gap<-frailtyPenal(Surv(time,event)~
```

```
as.factor(dukes)+cluster(id)+strata(sex),
n.knots=10,kappa=c(10000,10000),data=readmission)
```

The variable `time` corresponds to the survival times studied, and `event` is a censor indicator or a binary variable which indicates if the subject is censored or if he had the event at time `time`. In the previous model, the basic timescale selected is the time between two readmissions. The stratification option `strata(sex)` allows for two different baseline hazard functions for men and women. Baseline hazard functions are estimated by splines with 10 nodes and two smoothing parameters kappa1 and kappa2 corresponding to the two strata. The option `cluster(id)` specifies the variable where we want to put a random effect (`id`), here on the subjects. If one wishes to choose another timescale, for instance the time since inclusion into the study, a condition of left-truncation is induced and two times are necessary: `t.start` and `t.stop` for the beginning and the end of the at risk period.

```
### Shared frailty model ##
### baseline timescale =#
### calendar time or time since entry into the study. ##
### With an automatic research of the smoothing parameter ##

fit.cal<-frailtyPenal(Surv(t.start,t.stop,event)~
as.factor(sex)+as.factor(dukes)+
as.factor(charlson)+cluster(id),data=readmission,
n.knots=6,kappa=5000,recurrentAG=TRUE,cross.validation=TRUE)
```

The baseline hazard or survival functions can be represented graphically with the function `plot`.

```
### By default, smooth baseline hazard function,
### without confidence bands:
  plot(fit.cal,conf=FALSE)
### Survival function:
  plot(fit.cal,type="surv",conf=FALSE)
```

The R package `frailtypack` provides also a posteriori random effects predictions for each "group" or each "subject." This information is contained in the variable `frailty.pred` of each frailty model.

```
#=== Prediction of the random effects =========
```

```
pdf(file="res_frailty.pdf")

effectif <-as.vector(table(readmission$id))
valeur.frailty <- fit.cal$frailty.pred

plot(1:403,valeur.frailty,xlab="Number of events per patient",
ylab="Frailty predictions for each patient", type="p",
  axes=F,
  cex=effectif,
  pch=1,ylim=c(-0.1,5),xlim=c(-2,420))
  axis(1,round(seq(0,403,length=10),digit=0))
  axis(2,round(seq(0,5,length=10),digit=1))
```

In packages R survival and frailtypack, the distribution of the random effects is by default a gamma distribution. It is possible to specify a log-normal distribution, as follows:

```
#-------------- Package R SURVIVAL --------------------

### Gaussian frailty models ##
### with calendar timescale  ###

  fit1.cal.gauss<-coxph(Surv(t.start,t.stop,event)~
  as.factor(sex)+as.factor(dukes)+
  as.factor(charlson)+frailty(id,dist='gaussian'),data=readmission)

#-------------- Package R FRAILTYPACK --------------------

### Gaussian frailty models ##
### with calendar timescale  ###

  fit2.cal.gauss<-frailtyPenal(Surv(t.start,t.stop,event)~
  as.factor(sex)+as.factor(dukes)+
  as.factor(charlson)+cluster(id),RandDist='LogN',
  data=readmission,n.knots=6,kappa=5000,recurrentAG=TRUE)
```

10.4.4 Joint frailty models with the R package frailtypack and the SAS procedure NLMIXED

The R package frailtypack allows to estimate joint models with parametric form of basic hazard functions (Weibull or piecewise constant) or semiparametric (by splines). The random effect distribution may be gamma or log-normal, as shown in this example:

```
#-------------- Package R FRAILTYPACK --------------------------
```

```
library(frailtypack)
data(readmission)

### Gamma shared frailty models  ##
### with gap times ###

  modJoint_gap<-frailtyPenal(Surv(time,event)
  ~cluster(id)+sex+as.factor(dukes)
  +as.factor(charlson)+terminal(death),
  formula.terminalEvent=~sex+as.factor(dukes)+as.factor(charlson),
  data=readmission,n.knots=14,kappa=c(9550000000,1410000000000),
  recurrentAG=FALSE,hazard="Splines")


### Gaussian shared frailty models  ##
### with gap times ###

  modJoint_gap_normal<-frailtyPenal(Surv(time,event)
  ~cluster(id)+sex+as.factor(dukes)
  +as.factor(charlson)+terminal(death),
  formula.terminalEvent=~sex+as.factor(dukes)+as.factor(charlson),
  data=readmission,n.knots=14,kappa=c(9550000000,1410000000000),
  RandDist='LogN',recurrentAG=FALSE,hazard="Splines")
```

Here is an example of programming the joint random effects model in SAS NLMIXED for times between two events, with a Gaussian distribution of the random effects (default distribution). This procedure requires the programming of the expression of the log-likelihood associated with the model. In this example, we divide the follow-up period of observation in five time intervals according to quintiles in order to have constant stepwise hazard functions with the same number of events in each time interval. The random effect omega is here specific to each subject id.

```
#-------------- with the procedure SAS NLMIXED ------------------

/*** For a gaussian joint frailty model,
for recurrent events and a  terminal event,
 with gap times ***/

proc nlmixed data=Readmission qpoints=5;
parms r01=.1 r02=.1 r03=.1 r04=.1 r05=.1
  h01=.02 h02=.02 h03=.02 h04=.02 h05=.02
/* r0i and h0i are the period over each quantile interval  */
/* event_ri and event_di are event indicators*/
  beta1=1 beta2=.5 theta=2  alpha=.5 ;
```

```
bounds r01 r02 r03 r04 r05   h01 h02 h03 h04 h05 var >=0;

base_haz_r=r01 * event_r1 + r02 * event_r2 + r03 * event_r3
+ r04 * event_r4 + r05 * event_r5;
cum_base_haz_r=r01 * dur_r1 + r02 * dur_r2 + r03 * dur_r3
+ r04 * dur_r4 + r05 * dur_r5 ;

base_haz_d=h01 * event_d1 + h02 * event_d2 + h03 * event_d3
+ h04 * event_d4 + h05 * event_d5 ;
cum_base_haz_d=h01 * dur_d1 + h02 * dur_d2 + h03 * dur_d3
+ h04 * dur_d4 + h05 * dur_d5  ;

mu1= beta1 * X1 +  omega; /* for recurrent events */
mu2= beta2 * X1  + alpha * omega; /* fo death */

loglik1=-exp(mu1) * cum_base_haz_r;
loglik2=-exp(mu2) * cum_base_haz_d;
/*log likelihood for recurrences */
if event_all=1 then loglik = log(base_haz_r) + mu1 ;
/*log likelihood for death */
if event_all=2 then loglik = log(base_haz_d) + mu2 + loglik2 + loglik1;
/*log likelihood  or censoring */
if event_all=0 then loglik = loglik1 + loglik2;
model time ~ general(loglik);
random omega ~ normal(0, theta) subject=id;
run;
```

It is also possible in SAS with the NLMIXED procedure to program a joint
gamma frailty model with mean 1 and variance theta using the reformulation
of the likelihood proposed in Liu and Yu (2008).

```
/*****************************************************************/


proc nlmixed data=five qpoints=5;

parms r01=.1 r02=.1 r03=.1 r04=.1 r05=.1  beta1=-.5 theta=1
   h01=.02 h02=.02 h03=.02 h04=.02 h05=.02   alpha1=-.4 alpha=1;
bounds r01 r02 r03 r04 r05 r06 h01 h02 h03 h04 h05   theta >=0;

base_haz_r=r01 * event_r1 + r02 * event_r2 + r03 * event_r3
+ r04 * event_r4 + r05 * event_r5  ;
cum_base_haz_r=r01 * dur_r1 + r02 * dur_r2 + r03 * dur_r3
+ r04 * dur_r4 + r05 * dur_r5   ;
```

```
base_haz_d=h01 * event_d1 + h02 * event_d2 + h03 * event_d3
+ h04 * event_d4 + h05 * event_d5 ;
cum_base_haz_d=h01 * dur_d1 + h02 * dur_d2 + h03 * dur_d3
+ h04 * dur_d4 + h05 * dur_d5 ;


expa=exp(omega);
* Log Gamma density ;
* Here, shape=1/theta, scale=1/theta, donc mean=1 and var=theta;
loggammaden=(1/theta-1)*omega - 1/theta * expa
- 1/theta* log(theta) -lgamma(1/theta);
lognormalden=-omega*omega/2; /* Standard lognormal density */


mu1= beta1 * X1 +  omega; /* for recurrent events*/
mu2= alpha1 * X1  + alpha * omega; /* for death */


loglik1=-exp(mu1) * cum_base_haz_r;
loglik2=-exp(mu2) * cum_base_haz_d;
/*log likelihood for recurrent events */
if event_all=1 then loglik= log(base_haz_r) + mu1 ;
/*log likelihood for death */
if event_all=2 then loglik=loglik1 + log(base_haz_d) + mu2 + loglik
/*log likelihood for censoring*/
if event_all=0 then loglik=loglik1 + loglik2;
/* Reformulation  of a gamma distribution towards a gaussian */
if event_all=2 or event_all=0 then
loglik=loglik + loggammaden + omega - lognormalden;


model stoptime ~ general(loglik);
random omega ~ normal(0, 1) subject=id;
run;
```

10.4.5   Nested frailty models with the R package `frailtypack`

Here, we illustrate the use of the R package `frailtypack` to analyze data with multiple levels of clustering, by nested frailty models. In this example (data "CGD"), recurrent infection times on 128 patients from 13 hospitals were observed. These hierarchical data have two levels of clustering: the patient level `id` and hospital level `center`. In the program, we simply have to specify the instructions `cluster(center)` and `subcluster(id)`. It may be recommended initially to fit standard frailty models (with a single random effect) before fitting a nested frailty model. In the following illustrations, we present different possible choices for the baseline timescale for recurrent data (in gap times or in calendar timescale) and then with different choices for the baseline hazard functions (parametric in Weibull or semi-parametric with splines).

```
library(frailtypack)
data(cgd)

#======= Shared frailty models ==============================
#== with calendar timescale


shared.cgd.center.cal<-frailtyPenal(Surv(tstart,tstop,status)~
cluster(center)+treat,data=cgd,recurrentAG=T,
n.knots=8,kappa=1000,hazard="Splines")
shared.cgd.center.cal

shared.cgd.id.cal<-frailtyPenal(Surv(tstart,tstop,status)~
cluster(id)+treat,
data=cgd,recurrentAG=T,
n.knots=8,kappa=1000,hazard="Splines")#,cross.validation=T)
shared.cgd.id.cal

#======= Shared frailty models ==============================
#== with gap times

shared.cgd.center.gap<-frailtyPenal(Surv((tstop-tstart),status)~
cluster(center)+treat,data=cgd,
n.knots=8,kappa=1000,hazard="Splines")
shared.cgd.center.gap

shared.cgd.id.gap<-frailtyPenal(Surv((tstop-tstart),status)~
cluster(id)+treat,data=cgd,
n.knots=8,kappa=1000,hazard="Splines")
shared.cgd.id.gap


#======= Nested frailty models ==============================
#== with calendar timescales
#== and an hazard function estimated by  splines


nested.cgd.cal<-frailtyPenal(Surv(tstart,tstop,status)~
cluster(center)+subcluster(id)+treat,
data=cgd,recurrentAG=T,
n.knots=8,kappa=1000,hazard="Splines")
nested.cgd.cal


#======= Nested frailty models ==============================
```

```
#== with gap times and
#== a baseline hazard function estimated by splines

nested.cgd.gap<-frailtyPenal(Surv((tstop-tstart),status)~
cluster(center)+subcluster(id)+treat,
data=cgd, n.knots=8,kappa=1000,hazard="Splines")
nested.cgd.gap



#======= Nested frailty models ===============================
#== with gap times and
#== a baseline hazard function estimated
#== with a Weibull distribution

nested.cal.weib<-frailtyPenal(Surv(tstart,tstop,status)~
cluster(center)+ subcluster(id)+treatnum,
data=cgd,hazard="Weibull")

nested.cal.weib

#====== graphs: smooth baseline hazard functions

plot(nested.cgd.gap,conf.bands=F,ylim=c(0,0.014),xlim=c(0,350))
text(250,0.002,"gap time",cex=1.5)
par(new=T)
plot(nested.cgd.cal,conf.bands=F,ylim=c(0,0.014),xlim=c(0,350))
text(190,0.01,"calendar time",cex=1.5)
```

10.5   Appendix for Chapter 7: multistate models

10.5.1   The package `mstate`

Considerable effort has been made in recent years to develop software application especially for R to make inference in multistate models. In Example 7.5.6, we used the R package `mstate` developed by De Wreede et al. (2010) to perform non- and semi-parametric (Cox) estimation in the illness-death model for bone marrow transplantation data. The package covers all steps of the analysis of multistate models observed in continuous time, from model building and data preparation to estimation and graphical representation of

the results. A step-by-step guide of the use of the software can be found in
De Wreede et al. (2010). The illness-death model considered in Example 7.5.6
can be described by means of a 3-by-3 transition matrix. A number at entry
(h, j) of the matrix represents a possible transition from state h to state j.
These numbers range here from 1 to 3, because the model has 3 possible transitions. If a transition between two states is not allowed, the entry becomes
NA. The function `transMat()` creates the transition matrix `tmat`.

```
# loading mstate and the data set
library("mstate")
data("bmt")
# transition matrix
tmat <- transMat(x = list(c(2,3), c(3), c()),
        names = c("Transp", "PlaqRec", "Rel/death"))
tmat
```

The first step in data preparation is to recode data into a 'long format'
suitable for a multistate analysis. In this format, each individual has as many
rows as transitions for which he/she is at risk. The function `msprep()` transforms a data frame into long format.

```
msebmt <- msprep(data = bmt, trans = tmat, time = c(NA, "tp", "trd"),
        status = c(NA, "dp", "drd"),
        keep = c("group2", "group3", "agep", "aged", "ttt", "mtx"))
events(msebmt)
```

Arguments for `msprep()` are a `time` and `status` vector indicating the
time of entry in every state and the accompanying status indicator. The `keep`
argument contains the names of the covariates that will be used in the analysis.
The output is a data frame in long format, an object of class 'msdata'. The
numbers of transitions, both in terms of frequencies and percentages, are given
by the function `events()`.

It is possible to model different covariate effects on each transition. This
can be done by creating transition-specific covariates: each covariate Z is split
up into as many covariates Z_{hj} as there are transitions in the model; for the
transition from h to j, Z_{hj} is equal to Z; for all other transitions, $Z_{hj} = 0$.
The function `expand.covs()` expands the covariates specified by the user on
the basis of an object of class 'msdata'. For the analysis, we convert time in
days into years.

```
covs <- c("group2", "group3", "agep", "aged", "ttt", "mtx")
msebmt <- expand.covs(msebmt, covs, longnames = FALSE)
msebmt[, c("Tstart", "Tstop", "time")] <- msebmt[,
c("Tstart", "Tstop", "time")]/365.25
```

To obtain the estimators of the cumulative transition intensities $\hat{A}_{hj}(t)$ as
shown in Figure 7.5, the function `coxph()` from the `survival` package is used.

A Cox model is estimated with separate baseline hazards for each of the transitions and no covariates. Even if the transition intensities could be estimated separately, the combined use of long format data and a single stratified `coxph` object makes further calculations easier and useful in the multistate framework. The covariances of the estimated cumulative hazards can be computed by means of the Aalen estimator or by means of the Greenwood estimator. Finally, the `plot()` function produces a graph of all estimated cumulative hazards in different colors as illustrated in Figure 7.5.

```
c0 <- coxph(Surv(Tstart, Tstop, status) ~ strata(trans),
data = msebmt, method = "breslow")
msf0 <- msfit(object = c0, vartype = "greenwood", trans = tmat)
plot(msf0, las = 1, lwd=2, lty = 1:3,
legend = c("0->1", "0->2", "1->2"),
xlab = "Years since transplantation",
ylab = "Cumulative intensities",
legend.pos = c(3,2))
```

The function `probtrans()` calculates the estimated transition probabilities $\hat{P}_{hj}(s,t)$ for $s < t$, and optionally the standard errors and/or the covariances of the transition probabilities. The argument `predt` gives the starting time for prediction, that is, the starting time s for the calculation of the transition probabilities. The `plot()` method enables the user to show the transition probabilities in various ways.

```
pt0 <- probtrans(msf0, predt = 0, method = "greenwood")
summary(pt0, from 1)
library("colorspace")
statecols <- heat_hcl(6, c = c(80, 30), l = c(30, 90),
power = c(1/5, 2))[c(6, 5, 3, 4, 2, 1)]
ord <- c(2, 3, 1)
plot(pt0, lwd=2, lty=1:3, xlab = "Years since transplantation",
ylab = "Transition probabilities", las = 1, type = "single",
col = statecols[ord])
```

The result is shown in Figure 7.6. A similar result for the situation after 100 days can be created by choosing `predt=100`; this is displayed in Figure 7.7.

```
pt100 <- probtrans(msf0, predt = 100/365.25, method = "greenwood")
plot(pt100, lwd=2, lty=1:3, from=1,
xlab = "Years since transplantation",
ylab = "Transition probabilities",
las = 1, type = "single", col = statecols[ord])
plot(pt100, lwd=2, lty=1:3, from=2,
xlab = "Years since transplantation",
```

```
ylab = "Transition probabilities",
las = 1, type = "single", col = statecols[ord])
```

To investigate the role of three explanatory variables (type or group of disease, patient age, prophylaxis) on the transition intensities, we consider a proportional intensities model $\alpha_{hj}(t) = \alpha^0_{hj}(t) \exp(\beta_{hj} z_{hj})$, where the $\alpha^0_{hj}(t)$ are the baseline transition intensities and z_{hj} the vectors of explanatory variables. The function `coxph()` is used with expanded covariates to allow different covariate effects for the different transitions. To specify that each transition has its own baseline transition intensity, `+strata(trans)` has to be added to the covariates.

```
c6 <- coxph(Surv(Tstart, Tstop, status) ~ group2.1 + group2.2
+ group2.3 + group3.1 + group3.2 + group3.3
+ agep.1 + agep.2 + agep.3 + mtx.1 + mtx.2 + mtx.3
+ strata(trans), data = msebmt, method = "breslow")
c6
```

The results are presented in Table 7.1.

10.5.2 The package `SmoothHazard`

The `SmoothHazard` package for R (Touraine et al., 2013) provides estimates of the baseline transition intensities and of covariate effects for illness-death models. The case of left-truncated event times (delayed entry) is covered, as well as the case where for some subjects the transition time into the intermediate state is observed exactly and for others it is interval censored.

The package `SmoothHazard` allows to do predictions of transition probabilities, cumulative probabilities of event and life expectancies for a given set of covariates, based on estimated baseline transition intensities and on estimated covariates effects. The main functions of `SmoothHazard` are:

- `idm`: for fitting illness-death regression models based on possibly interval-censored disease times and right censored times.

A fitted illness-death model as produced by `idm` can be used in the following functions to calculate predictions:

- `predict`: for estimating transition probabilities and cumulative probabilities of event for a given set of covariates;

- `lifexpect`: for estimating life expectancies for a given set of covariates.

To obtain results presented in Table 7.2 with `SmoothHazard`, the syntax is:

```
fit.weib <- idm(formula01=Hist(time=list(l,r),
          event=dementia,entry=e)~ gender+certif,
```

```
       formula02=Hist(time=t,event=death,entry=e)~gender+certi:
       data=Paq1000)
fit.weib
```

Here, as no approach is specified, it is a Weibull parametric model (by default). The data are left-truncated as specified by the statement `entry=` and interval censored for the transition to the state 1 by the statement `list(l,r)`. To do the same with a penalized likelihood approach, the syntax is:

```
fit.pl <- idm(formula01=Hist(time=list(l,r),event=dementia,entry=e)~
       gender+certif,
       formula02=Hist(time=t,event=death,entry=e)~gender+certif,
       method="Splines",CV=1,kappa=c(100000,10000,10000),
       data=Paq1000)
fit.pl
```

Here, the penalized likelihood approach is specified by the `method="Splines"` statement and the smoothing parameter is estimated by cross-validation (statement `CV=1`).

The function `predict` is used for estimating transition probabilities and cumulative probabilities. To obtain results presented in Figures 7.10 and 7.13, the syntax is:

```
fem <- Paq1000[Paq1000$gender==0,]
fit.plf <- idm(formula01=Hist(time=list(l,r),event=dementia,entry=e
               formula02=Hist(time=t,event=death,entry=e)~1,
               method="Splines",CV=1,kappa=c(100000,10000,10000),
               data=fem)
fit.plf
p_f <- predict(fit.plf,s=65,t=70)
p_f
```

Here, estimators of probabilities $F_{01}(65, 70)$, $P_{00}(65, 70)$, $P_{01}(65, 70)$, $P_{02}^1(65, 70)$ and $P_{02}^0(65, 70)$ for women, with a penalized likelihood approach are given.

Finally, the function `lifexpect` is used for estimating life expectancies as illustrated in Figure 7.15:

```
le.plf <- lifexpect(fit.plf,s=65,CI=FALSE)
le.plf
```

10.6 Appendix for Chapter 8: joint models for longitudinal data and time to events

10.6.1 Joint models with shared random effects

As evoked in Chapter 8, three packages are currently available to fit joint models with shared random effects (JM, JMbayes and joineR) as well as a stata program stjm. Shared random-effect joint models can also be fitted in SAS with the macro JMfit and the procedure NLMIXED. However, NLMIXED requires the complete specification of the joint log-likelihood conditional to the random effects and is thus quite troublesome compared to the other available programs.

In this appendix, we describe only the use of the function jointModel of package JM. The trick of this package is that implementation of the joint model is done in two steps.

First, the user initializes the model and specifies the two sub-models (longitudinal and survival) by calling:

- function lme to fit the linear mixed model. In this call, all the functions of time used to define the shape of the trajectory with time have to be defined directly as functions of the unique time-scale variable.

- function coxph to fit the proportional hazard model without the shared random effects.

Then, the shared random-effect joint model is defined in function jointModel according to these two objects (lme and coxph) as well as the arguments defining the association structure between the two sub-models.

To illustrate this implementation, we use the joint model defined in Application 8.2.4 with a dependency on the current level of the marker. For the sake of simplicity, the effect of covariates in the longitudinal part were removed. The model is:

$$\log(\text{PSA}_{ij} + 0.1) = \tilde{Y}_i(\text{time}_{ij}) + \epsilon_{ij}$$
$$= (\mu_0 + b_{0i}) + (\mu_1 + b_{1i}) f_1(\text{time}_{ij}) + (\mu_2 + b_{2i}) \text{time}_{ij} + \epsilon_{ij}$$
$$(10.2)$$

$$\lambda_i(t) = \lambda_0(t) \exp(\text{iPSA}_i \gamma_1 + \text{tstage}_i \gamma_2 + \text{gleason7}_i \gamma_3 + \text{gleason\_sup7}_i \gamma_4 + \tilde{Y}_i(t)\eta_1 + (\partial \tilde{Y}_i(t)/\partial t)\eta_2)$$
$$(10.3)$$

where $\epsilon_{ij} \sim \mathcal{N}(0, \sigma^2)$ et $b_i = (b_{0i}, b_{1i}, b_{2i})^T \sim \mathcal{N}(0, B)$.

This model is implemented by first fitting the two sub-model functions under the independence assumption on respectively the data in vertical format UM for the longitudinal part, and on the data with one row per subject UMdemo for the survival part:

```
library(JM)
fitLME <- lme(logPSA ~ I((time+1)^(-1.5) - 1) + time,
           random =~ 1 + I((time+1)^(-1.5) - 1) + time | ID,
           data = UM, method = "ML")
UMdemo <- UM[!duplicated(UM$ID), ]
fitCOX <- coxph(Surv(Tsurv, event) ~ ipsa + tstage + gleason7 +
           gleason_sup7, data = UMdemo, x = TRUE)
```

Then, the structure of the joint model is defined through the call of jointModel. When $\eta_2 = 0$, the call is:

```
fitJOINT1 <- jointModel(fitLME, fitCOX, timeVar = "time",
              method = "spline-PH-aGH", parameterization = "value",
              control = list(GHk = 9))
```

When a dependency on the current level and the slope is assumed, the user has to specify first the derivative form of the modelled marker in derForm:

```
derForm <- list(fixed =~ I(-1.5*(time + 1)^(-2.5)) + 1,
           indFixed = c(2, 3),
           random= ~ I(-1.5*(time + 1)^(-2.5)) + 1,
           indRandom = c(2, 3))
fitJOINT2 <- jointModel(fitLME, fitCOX, timeVar = "time",
              method = "spline-PH-aGH", parameterization = "both",
              derivForm = derForm, control = list(GHk = 9))
```

In these two calls, the first two arguments are the lme and coxph objects that were previously fitted. Then timeVar gives the variable that corresponds to the time-scale. This variable is the unique indicator of time in the whole function. In particular, in the call of lme, the function of time $f_1(t)$ was defined as a function of the time-scale (time). Argument method defines simultaneously the parametric family for the baseline risk function λ_0, the type of survival model (proportional hazards or accelerated failure time) and the integration technique. Thus, method="spline-PH-GH" fits a model with proportional hazards (PH), a Gauss-Hermite quadrature (GH) and a baseline risk function approximated by splines (the logarithm of the baseline risk is a linear combination of B-splines) while method="weibull-AFT-GH" fits an accelerated failure time model (AFT) with a Gauss-Hermite quadrature (GH) and a Weibull baseline risk function. An essential point in the specification of the model is the type of dependency assumed between the longitudinal marker and the time-to-event. Argument parameterization="value" assumes a dependency on the current level of the marker only (with η_1) while parameterization="both" assumes a dependency on the current level and the current slope (with η_1 and η_2). In the latter case, the derivative of the marker at the current time is given in argument derivForm as described above. It is possible to assume a dependency through the current slope (η_2) only by specifying parameterization="slope". Finally, many options not detailed here can be provided in control.

Functions to perform post-fit analyses from a fitted model are available, including plot, residuals, fitted or survfitJM. Details on this function can be found online and in the dedicated book (Rizopoulos, 2012b) and the companion paper (Rizopoulos, 2010). We note that JM also handles events defined in a competing setting, and external time-dependent covariates.

10.6.2 Latent class joint models

Joint latent class models are implemented in lcmm package with function Jointlcmm. This function makes use of the syntax of hlme function for the specifications of the latent class linear mixed sub-model and the multinomial logistic model for the class-membership. Added in Jointlcmm is the specification of the survival sub-model which is conditional to the latent class.

To illustrate the call to function Jointlcmm, we use the joint latent class model described in the application in Section 8.3.4, except that we do not include covariates in the longitudinal model for the sake of simplicity. The probability of latent class membership is not modelled according to covariates, and the longitudinal and survival are defined in each latent class g by:

$$
\begin{aligned}
\log(\text{PSA}_{ij} + 0.1) = (\mu_{0g} + b_{0i}) + (\mu_{1g} + b_{1i})\, f_1(\text{time}_{ij}) \\
+ (\mu_{2g} + b_{2i})\, \text{time}_{ij} + \epsilon_{ij}
\end{aligned} \tag{10.4}
$$

$$
\lambda_i(t) = \lambda_{0g}(t) \exp(\text{iPSA}_i \gamma_1 + \text{tstage}_i \gamma_2 + \text{gleason7}_i \gamma_3 + \text{gleason\_sup7}_i \gamma_4) \tag{10.5}
$$

with $\epsilon_{ij} \sim \mathcal{N}(0, \sigma^2)$ and $b_i = (b_{0i}, b_{1i}, b_{2i})^T \sim \mathcal{N}(0, \omega_g^2 B)$ in latent class g and $\omega_G = 1$. We assume here class-specific Weibull baseline risk functions for $\lambda_{0g}(t)$.

The call with function Jointlcmm for this model and $G = 4$ is:

```
library(lcmm)
jlcm4 <- Jointlcmm(fixed = logPSA ~ time + f1t, mixture =~ time
            + f1t, random =~ time + f1t, ng = 4, subject = "ID",
            survival = Surv(Tsurv, event) ~ iPSA + tstage +
            gleason7 + gleason\_sup7, hazard = "Weibull",
            hazardtype = "Specific", nwg = T, data = UM)
summary(jlcm4)
```

As in `hlme` function, parts `fixed` and `random` specify, respectively, the mean effects and the individual random effects included in the model (according to the grouping variable defined in `subject`). The number of latent classes is indicated in argument `ng`. Argument `survival` completes the call with the specification of the survival sub-model. In this survival part, function `surv` (of package `survival` described for standard survival models) is used to define the right-censored (possibly left-truncated and of possible multiple causes) survival data. Here, the observed time is `Tsurv` and the indicator of event is `event` (there is no delayed entry). Covariates included in the sub-model are entered on the right-hand side of $\sim$. In order to define class-specific effects for covariate `X`, the user can specify `mixture(X)` rather than `X`. In addition, the user needs to specify the parametric family used for the baseline risk functions with option `hazard` and the possible proportionality assumption over latent classes with `hazardtype`. Implemented families are `hazard=Weibull` (by default) for Weibull baseline risk functions, `hazard=piecewise` for baseline risk functions that are approximated by step functions and `hazard=splines` for baseline risks approximated by a limited number of M-splines. For the last two, the number and position of the knots can be entered. By default, the baseline risk functions are specific to each latent class (`hazardtype="Specific"`) but proportional risks over classes (`hazardtype="PH"`) or common risks over classes (`hazardtype="Common"`) can also be defined. We note that the data set `data` should be displayed in the vertical way (1 row is one repeated observation) as in any function for longitudinal model.

From a fitted `Jointlcmm` object (`jlcm4` here), a series of postfit analyses and outputs can be obtained. Most functions available for objects `hlme` and `lcmm` also work with `Jointlcmm` such as `postprob`. For example, `plot` function provides a series of plots (residuals, predictions *vs.* observations, as well as the predicted baseline risk functions and the survival functions) and predicted mean trajectories in each latent class are computed with `predictY`. In addition, the predicted baseline risks and survival functions are given in `jlcm4$predSurv`, and individual dynamic predictions can be computed with function `dynpred` and plotted with `plot.dynpred`. The predictive power of a joint latent class model can finally be directly evaluated by function `epoce` or by the use of other packages (as `timeroc`) from the individual dynamic predictions computed in `dynpred`.

Extensions of the joint latent class mixed model are proposed in `Jointlcmm` such as joint models with a curvilinear mixed sub-model, or joint latent class models in the presence of competing risks. Details are available online and in the companion paper (Proust-Lima et al., 2015).

Bibliography

Aalen, O. O. (1978). Nonparametric inference for a family of counting processes. *The Annals of Statistics* pages 701–726.

Aalen, O. O. (1987). Dynamic modelling and causality. *Scandinavian Actuarial Journal* pages 177–190.

Aalen, O. O. (1989). A linear regression model for the analysis of life times. *Statistics in Medicine* **8**, 907–925.

Aalen, O. O., Borgan, Ø., and Fekjaer, H. (2001). Covariate adjustment of event histories estimated from Markov chains: the additive approach. *Biometrics* **57**, 993–1001.

Aalen, O. O., Borgan, O., and Gjessing, H. (2008). *Survival and event history analysis: a process point of view.* Springer.

Aalen, O. O., Farewell, V. T., de Angelis, D., Day, N. E., and Gill, O. N. (1997). A Markov model for HIV disease progression including the effect of HIV diagnosis and treatment: application to AIDS prediction in England and Wales. *Statistics in Medicine* **16**, 2191–2210.

Aalen, O. O., Røysland, K., Gran, J. M., and Ledergerber, B. (2012). Causality, mediation and time: a dynamic viewpoint. *Journal of the Royal Statistical Society: Series A (Statistics in Society)* **175**, 831–861.

Abramowitz, M. and Stegun, I. A. (1972). Handbook of mathematical functions with formulas, graphs, and mathematical tables. *National Bureau of Standards Applied Mathematics Series 55. Tenth Printing.*

Akaike, H. (1973). Information theory as an extension of the maximum likelihood principle. In Petrov, B. N. and Csaki, F., editors, *Second International Symposium on Information Theory,* pages 267–281. Akademiai Kiado.

Albert, P. S. and Shih, J. H. (2010). On estimating the relationship between longitudinal measurements and time-to-event data using a simple two-stage procedure. *Biometrics* **66**, 983–987.

Alioum, A. and Commenges, D. (2001). MKVPCI: a computer program for Markov models with piecewise constant intensities and covariates. *Computer Methods and Programs in Biomedicine* **64**, 109–119.

Alioum, A., Commenges, D., Thiébaut, R., and Dabis, F. (2005). A multistate approach for estimating the incidence of human immunodeficiency virus by using data from a prevalent cohort study. *Journal of the Royal Statistical Society: Series C (Applied Statistics)* **54**, 739–752.

Allison, P. (2012). *Survival Analysis Using SAS: A Practical Guide.* SAS Institute.

Andersen, P. K., Borch-Johnsen, K., Deckert, T., Green, A., Hougaard, P., Keiding, N., and Kreiner, S. (1985). A Cox regression model for the relative mortality and its application to diabetes mellitus survival data. *Biometrics* **41**, 921–932.

Andersen, P. K., Borgan, Ø., Gill, R. D., and Keiding, N. (1993). *Statistical methods based on counting processes.* Springer: New York.

Andersen, P. K. and Gill, R. D. (1982). Cox's regression model for counting processes: a large sample study. *Annals of statistics* **10**, 1100–1120.

Andersen, P. K. and Keiding, N. (2002). Multistate models for event history analysis. *Statistical Methods in Medical Research* **11**, 91–115.

Andersen, P. K. and Keiding, N. (2006). *Survival and event history analysis.* Wiley.

Andersen, P. K. and Keiding, N. (2012). Interpretability and importance of functionals in competing risks and multistate models. *Statistics in Medicine* **31**, 1074–1088.

Andersen, P. K. and Klein, J. P. (2007). Regression analysis for multistate models based on a pseudo-value approach, with applications to bone marrow transplantation studies. *Scandinavian Journal of Statistics* **34**, 3–16.

Andersen, P. K. and Perme, M. P. (2008). Inference for outcome probabilities in multistate models. *Lifetime data analysis* **14**, 405–431.

Andersen, P. K. and Perme, M. P. (2010). Pseudo-observations in survival analysis. *Statistical Methods in Medical Research* **19**, 71–99.

Andrinopoulou, E.-R., Rizopoulos, D., Takkenberg, J. J. M., and Lesaffre, E. (2014). Joint modeling of two longitudinal outcomes and competing risk data. *Statistics in medicine* **33**, 3167–3178.

Arjas, E. Time to consider time, and time to predict? *Statistics in Biosciences*
.

Arjas, E. and Parner, J. (2004). Causal reasoning from longitudinal data. *Scandinavian Journal of Statistics* **31**, 171–187.

Bailey, N. T. J. (1975). *The mathematical theory of infectious diseases and its applications.* Charles Griffin.

Bates, D., Mächler, M., Bolker, B., and Walker, S. (2014). Fitting linear mixed-effects models using lme4. *arXiv preprint arXiv:1406.5823*.

Bauer, D. J. and Curran, P. J. (2003). Distributional assumptions of growth mixture models: implications for overextraction of latent trajectory classes. *Psychological Methods* **8**, 338–63.

Beal, S. L. and Sheiner, L. B. (1982). Estimating population kinetics. *Critical Reviews in Biomedical Engineering* **8**, 195–222.

Belot, A., Abrahamowicz, M., Remontet, L., and Giorgi, R. (2010). Flexible modeling of competing risks in survival analysis. *Statistics in Medicine* **29**, 2453–2468.

Berndt, E. K., Hall, B. H., and Hall, R. E. (1974). Estimation and inference in nonlinear structural models. In *Annals of Economic and Social Measurement*, 3, 103–116.

Berzuini, C., Dawid, P., and Didelez, V. (2012). Assessing dynamic treatment strategies. In Berzuini, C., Dawid, P., and Bernadinelli, L., editors, *Causality: Statistical perspectives and applications*. Wiley.

Blanche, P., Proust-Lima, C., Loubère, L., Berr, C., Dartigues, J.-F., and Jacqmin-Gadda, H. (2015). Quantifying and comparing dynamic predictive accuracy of joint models for longitudinal marker and time-to-event in presence of censoring and competing risks. *Biometrics* **71**, 102–113.

Box-Steffensmeier, J. M. and De Boef, S. (2006). Repeated events survival models: The conditional frailty model. *Statistics in Medicine* **25**, 3518–3533.

Brémaud, P. (1999). *Markov Chains: Gibbs measures, Montecarlo simulation and queues*. Springer.

Britton, T. (2010). Stochastic epidemic models: a survey. *Mathematical biosciences* **225**, 24–35.

Broadbent, A. (2013). *Philosophy of epidemiology*. Palgrave Macmillan.

Brown, E. and Ibrahim, J. (2003). A bayesian semi-parametric joint hierarchical model for longitudinal and survival data. *Biometrics* **59**, 221–228.

Brown, E. R., Ibrahim, J. G., and DeGruttola, V. (2005). A flexible b-spline model for multiple longitudinal biomarkers and survival. *Biometrics* **61**, 64–73.

Brown, E. R., MaWhinney, S., Jones, R. H., Kafadar, K., and Young, B. (2001). Improving the fit of bivariate smoothing splines when estimating longitudinal immunological and virological markers in HIV patients with individual antiretroviral treatment strategies. *Statistics in Medicine* **20**, 2489–2504.

Bunge, M. (1979). *Causality and modern science.* Courier Corporation.

Cartwright, N. (1979). Causal laws and effective strategies. *Noûs* **13**, 419–437.

Celeux, G., Chauveau, D., and Diebolt, J. (1996). Stochastic versions of the EM algorithm: an experimental study in the mixture case. *Journal of Statistical Computation and Simulation* **55**, 287–314.

Chatterjee, N. and Shih, J. (2001). A Bivariate Cure-Mixture Approach for Modeling Familial Association in Diseases. *Biometrics* **57**, 779–786.

Chi, Y.-Y. and Ibrahim, J. G. (2006). Joint models for multivariate longitudinal and multivariate survival data. *Biometrics* **62**, 432–445.

Clayton, D. G. (1991). A Monte Carlo method for Bayesian inference in frailty models. *Biometrics* **47**, 467–485.

Cole, S. R. and Hernán, M. A. (2008). Constructing inverse probability weights for marginal structural models. *American Journal of Epidemiology* **168**, 656–664.

Cole, S. R., Hernán, M. A., Margolick, J. B., Cohen, M. H., and Robins, J. M. (2005). Marginal structural models for estimating the effect of highly active antiretroviral therapy initiation on CD4 cell count. *American Journal of Epidemiology* **162**, 471–478.

Commenges, D. and Gégout-Petit, A. (2005). Likelihood inference for incompletely observed stochastic processes: ignorability conditions. *arXiv preprint math/0507151* .

Commenges, D. and Gégout-Petit, A. (2007). Likelihood for generally coarsened observations from multistate or counting process models. *Scandinavian journal of statistics* **34**, 432–450.

Commenges, D. and Gégout-Petit, A. (2009). A general dynamical statistical model with causal interpretation. *Journal of the Royal Statistical Society: Series B (Statistical Methodology)* **71**, 719–736.

Commenges, D. and Gégout-Petit, A. (2015). The stochastic system approach for estimating dynamic treatments effect. *Lifetime Data Analysis* **in press**.

Commenges, D. and Hejblum, B. P. (2013). Evidence synthesis through a degradation model applied to myocardial infarction. *Lifetime data analysis* **19**, 1–18.

Commenges, D. and Jacqmin-Gadda, H. (1997). Generalized score test of homogeneity based on correlated random effects models. *Journal of the Royal Statistical Society: Series B (Statistical Methodology)* **59**, 157–171.

Commenges, D., Jacqmin-Gadda, H., Proust, C., and Guedj, J. (2006). A Newton-like algorithm for likelihood maximization: the robust-variance scoring algorithm. *Arxiv preprint arXiv:Math/0610402* .

Commenges, D., Joly, P., Gégout-Petit, A., and Liquet, B. (2007). Choice between semi-parametric estimators of Markov and non-Markov multistate models from coarsened observations. *Scandinavian Journal of Statistics* **34**, 33–52.

Commenges, D., Proust-Lima, C., Samieri, C., and Liquet, B. (2015). A universal approximate cross-validation criterion for regular risk functions. *International Journal of Biostatistics* **11**, 51–67.

Commenges, D., Sayyareh, A., Letenneur, L., Guedj, J., and Bar-Hen, A. (2008). Estimating a difference of Kullback-Leibler risks using a normalized difference of AIC. *The Annals of Applied Statistics* **2**, 1123–1142.

Cook, R. J. and Lawless, J. F. (2007). *The statistical analysis of recurrent events*. Springer: New York.

Corbière, F. and Joly, P. (2007). A SAS macro for parametric and semi-parametric mixture cure models. *Computer Methods and Programs in Biomedicine* **85**, 173–180.

Cox, D. R. (1972). Regression models and life-tables. *Journal of the Royal Statistical Society. Series B (Methodological)* **34**, 187–220.

Cox, D. R. (1975). Partial likelihood. *Biometrika* **62**, 269–276.

Cox, D. R. and Hinkley, D. V. (1979). *Theoretical statistics*. CRC Press.

Craver, C. F. and Darden, L. (2013). *In search of mechanisms: Discoveries across the life sciences*. University of Chicago Press.

Crowther, M. J., Abrams, K. R., and Lambert, P. C. (2013). Joint modeling of longitudinal and survival data. *Stata Journal* **13**, 165–184.

Dafni, U. G. and Tsiatis, A. A. (1998). Evaluating surrogate markers of clinical outcome when measured with error. *Biometrics* **54**, 1445–1462.

Danieli, C., Remontet, L., Bossard, N., Roche, L., and Bélot, A. (2012). Estimating net survival: the importance of allowing for informative censoring. *Statistics in Medicine* **31**, 775–86.

Dantan, E., Joly, P., Dartigues, J.-F., and Jacqmin-Gadda, H. (2011). Joint model with latent state for longitudinal and multistate data. *Biostatistics* **12**, 723–736.

Dartigues, J. F., Gagnon, M., Barberger-Gateau, P., Letenneur, L., Commenges, D., Sauvel, C., Michel, P., and Salamon, R. (1992). The paquid epidemiological program on brain ageing. *Neuroepidemiology* **11 Suppl 1,** 14–8.

DasGupta, A. (2008). *Asymptotic theory of statistics and probability.* Springer Science & Business Media.

Dawid, A. P. (2000). Causal inference without counterfactuals. *Journal of the American Statistical Association* **95,** 407–424.

De Wreede, L. C., Fiocco, M., and Putter, H. (2010). The mstate package for estimation and prediction in non-and semi-parametric multistate and competing risks models. *Computer Methods and Programs in Biomedicine* **99,** 261–274.

Delattre, M., Genon-Catalot, V., and Samson, A. (2013). Maximum likelihood estimation for stochastic differential equations with random effects. *Scandinavian Journal of Statistics* **40,** 322–343.

Dempster, A. P., Laird, N. M., and Rubin, D. B. (1977). Maximum likelihood from incomplete data via the EM algorithm. *Journal of the Royal Statistical Society. Series B (Methodological)* pages 1–38.

Dickman, P. W., Sloggett, A., Hills, M., Hakulinen, T., et al. (2004). Regression models for relative survival. *Statistics in Medicine* **23,** 51–64.

Didelez, V. (2008). Graphical models for marked point processes based on local independence. *Journal of the Royal Statistical Society: Series B (Statistical Methodology)* **70,** 245–264.

Dietz, K. (1993). The estimation of the basic reproduction number for infectious diseases. *Statistical Methods in Medical Research* **2,** 23–41.

Diggle, P. J. (1988). An approach to the analysis of repeated measurements. *Biometrics* **44,** 959–971.

Drylewicz, J., Commenges, D., and Thiébaut, R. (2012). Maximum a posteriori estimation in dynamical models of primary HIV infection. *Statistical Communications in Infectious Diseases* **4,** 1–34.

Duchateau, L. and Janssen, P. (2008). *The frailty model.* Springer: New York.

Ducrocq, V. and Casella, G. (1996). A Bayesian analysis of mixed survival models. *Genetics, Selection, Evolution: GSE* **28,** 505.

Ederer, F., Axtell, L. M., and Cutler, S. J. (1961). The relative survival rate: A statistical methodology. *National Cancer Institute Monograph* **6,** 101–121.

Ederer, F. and Heise, H. (1959). *Instructions to IBM 650 programmers in processing survival computations.* Methodological note 100. National Cancer Institute, Bethesda MD.

Edgington, E. S. (1995). *Randomisation Tests.* New York: Marcel Dekker.

Efron, B. (1977). The efficiency of Cox's likelihood function for censored data. *Journal of the American Statistical Association* **72**, 557–565.

Efron, B. and Tibshirani, R. J. (1994). *An introduction to the bootstrap.* CRC press.

Elashoff, R. M., Li, G., and Li, N. (2008). A joint model for longitudinal measurements and survival data in the presence of multiple failure types. *Biometrics* **64**, 762–771.

Elliott, M. R., Ten Have, T. R., Gallo, J., Bogner, H. R., and Katz, I. R. (2005). Using a Bayesian latent growth curve model to identify trajectories of positive affect and negative events following myocardial infarction. *Biostatistics* **6**, 119–143.

Estève, J., Benhamou, E., Croasdale, M., and Raymond, L. (1990). Relative survival and the estimation of net survival: elements for further discussion. *Statistics in Medicine* **9**, 529–538.

Falcon, A. (2014). Aristotle on causality. *The Stanford Encyclopedia of Philosophy.*

Ferrer, L., Dignam, J., Rondeau, V., Pickles, T., and Proust-Lima, C. (2015). Joint modelling of longitudinal and multistate processes: application to clinical progressions in prostate cancer. *submitted.* http://arxiv.org/abs/1506.07496

Fieuws, S. and Verbeke, G. (2006). Pairwise fitting of mixed models for the joint modeling of multivariate longitudinal profiles. *Biometrics* **62**, 424–431.

Fine, J. P. and Gray, R. J. (1999). A proportional hazards model for the subdistribution of a competing risk. *Journal of the American Statistical Association* **94**, 496–509.

Fleming, T. R. and Harrington, D. P. (1991). *Counting processes and survival analysis.* Wiley Series in Probability and Mathematical Statistics: Applied Probability and Statistics Section.

Fletcher, R. (2013). *Practical methods of optimization.* John Wiley & Sons.

Florens, J. P. and Fougère, D. (1996). Noncausality in continuous time. *Econometrica* **64**, 1195–1212.

Fosen, J., Ferkingstad, E., Borgan, Ø., and Aalen, O. O. (2006). Dynamic path analysis-a new approach to analyzing time-dependent covariates. *Lifetime data analysis* **12**, 143–67.

Foulley, J. L., San Cristobal, M., Gianola, D., and Im, S. (1992). Marginal likelihood and bayesian approaches to the analysis of heterogeneous residual variances in mixed linear Gaussian models. *Computational Statistics & Data Analysis* **13**, 291–305.

Frydman, H. (1995). Nonparametric estimation of a Markov "illness-death process" from interval-censored observations, with application to diabetes survival data. *Biometrika* **82**, 773–789.

Frydman, H. and Szarek, M. (2009). Nonparametric estimation in a Markov "illness–death" process from interval censored observations with missing intermediate transition status. *Biometrics* **65**, 143–151.

Gallant, A. R. and Nychka, D. W. (1987). Semi-nonparametric maximum likelihood estimation. *Econometrica* **55**, 363–390.

Gégout-Petit, A. and Commenges, D. (2010). A general definition of influence between stochastic processes. *Lifetime data analysis* **16**, 33–44.

Geneletti, S. and Dawid, A. P. (2011). Defining and identifying the effect of treatment on the treated. In Illari, P. M., Russo, F., and Williamson, J., editors, *Causality in the Sciences*. Oxford University Press.

Genz, A. and Keister, B. D. (1996). Fully symmetric interpolatory rules for multiple integrals over infinite regions with Gaussian weight. *Journal of Computational and Applied Mathematics* **71**, 299–309.

Ghosh, D. and Lin, D.-Y. (2003). Semi-parametric analysis of recurrent events data in the presence of dependent censoring. *Biometrics* **59**, 877–885.

Gill, R. D. and Schumacher, M. (1987). A simple test for the proportional hazards assumption. *Biometrika* **74**, 289–300.

Gill, R. D., Van Der Laan, M. J., and Robins, J. M. (1997). Coarsening at random: Characterizations, conjectures, counter-examples. In *Proceedings of the First Seattle Symposium in Biostatistics*, pages 255–294. Springer.

Giorgi, R., Abrahamowicz, M., Quantin, C., Bolard, P., Esteve, J., Gouvernet, J., and Faivre, J. (2003). A relative survival regression model using B-spline functions to model non-proportional hazards. *Statistics in Medicine* **22**, 2767–2784.

González, J. R., Fernandez, E., Moreno, V., Ribes, J., Peris, M., Navarro, M., Cambray, M., and Borràs, J. M. (2005). Sex differences in hospital readmission among colorectal cancer patients. *Journal of epidemiology and community health* **59**, 506–511.

Good, P. (2000). *Permutation tests*. Springer.

Granger, C. W. J. (1969). Investigating causal relations by econometric models and cross-spectral methods. *Econometrica* **37**, 424–438.

Gray, R. J. (1988). A class of k-sample tests for comparing the cumulative incidence of a competing risk. *Annals of Statistics* **16**, 1141–1154.

Grégoire, T. G., Schabenberger, O., and Barrett, J. P. (1995). Linear modelling of irregularly spaced, unbalanced, longitudinal data from permanent-pbot measurements. *Canadian Journal of Forest Research* **25**, 137–156.

Guedj, J., Thiébaut, R., and Commenges, D. (2007). Maximum likelihood estimation in dynamical models of HIV. *Biometrics* **63**, 1198–1206.

Guo, X. and Carlin, B. P. (2004). Separate and joint modeling of longitudinal and event time data using standard computer packages. *The American Statistician* **58**, 16–24.

Ha, I. D., Sylvester, R., Legrand, C., and MacKenzie, G. (2011). Frailty modelling for survival data from multi-centre clinical trials. *Statistics in Medicine* **30**, 2144–2159.

Hakulinen, T. (1982). Cancer survival corrected for heterogeneity in patient withdrawal. *Biometrics* **38**, 933–942.

Hakulinen, T. and Tenkanen, L. (1987). Regression analysis of relative survival rates. *Applied Statistics* **36**, 309–317.

Han, J., Slate, E. H., and Pena, E. A. (2007). Parametric latent class joint model for a longitudinal biomarker and recurrent events. *Statistics in Medicine* **26**, 5285–5302.

Hanagal, D. D. (2011). *Modeling survival data using frailty models.* Chapman & Hall, CRC press.

Harville, D. A. (1974). Bayesian inference for variance components using only error contrasts. *Biometrika* **61**, 383–385.

Harville, D. A. (1977). Maximum likelihood approaches to variance component estimation and to related problems. *Journal of the American Statistical Association* **72**, 320–338.

Heitjan, D. F. and Rubin, D. B. (1991). Ignorability and coarse data. *The Annals of Statistics* **19**, 2244–2253.

Henderson, R., Diggle, P., and Dobson, A. (2000). Joint modelling of longitudinal measurements and event time data. *Biostatistics* **1**, 465–80.

Hess, K. R. (1995). Graphical methods for assessing violations of the proportional hazards assumption in Cox regression. *Statistics in Medicine* **14**, 1707–1723.

Hill, B. (1965). The Environment and Disease: Association or Causation? *Proceedings of the Royal Society of Medicine* **58**, 295–300.

Hindmarsh, A. C. (1983). ODEPACK, a systematized collection of ODE solvers. *IMACS transactions on scientific computation* **1**, 55–64.

Hipp, J. R. and Bauer, D. J. (2006). Local solutions in the estimation of growth mixture models. *Psychological Methods* **11**, 36–53.

Ho, D. D., Neumann, A. U., Perelson, A. S., Chen, W., Leonard, J. M., Markowitz, M., et al. (1995). Rapid turnover of plasma virions and cd4 lymphocytes in HIV-1 infection. *Nature* **373**, 123–126.

Hosmer Jr, D. W., Lemeshow, S., and May, S. (2011). *Applied survival analysis: regression modeling of time to event data.* Wiley-Interscience.

Hougaard, P. (2000). *Analysis of multivariate survival data.* Springer Verlag.

Hu, W., Li, G., and Li, N. (2009). A Bayesian approach to joint analysis of longitudinal measurements and competing risks failure time data. *Statistics in medicine* **28**, 1601–1619.

Hubbard, A. E., Ahern, J., Fleischer, N. L., Van der Laan, M., Lippman, S. A., Jewell, N., Bruckner, T., and Satariano, W. A. (2010). To gee or not to gee: comparing population average and mixed models for estimating the associations between neighborhood risk factors and health. *Epidemiology* **21**, 467–474.

Hume, D. (2011). *An enquiry concerning human understanding.* Broadview Press.

Jackson, C. H. (2011). Multistate models for panel data: the msm package for R. *Journal of Statistical Software* **38**, 1–29.

Jacobsen, M. and Keiding, N. (1995). Coarsening at random in general sample spaces and random censoring in continuous time. *The Annals of Statistics* **23**, 774–786.

Jacod, J. and Shiryaev, A. N. (2003). *Limit Theorems for Stochastic Processes, ser. A Series of Comprehensive Studies in Mathematics.* Springer.

Jacqmin-Gadda, H., Fabrigoule, C., Commenges, D., and Dartigues, J.-F. (1997). A 5-year longitudinal study of the mini-mental state examination in normal aging. *American Journal of Epidemiology* **145**, 498–506.

Jacqmin-Gadda, H., Proust-Lima, C., Taylor, J. M. G., and Commenges, D. (2010). Score test for conditional independence between longitudinal outcome and time to event given the classes in the joint latent class model. *Biometrics* **66**, 11–19.

Jacqmin-Gadda, H., Sibillot, S., Proust, C., Molina, J., and Thiébaut, R. (2007). Robustness of the linear mixed model to misspecified error distribution. *Computational Statistics & Data Analysis* **51**, 5142–5154.

Jacqmin-Gadda, H., Thiébaut, R., Chêne, G., and Commenges, D. (2000). Analysis of left-censored longitudinal data with application to viral load in HIV infection. *Biostatistics* **1**, 355–368.

Jazwinski, A. H. (1970). *Stochastic Process and Filtering Theory*. Academic Press.

Joly, P. and Commenges, D. (1999). A penalized likelihood approach for a progressive three-state model with censored and truncated data: Application to AIDS. *Biometrics* **55**, 887–890.

Joly, P., Commenges, D., Helmer, C., and Letenneur, L. (2002). A penalized likelihood approach for an illness–death model with interval-censored data: application to age-specific incidence of dementia. *Biostatistics* **3**, 433–443.

Joly, P., Commenges, D., and Letenneur, L. (1998). A penalized likelihood approach for arbitrarily censored and truncated data: application to age-specific incidence of dementia. *Biometrics* **54**, 185–194.

Joly, P., Durand, C., Helmer, C., and Commenges, D. (2009). Estimating life expectancy of demented and institutionalized subjects from interval-censored observations of a multistate model. *Statistical Modelling* **9**, 345–360.

Joly, P., Gerds, T. A., Qvist, V., Commenges, D., and Keiding, N. (2012). Estimating survival of dental fillings on the basis of interval-censored data and multistate models. *Statistics in Medicine* **31**, 1139–1149.

Jones, D. S., Plank, M., and Sleeman, B. D. (2011). *Differential equations and mathematical biology*. CRC press.

Jones, R. H. and Boadi-Boateng, F. (1991). Unequally spaced longitudinal data with ar (1) serial correlation. *Biometrics* pages 161–175.

Jöreskog, K. G., Sörbom, D., and Du Toit, S. H. C. (2001). *LISREL 8: New statistical features*. Scientific Software International.

Kalbfleisch, J. D. (1978). Likelihood methods and nonparametric tests. *Journal of the American Statistical Association* **73**, 167–170.

Kalbfleisch, J. D. and Prentice, R. L. (2002). *The statistical analysis of failure time data*. Wiley-Interscience: NJ.

Kalman, R. E. and Bucy, R. S. (1961). New results in linear filtering and prediction theory. *Journal of Basic Engineering* **83**, 95–108.

Kaplan, E. L. and Meier, P. (1958). Nonparametric estimation from incomplete observations. *Journal of the American statistical association* **53**, 457–481.

Kay, R. (1986). Treatment effects in competing-risks analysis of prostate cancer data. *Biometrics* **42**, 203–211.

Keiding, N., Klein, J. P., and Horowitz, M. M. (2001). Multistate models and outcome prediction in bone marrow transplantation. *Statistics in Medicine* **20**, 1871–1885.

Kendall, M. G. (1938). A new measure of rank correlation. *Biometrika* **30**, 81–93.

Klebaner, F. C. (2005). *Introduction to stochastic calculus with applications.* World Scientific Publishing Company.

Klein, J. P. (1992). Semi-parametric estimation of random effects using the Cox model based on the EM algorithm. *Biometrics* **48**, 795–806.

Klein, J. P. and Andersen, P. K. (2005). Regression modeling of competing risks data based on pseudovalues of the cumulative incidence function. *Biometrics* **61**, 223–229.

Klein, J. P. and Moeschberger, M. L. (2003). *Survival Analysis: Techniques for Censored and Truncated Data.* Statistics for Biology and Health. Springer.

Klein, J. P. and Shu, Y. (2002). Multistate models for bone marrow transplantation studies. *Statistical Methods in Medical Research* **11**, 117–139.

Komarek, A. (2009). A new R package for bayesian estimation of multivariate normal mixtures allowing for selection of the number of components and interval-censored data. *Computational Statistics and Data Analysis* **53**, 3932–3947.

Konishi, S. and Kitagawa, G. (1996). Generalised information criteria in model selection. *Biometrika* **83**, 875–890.

Kooperberg, C. and Clarkson, D. B. (1997). Hazard regression with interval-censored data. *Biometrics* **61**, 1485–1494.

Kuhn, E. and Lavielle, M. (2004). Coupling a stochastic approximation version of EM with an MCMC procedure. *ESAIM: Probability and Statistics* **8**, 115–131.

Kuhn, E. and Lavielle, M. (2005). Maximum likelihood estimation in nonlinear mixed effects models. *Computational Statistics & Data Analysis* **49**, 1020–1038.

Laird, N. M. and Ware, J. H. (1982). Random-effects models for longitudinal data. *Biometrics* **38**, 963–974.

Lavielle, M. (2014). *Mixed Effects Models for the Population Approach: Models, Tasks, Methods and Tools*. CRC Press.

Lee, E. W., Wei, L., Amato, D. A., and Leurgans, S. (1992). Cox-type regression analysis for large numbers of small groups of correlated failure time observations. In *Survival analysis: state of the art*, pages 237–247. Springer.

Leffondré, K., Touraine, C., Helmer, C., and Joly, P. (2013). Interval-censored time-to-event and competing risk with death: is the illness-death model more accurate than the Cox model? *International journal of epidemiology* **42**, 1177–1186.

Legrand, C., Ducrocq, V., Janssen, P., Sylvester, R., and Duchateau, L. (2005). A Bayesian approach to jointly estimate centre and treatment by centre heterogeneity in a proportional hazards model. *Statistics in Medicine* **24**, 3789–3804.

Lesaffre, E. and Lawson, A. B. (2012). *Bayesian biostatistics*. John Wiley & Sons.

Lesaffre, E. and Spiessens, B. (2001). On the effect of the number of quadrature points in a logistic random effects model: an example. *Journal of the Royal Statistical Society: Series C (Applied Statistics)* **50**, 325–335.

Lewis, D. (1973). Causation. *The journal of philosophy* **70**, 556–567.

Li, N., Elashoff, R. M., Li, G., and Tseng, C.-H. (2012). Joint analysis of bivariate longitudinal ordinal outcomes and competing risks survival times with nonparametric distributions for random effects. *Statistics in medicine* **31**, 1707–1721.

Liang, K. Y. and Zeger, S. L. (1986). Longitudinal data analysis using generalized linear models. *Biometrika* **73**, 13–22.

Lin, D. and Wei, L.-J. (1989). The robust inference for the Cox proportional hazards model. *Journal of the American Statistical Association* **84**, 1074–1078.

Lin, D. Y., Wei, L. J., and Ying, Z. (1993). Checking the Cox model with cumulative sums of martingale-based residuals. *Biometrika* **80**, 557–572.

Lin, H., McCulloch, C. E., and Mayne, S. T. (2002). Maximum likelihood estimation in the joint analysis of time-to-event and multiple longitudinal variables. *Statistics in Medicine* **21**, 2369–2382.

Lin, H., McCulloch, C. E., and Rosenheck, R. A. (2004). Latent pattern mixture models for informative intermittent missing data in longitudinal studies. *Biometrics* **60**, 295–305.

Lin, H., McCulloch, C. E., Turnbull, B. W., Slate, E. H., and Clark, L. C. (2000). A latent class mixed model for analysing biomarker trajectories with irregularly scheduled observations. *Statistics in medicine* **19**, 1303–1318.

Lin, H., Turnbull, B. W., McCulloch, C. E., and Slate, E. H. (2002). Latent class models for joint analysis of longitudinal biomarker and event process data: application to longitudinal prostate-specific antigen readings and prostate cancer. *Journal of the American Statistical Association* **97**, 53–65.

Lindstrom, M. J. and Bates, D. M. (1990). Nonlinear mixed effects models for repeated measures data. *Biometrics* **46**, 673–687.

Little, R. J. A. (1993). Pattern-mixture models for multivariate incomplete data. *Journal of the American Statistical Association* **88**, 125–134.

Little, R. J. A. and Rubin, D. B. (1987). *Statistical analysis with missing data*. Wiley: New York.

Liu, L. and Huang, X. (2009). Joint analysis of correlated repeated measures and recurrent events processes in the presence of death, with application to a study on acquired immune deficiency syndrome. *Journal of the Royal Statistical Society: Series C (Applied Statistics)* **58**, 65–81.

Liu, L., Wolfe, R. A., and Huang, X. (2004). Shared frailty models for recurrent events and a terminal event. *Biometrics* **60**, 747–756.

Liu, L. and Yu, Z. (2008). A likelihood reformulation method in non-normal random effects models. *Statistics in Medicine* **27**, 3105–3124.

Locatelli, I., Rosina, A., Lichtenstein, P., and Yashin, A. I. (2007). A correlated frailty model with long-term survivors for estimating the heritability of breast cancer. *Statistics in Medicine* **26**, 3722–3734.

Louis, T. A. (1982). Finding the observed information matrix when using the EM algorithm. *Journal of the Royal Statistical Society. Series B (Methodological)* **44**, 226–233.

Lyles, R. H., Lyles, C. M., and Taylor, D. J. (2000). Random regression models for human immunodeficiency virus ribonucleic acid data subject to left censoring and informative drop-outs. *Journal of the Royal Statistical Society: Series C (Applied Statistics)* **49**, 485–497.

Machamer, P. (2004). Activities and Causation: The Metaphysics and Epistemology of Mechanisms. *International Studies in the Philosophy of Science* **18**, 27–39.

Mandel, M. (2013). Simulation-based confidence intervals for functions with complicated derivatives. *The American Statistician* **67**, 76–81.

Marquardt, D. W. (1963). An algorithm for least-squares estimation of non-linear parameters. *Journal of the society for Industrial and Applied Mathematics* **11**, 431–441.

Martinussen, T. and Scheike, T. H. (2006). *Dynamic regression models for survival data.* Springer.

McGilchrist, C. A. and Aisbett, C. W. (1991). Regression with frailty in survival analysis. *Biometrics* **47**, 461–466.

Michiels, B., Molenberghs, G., Bijnens, L., Vangeneugden, T., and Thijs, H. (2002). Selection models and pattern-mixture models to analyse longitudinal quality of life data subject to drop-out. *Statistics in Medicine* **21**, 1023–1041.

Molenberghs, G. and Verbeke, G. (2007). Likelihood ratio, score, and Wald tests in a constrained parameter space. *The American Statistician* **61**, 22–27.

Molina, J. M., Chêne, G., et al. (1999). The ALBI trial: A randomized controlled trial comparing stavudine plus didanosine with zidovudine plus lamivudine and a regimen alternating both combinations in previously untreated patients infected with human immunodeficiency virus. *The Journal of Infectious Diseases* **180**, 351–358.

Murray, J. D. (2002). *Mathematical Biology I: An Introduction.* Springer.

Muthén, B. O. (2002). Beyond SEM : General latent variable modeling. *Behaviormetrika* **29**, 81–117.

Muthén, B. O. (2003). Statistical and substantive checking in growth mixture modeling: comment on Bauer and Curran (2003). *Psychological Methods* **8**, 369–377; discussion 384–393.

Muthén, B. O. and Shedden, K. (1999). Finite mixture modeling with mixture outcomes using the EM algorithm. *Biometrics* **55**, 463–469.

Muthén, L. K. and Muthén, B. (2007). *Mplus user's guide. 5th.* Muthén & Muthén, Los Angeles, CA.

Nelder, J. A. and Mead, R. (1965). A simplex method for function minimization. *Computer Journal* **7**, 308–313.

Nelder, J. A. and Wedderburn, R. W. M. (1972). Generalized linear models. *Journal of the Royal Statistical Society A* **135**, 370–384.

Neuhaus, J. M., Kalbfleisch, J. D., and Hauck, W. W. (1991). A comparison of cluster-specific and population-averaged approaches for analyzing correlated binary data. *International Statistical Review* **59**, 25–35.

Nielsen, G. G., Gill, R. D., Andersen, P. K., and Sørensen, T. I. A. (1992). A counting process approach to maximum likelihood estimation in frailty models. *Scandinavian Journal of Statistics* **19**, 25–43.

Nowak, M. A. and May, R. M. (2000). *Virus dynamics*. Oxford University Press.

Oehlert, G. W. (1992). A note on the delta method. *The American Statistician* **46**, 27–29.

Øksendal, B., Øksendal, B., and Ksendal, B. K. (1992). *Stochastic differential equations: an introduction with applications*, volume 5. Springer New York.

O'Sullivan, F. (1988). Fast computation of fully automated log-density and log-hazard estimators. *SIAM Journal on scientific and statistical computing* **9**, 363–379.

Park, T. and Lee, S. Y. (2004). Model diagnostic plots for repeated measures data. *Biometrical Journal* **46**, 441–452.

Pearl, J. (2000). *Causality: Models, reasoning, and inference*. Cambridge Univ Press.

Peng, Y. and Carriere, K. C. (2002). An empirical comparison of parametric and semi-parametric cure models. *Biometrical journal* **44**, 1002–1014.

Peng, Y. and Zhang, J. (2008). Estimation method of the semi-parametric mixture cure gamma frailty model. *Statistics in Medicine* **27**, 5177–5194.

Pepe, M. S. and Anderson, G. L. (1994). A cautionary note on inference for marginal regression models with longitudinal data and general correlated response data. *Communications in Statistics-Simulation and Computation* **23**, 939–951.

Perelson, A. S., Neumann, A. U., Markowitz, M., Leonard, J. M., and Ho, D. D. (1996). HIV-1 dynamics in vivo: virion clearance rate, infected cell life-span, and viral generation time. *Science* **271**, 1582–1586.

Perme, M. P., Henderson, R., and Stare, J. (2009). An approach to estimation in relative survival regression. *Biostatistics* **10**, 136–146.

Perme, M. P., Stare, J., and Estève, J. (2012). On estimation in relative survival. *Biometrics* **68**, 113–120.

Peto, R. (1973). Experimental survival curves for interval-censored data. *Journal of the Royal Statistical Society. Series C (Applied Statistics)* **22**, 86–91.

Philipps, V., Amieva, H., Andrieu, S., Dufouil, C., Berr, C., Dartigues, J., Jacqmin-Gadda, H., and Proust-Lima, C. (2014). Normalized MMSE for assessing cognitive change in population-based brain aging studies. *Neuroepidemiology* **43**, 15–25.

Picchini, U., Gaetano, A., and Ditlevsen, S. (2010). Stochastic differential mixed-effects models. *Scandinavian Journal of Statistics* **37**, 67–90.

Pinheiro, J. C. and Bates, D. M. (1995). Approximations to the log-likelihood function in the nonlinear mixed-effects model. *Journal of computational and Graphical Statistics* **4**, 12–35.

Pocock, S., Gore, S., and Kerr, G. (1982). Long-term survival analysis: the curability of breast cancer. *Statistics in Medicine* **1**, 93–104.

Pohar, M. and Stare, J. (2006). Relative survival analysis in R. *Computer Methods and Programs in Biomedicine* **81**, 272–278.

Prague, M., Commenges, D., Drylewicz, J., and Thiébaut, R. (2012). Treatment monitoring of HIV-infected patients based on mechanistic models. *Biometrics* **68**, 902–911.

Prague, M., Commenges, D., Guedj, J., Drylewicz, J., and Thiébaut, R. (2013). NIMROD: A program for inference via normal approximation of the posterior in models with random effects based on ordinary differential equations. *Computer Methods and Programs in Biomedicine* **111**, 447 – 458.

Prague, M., Commenges, D., and Thièbaut, R. (2015). Dynamic approach and marginal structural models to estimate the effect of HAART on CD4 counts in observational studies. *arXiv:1503.08658 [stat.ME]* .

Prentice, R. (1982). Covariate measurement errors and parameter estimation in a failure time regression model. *Biometrika* **69**, 331–42.

Price, D. L. and Manatunga, A. K. (2001). Modelling survival data with a cured fraction using frailty models. *Statistics in Medicine* **20**, 1515–1527.

Proust, C. and Jacqmin-Gadda, H. (2005). Estimation of linear mixed models with a mixture of distribution for the random-effects. *Computer Methods and Programs in Biomedicine* **78**, 165–173.

Proust, C., Jacqmin-Gadda, H., Taylor, J. M. G., Ganiayre, J., and Commenges, D. (2006). A nonlinear model with latent process for cognitive evolution using multivariate longitudinal data. *Biometrics* **62**, 1014–1024.

Proust-Lima, C., Amieva, H., Jacqmin-Gadda, H., and Commenges, D. (2013). Analysis of multivariate mixed longitudinal data: a flexible latent process approach. *British Journal of Mathematical and Statistical Psychology* **66**, 470–487.

Proust-Lima, C., Dartigues, J.-F., and Jacqmin-Gadda, H. (2011). Misuse of the linear mixed model when evaluating risk factors of cognitive decline. *American Journal of Epidemiology* **174**, 1077–1088.

Proust-Lima, C., Dartigues, J.-F., and Jacqmin-Gadda, H. (2015). Joint modelling of repeated multivariate cognitive measures and competing risks of dementia and death: a latent process and latent class approach. *Statistics in Medicine*, in press.

Proust-Lima, C., Joly, P., Dartigues, J.-F., and Jacqmin-Gadda, H. (2009). Joint modelling of multivariate longitudinal outcomes and a time-to-event: A nonlinear latent class approach. *Computational Statistics & Data Analysis* **53**, 1142–1154.

Proust-Lima, C., Philipps, V., and Liquet, B. (2015). Estimation of extended mixed models using latent classes and latent processes: the R package lcmm. *arXiv:1503.00890 [stat]* arXiv: 1503.00890.

Proust-Lima, C., Sene, M., Taylor, J. M. G., and Jacqmin-Gadda, H. (2014). Joint latent class models for longitudinal and time-to-event data: A review. *Statistical Methods in Medical Research* **23**, 74–90.

Proust-Lima, C. and Taylor, J. M. G. (2009). Development and validation of a dynamic prognostic tool for prostate cancer recurrence using repeated measures of post-treatment PSA: a joint modelling approach. *Biostatistics* **10**, 535–549.

Putter, H., Fiocco, M., and Geskus, R. B. (2007). Tutorial in biostatistics: competing risks and multistate models. *Statistics in Medicine* **26**, 2389–2430.

Rabe-Hesketh, S., Skrondal, A., and Pickles, A. (2004). Generalized multilevel structural equation modelling. *Psychometrika* **69**, 167–190.

Rabiner, L. R. (1989). A tutorial on hidden Markov models and selected applications in speech recognition. *Proceedings of the IEEE* **77**, 257–286.

Ramlau-Hansen, H. (1983). The choice of a kernel function in the graduation of counting process intensities. *Scandinavian Actuarial Journal* **3**, 165–182.

Ramsay, J. O. (1988). Monotone Regression Splines in Action. *Statistical Science* **3**, 425–461.

Ramsay, J. O., Hooker, G., Campbell, D., and Cao, J. (2007). Parameter estimation for differential equations: a generalized smoothing approach. *Journal of the Royal Statistical Society: Series B (Statistical Methodology)* **69**, 741–796.

Reichenbach, H. (1956). *The direction of time.* University of California Press.

Remontet, L., Bossard, N., Belot, A., and Esteve, J. (2006). An overall strategy based on regression models to estimate relative survival and model the effects of prognostic factors in cancer survival studies. *Statistics in Medicine* **26**, 2214–2228.

Richardson, T. S., Rotnitzky, A., et al. (2014). Causal etiology of the research of James M. Robins. *Statistical Science* **29**, 459–484.

Ripatti, S. and Palmgren, J. (2000). Estimation of multivariate frailty models using penalized partial likelihood. *Biometrics* **56**, 1016–1022.

Rizopoulos, D. (2010). JM: An R package for the joint modelling of longitudinal and time-to-event data. *Journal of Statistical Software* **35**, 1–33.

Rizopoulos, D. (2011). Dynamic predictions and prospective accuracy in joint models for longitudinal and time-to-event data. *Biometrics* **67**, 819–829.

Rizopoulos, D. (2012a). Fast fitting of joint models for longitudinal and event time data using a pseudo-adaptive gaussian quadrature rule. *Computational Statistics & Data Analysis* **56**, 491–501.

Rizopoulos, D. (2012b). *Joint Models for Longitudinal and Time-to-event Data: With Applications in R*. CRC Press.

Rizopoulos, D. and Ghosh, P. (2011). A Bayesian semi-parametric multivariate joint model for multiple longitudinal outcomes and a time-to-event. *Statistics in Medicine* **30**, 1366–1380.

Rizopoulos, D., Verbeke, G., and Lesaffre, E. (2009). Fully exponential Laplace approximations for the joint modelling of survival and longitudinal data. *Journal of the Royal Statistical Society: Series B (Statistical Methodology)* **71**, 637–654.

Robbins, H. and Monro, S. (1951). A stochastic approximation method. *The Annals of Mathematical Statistics* **22**, 400–407.

Roberts, G. O. and Stramer, O. (2001). On inference for partially observed nonlinear diffusion models using the Metropolis–Hastings algorithm. *Biometrika* **88**, 603–621.

Robins, J. M. (1986). A new approach to causal inference in mortality studies with a sustained exposure period: application to control of the healthy worker survivor effect. *Mathematical Modelling* **7**, 1393–1512.

Robins, J. M. and Hernán, M. A. (2009). Estimation of the causal effects of time-varying exposures, in Fitzmaurice, Davidian, Verbeke, Molenberghs (Eds), *Longitudinal data analysis*, pages 553–599.

Robins, J. M., Rotnitzky, A., and Zhao, L. P. (1995). Analysis of semiparametric regression models for repeated outcomes in the presence of missing data. *Journal of the American Statistical Association* **90**, 106–121.

Rondeau, V., Commenges, D., and Joly, P. (2003). Maximum penalized likelihood estimation in a gamma-frailty model. *Lifetime Data Analysis* **9**, 139–153.

Rondeau, V., Filleul, L., and Joly, P. (2006). Nested frailty models using maximum penalized likelihood estimation. *Statistics in Medicine* **25,** 4036–4052.

Rondeau, V., Mathoulin-Pelissier, S., Jacqmin-Gadda, H., Brouste, V., and Soubeyran, P. (2007). Joint frailty models for recurring events and death using maximum penalized likelihood estimation: application on cancer events. *Biostatistics* **8,** 708–721.

Rondeau, V., Michiels, S., Liquet, B., and Pignon, J. P. (2008). Investigating trial and treatment heterogeneity in an individual patient data meta-analysis of survival data by means of the penalized maximum likelihood approach. *Statistics in Medicine* **27,** 1894–1910.

Rondeau, V., Schaffner, E., Corbière, F., Mathoulin-Pélissier, S., and Gonzalez, J. (2013). Cure frailty models for survival data: an application to breast cancer recurrences. *Statistical Methods in Medical Research* **22,** 243–260.

Rosenbaum, S. E. (2011). *Basic pharmacokinetics and pharmacodynamics: An integrated textbook and computer simulations.* John Wiley & Sons.

Rouanet, A., Joly, P., Dartigues, J.-F., Proust-Lima, C., and Jacqmin-Gadda, H. (2015). Joint latent class model for longitudinal data and interval-censored semi-competing events: Application to Alzheimer's disease. *submitted.* http://arxiv.org/abs/1506.07415

Rubin, D. B. (1974). Estimating causal effects of treatments in randomized and nonrandomized studies. *Journal of Educational Psychology* **66,** 688.

Rubin, D. B. (1976). Inference and missing data. *Biometrika* **63,** 581–592.

Rue, H., Martino, S., and Chopin, N. (2009). Approximate Bayesian inference for latent Gaussian models by using integrated nested Laplace approximations. *Journal of the Royal Statistical Society: Series B (statistical methodology)* **71,** 319–392.

Sastry, N. (1997). A nested frailty model for survival data, with an application to the study of child survival in Northeast Brazil. *Journal of the American Statistical Association* **92,** 426–435.

Schoenfeld, D. (1982). Partial residuals for the proportional hazards regression model. *Biometrika* **69,** 239–241.

Schwarz, G. (1978). Estimating the dimension of a model. *The Annals of Statistics* **6,** 461–464.

Seaman, S., Galati, J., Jackson, D., Carlin, J., et al. (2013). What is meant by missing at random? *Statistical Science* **28,** 257–268.

Sene, M., Bellera, C., and Cecile, P.-L. (2014). Shared random-effect models for the joint analysis of longitudinal and time-to-event data: application to the prediction of prostate cancer recurrence. *Journal de la Société Francaise de Statistique* **155**, 134–155.

Song, X., Davidian, M., and Tsiatis, A. A. (2002). An estimator for the proportional hazards model with multiple longitudinal covariates measured with error. *Biostatistics* **3**, 511–528.

Spiegelhalter, D. J., Abrams, K. R., and Myles, J. P. (2004). *Bayesian approaches to clinical trials and health-care evaluation.* Wiley: New York.

Spirtes, P., Glymour, C. N., and Scheines, R. (2000). *Causation, prediction, and search*, volume 81. MIT press.

Splawa-Neyman, J. (1990). On the application of probability theory to agricultural experiments. Essay on principles. Section 9. *Statistical Science* **5**, 472–480.

Stiratelli, R., Laird, N., and Ware, J. H. (1984). Random-effects models for serial observations with binary response. *Biometrics* **40**, 961–971.

Stram, D. O. and Lee, J. W. (1994). Variance components testing in the longitudinal mixed effects model. *Biometrics* **50**, 1171–1177.

Strevens, M. (2005). How are the sciences of complex systems possible? *Philosophy of Science* **72**, 531–556.

Suppes, P. (1970). *A Probabilistic Theory or Causality.* North Holland Publishing Co: Amsterdam.

Sy, J. P. and Taylor, J. M. G. (2000). Estimation in a Cox proportional hazards cure model. *Biometrics* **56**, 227–236.

Sy, J. P., Taylor, J. M. G., and Cumberland, W. G. (1997). A stochastic model for the analysis of bivariate longitudinal AIDS data. *Biometrics* **53**, 542–555.

Therneau, T. M. and Grambsch, P. M. (2000). *Modeling survival data: extending the Cox model.* Springer Verlag: New York.

Therneau, T. M., Grambsch, P. M., and Pankratz, V. S. (2003). Penalized survival models and frailty. *Journal of Computational and Graphical Statistics* **12**, 156–175.

Thiébaut, R. and Jacqmin-Gadda, H. (2004). Mixed models for longitudinal left-censored repeated measures. *Computer Methods and Programs in Biomedicine* **74**, 255–260.

Thiébaut, R., Jacqmin-Gadda, H., Chêne, G., Leport, C., and Commenges, D. (2002). Bivariate linear mixed models using SAS proc MIXED. *Computer Methods and Programs in Biomedicine* **69**, 249–256.

Thiébaut, R., Jacqmin-Gadda, H., Leport, C., Katlama, C., Costagliola, D., Le Moing, V., Morlat, P., Chêne, G., Group, A. S., et al. (2003). Bivariate longitudinal model for the analysis of the evolution of HIV RNA and CD4 cell count in HIV infection taking into account left censoring of HIV RNA measures. *Journal of Biopharmaceutical Statistics* **13**, 271–282.

Thijs, H., Molenberghs, G., Michiels, B., Verbeke, G., and Curran, D. (2002). Strategies to fit pattern-mixture models. *Biostatistics* **3**, 245–265.

Touraine, C., Helmer, C., and Joly, P. (2013). Predictions in an illness-death model. *Statistical Methods in Medical Research*.

Touraine, C., Thomas, G., and Joly, P. (2013). The smoothhazard package for R: Fitting regression models to interval-censored observations of illness-death models. *Research report 13/12. Department of Biostatistics*, Copenhagen University.

Tsiatis, A. A. and Davidian, M. (2001). A semi-parametric estimator for the proportional hazards model with longitudinal covariates measured with error. *Biometrika* **88**, 447–458.

Tsiatis, A. A. and Davidian, M. (2004). Joint modeling of longitudinal and time-to-event data: an overview. *Statistica Sinica* **14**, 809–834.

Tsiatis, A. A., Degruttola, V., and Wulfsohn, M. S. (1995). Modeling the relationship of survival to longitudinal data measured with error. Applications to survival and CD4 counts in patients with AIDS. *Journal of the American Statistical Association* **90**, 27–37.

Turnbull, B. W. (1976). The empirical distribution function with arbitrarily grouped, censored and truncated data. *Journal of the Royal Statistical Society. Series B (Methodological)* **38**, 290–295.

Vaida, F. and Xu, R. (2000). Proportional hazards model with random effects. *Statistics in Medicine* **19**, 3309–3324.

Van Buuren, S. and Groothuis-Oudshoorn, K. (2011). MICE: Multiple imputation by chained equations in R. *Journal of Statistical Software* **45**, (3).

Van der Vaart, A. W. (2000). *Asymptotic Statistics*. Cambridge University Press.

van Houwelingen, H. C. and Putter, H. (2008). Dynamic predicting by landmarking as an alternative for multistate modeling: an application to acute lymphoid leukemia data. *Lifetime data analysis* **14**, 447–463.

Verbeke, G. and Lesaffre, E. (1996). A linear mixed-effects model with heterogeneity in the random-effects population. *Journal of the American Statistical Association* **91**, 217–221.

Verbeke, G. and Molenberghs, G. (2009). *Linear mixed models for longitudinal data*. Springer.

Verbeke, G., Molenberghs, G., Thijs, H., Lesaffre, E., and Kenward, M. G. (2001). Sensitivity analysis for nonrandom dropout: a local influence approach. *Biometrics* **57**, 7–14.

Wahba, G. (1983). Bayesian "confidence intervals" for the cross-validated smoothing spline. *Journal of the Royal Statistical Society. Series B (Methodological)* **45**, 133–150.

Wang, Y. (2007). Derivation of various nonmem estimation methods. *Journal of Pharmacokinetics and pharmacodynamics* **34**, 575–593.

Wei, L.-J., Lin, D. Y., and Weissfeld, L. (1989). Regression analysis of multivariate incomplete failure time data by modeling marginal distributions. *Journal of the American statistical association* **84**, 1065–1073.

White, H. (1982). Maximum likelihood estimation of misspecified models. *Econometrica* **50**, 1–25.

Wienke, A. (2010). *Frailty models in survival analysis*. Chapman & Hall, CRC Biostatistics series.

Wienke, A., Lichtenstein, P., and Yashin, A. I. (2003). A bivariate frailty model with a cure fraction for modeling familial correlations in diseases. *Biometrics* **59**, 1178–1183.

Williams, D. (1991). *Probability with martingales*. Cambridge University Press.

Williamson, P., Kolamunnage-Dona, R., Philipson, P., and Marson, A. (2008). Joint modelling of longitudinal and competing risks data. *Statistics in medicine* **27**, 6426–6438.

Wimsatt, W. C. (1994). The ontology of complex systems: levels of organization, perspectives, and causal thickets. *Canadian Journal of Philosophy* **20**, 207–274.

Wolfinger, R. (1993). Laplace's approximation for nonlinear mixed models. *Biometrika* **80**, 791–795.

Woodward, J. (2014). A functional account of causation. *Philosophy of Science* **81**, 691–713.

Wright, S. (1921). Correlation and causation. *Journal of agricultural research* **20**, 557–585.

Wu, H. and Ding, A. A. (1999). Population HIV-1 dynamics in vivo: Applicable models and inferential tools for virological data from AIDS clinical trials. *Biometrics* **55**, 410–418.

Wulfsohn, M. S. and Tsiatis, A. A. (1997). A joint model for survival and longitudinal data measured with error. *Biometrics* **53**, 330–339.

Xu, J. and Zeger, S. L. (2001). The evaluation of multiple surrogate endpoints. *Biometrics* **57**, 81–87.

Yamaguchi, T. and Ohashi, Y. (1999). Investigating centre effects in a multicentre clinical trial of superficial bladder cancer. *Statistics in Medicine* **18**, 1961–1971.

Ye, W., Lin, X., and Taylor, J. M. (2008). Semi-parametric modeling of longitudinal measurements and time-to-event data—a two-stage regression calibration approach. *Biometrics* **64**, 1238–1246.

Yu, B. and Ghosh, P. (2010). Joint modeling for cognitive trajectory and risk of dementia in the presence of death. *Biometrics* **66**, 294–300.

Index